The Great Covid Deception

FIRST PRINTING

Billy Crone

Cover Design:
CHRIS TAYLOR

To my family, Church family,
and all those around the world
who have had loved ones
murdered from this viral agenda.

God will have the last word
on this evil and suffering
and satanic behavior.

If these people
do not ask for forgiveness
and get saved
through Jesus Christ,

Hell will be there
awaiting them
with open arms.

Contents

Preface

Like many of us, when the covid plandemic first hit, we had no idea of the true deceptive global agenda that was being thrust upon us. However, in a few weeks, when the emotional shock began to wear off from the media generated fear that was being jammed into our eyes every single day, some of us, who knew our Bible and Constitution all too well, began to awaken to the reality of an obvious rat. First it was the two weeks to flatten the curve in order to justify the lockdowns. Then it was wearing a mask, to two masks, to no masks, to now endless masks. Then came the poison death shots. First one, then two, then three, then four, to now never-ending boosters. Finally, the stark sick satanic murderous agenda began to emerge its ugly head. Death on a massive global scale never before seen since the days of Adolf Hitler. First a few, then thousands, to tens of thousands, to now untold millions, all the while knowing these are not even the true numbers that are being deliberately kept from us. In fact, just about everyone I know has a personal story of some loved one, coworker, neighbor, friend, you name it, that have all died as a direct result of these deadly jabs that are not even real vaccines. I myself have a family member that was pronounced cancer free, who then unfortunately took the shot and in just a couple of weeks was told the cancer was not only back but so aggressive it was untreatable and they died just a couple months later. I also know of several Christian brothers and sisters including Pastors who came down with covid, or so it was said, who then unfortunately went to the hospital that deliberately refused them known safe effective treatments only to give them a deadly course of care that led to their demise all the while raking in millions of dollars. If ever there was a time for us to speak up and speak out including the Gospel of Jesus Christ, it is now. One last piece of advice; when you are through reading this book, will you please READ YOUR BIBLE? I mean that in the nicest possible way. Enjoy, and I'm looking forward to seeing you someday!

Billy Crone
Las Vegas, Nevada
2022

Chapter One

The Statistics & Ingredients of Covid

The purpose for this book is because we want to be equipped as the church. I'm not a doctor nor do I play one on TV, believe it or not, but I am going to share with you what I know, including Biblically and then my duty will be done. My job as the shepherd is to get you equipped and then you can make your own decisions. Prayerful, Biblical, decisions.

As you know this whole year and a half, everybody has been freaked out and afraid. I'm not talking about just in the world, I'm talking about the church. There are churches who still have their doors closed. And there are Christians who still refuse to come to church services. As we will see, in my personal opinion, I believe it is unfounded in two different ways, Biblically, and I think it is also unfounded factually. Is this something that we should be afraid of?

Now let's look at the Biblical aspect. Number one: **Hebrews 10:25** tells us, do not forsake the assembling together as some are in the habit of doing. What does the Greek say? As some are in the habit of doing, the Greek means, as prescribed by law. Every time that Greek word is used in the New Testament it's always speaking of one of two things. It's speaking of Jewish Law or Roman Law, religious or civil law. God tells us in that context, certainly as the day approaches, we are getting close to the return of Jesus. He says whatever you do, don't stop meeting together.

No matter if it is a religious law or other churches tell you not to or it's a civil law and the government tells you not to, what's the balancing point? **Romans 13**. Yeah, **Romans 13,** of course, we submit to authority, but what is the caveat? They tell us to do something contrary to God's word. That's why we Christians, even though the laws on the books say you can go out and murder children in the womb, we don't support that. We don't submit to that. Why? Because that is going contrary to God's Law that says you shall not murder, that's murdering children. So that's wrong.

Same thing, when God tells us don't forsake meeting together, I don't care what the law says, what should we do as Christians? We need to meet together. But what has been the excuse for people to violate that command scripturally, and I'm not just talking about the church? FEAR! But you don't understand, we've got to do what they tell us, we're going to die. This is just horrible, it's a pandemic.

Well, let's deal with the Biblical aspect of this first. Is that how we are supposed to live as Christians in a constant state of fear? No!

Matthew 6:25-34 "Therefore I tell you, do not worry about your life, what you will eat or drink, or about your body, what you will wear. Is not life more important than food, and the body more important than clothes? Look at the birds of the air; they do not sow or reap or store away in barns, and yet your heavenly Father feeds them. Are you not much more valuable than they? Who of you by worrying can add a single hour to his life?

And why do you worry about clothes? See how the lilies of the field grow. They do not labor or spin. Yet I tell you that not even Solomon in all his splendor was dressed like one of these. If that is how God clothes the grass of the field, which is here today and tomorrow is thrown into the fire, will he not much more clothe you, O you of little faith? So do not worry, saying, 'What shall we eat?' Or 'What shall we drink?' Or 'What shall we wear?' For the pagans run after all these things, and your heavenly Father knows that you need them. But seek first his righteousness, and all these things will be given to you as well. Therefore, do not worry about tomorrow, for tomorrow will worry about itself. Each day has enough trouble of its own."

Don't worry about your life, would that include Covid-19? Now notice he didn't say ponder about it, think about what I am telling you. He gives a command. It's the same as do not murder, do not steal, it's what? Do not worry! So, he didn't say, with this whole Covid thing, just stay home and stare at the wall and grit your teeth and just don't worry. He gives you marching orders. What's the marching orders? That's not your focus Christian, your focus is on the Father, on His provision. If He takes care of the birds and they're not freaking out, He'll take care of you. Number two, you seek first His Kingdom and His righteousness, and it will all work out.

Philippians 4:4-7: "Rejoice in the Lord always, I will say it again: Rejoice! Let your gentleness be evident to all. The Lord is near. Do not be anxious about anything, but in everything, by prayer and petition, with thanksgiving present your requests to God. And the peace of God, which transcends all understanding, will guard your hearts and your minds in Christ Jesus."

What did he say? Rejoice in the Lord until Covid-19 comes along. No, I'm sorry, wrong translation, just read the Bible. And did you notice he said it twice? Rejoice, with an exclamation mark. Why does He want you to have a good countenance on your face? So, people can see that and when they are freaking out and they see you aren't freaking out, it's called a positive witness. When Jesus Christ comes again at the Rapture, which is the best-case scenario, we are out of here. We're not going through the 7-year Tribulation. We're in Heaven. We are going to be part of the Millennial Kingdom; we are going to rule and reign with Jesus Christ. The planet is going to be renovated to Garden of Eden conditions. We get to have peace with nature. And then after that we have the New Heavens and the New Earth, so shall it always be. No more satan, no more demons, awesome! The Lord's near, it's okay to smile!

So, He gives you marching orders. You don't just sit there and say, "I'm not anxious, I'm not anxious!" He says what? You have a concern, maybe you are concerned about your health, what do you do? Pray, trust God, enjoy his peace and have a great day. Now, as I have shared before many times, in **Matthew 6** the word worry, and in **Philippians 4** the word anxious, is the same Greek word. The root meaning of that word means "consumed with self."

And that's a bombshell because, when do we worry and when do we get anxious? When you do the opposite of what God tells you to do. When you get consumed with "self", self-problems, self-health, self-finances, self-situations, self-sin, self-satanic attacks, you're always going to worry. But what does He say about all these things? Your marching orders are, "Seek His kingdom and righteousness and pray. What's your focus? Your focus isn't on yourself. If you get consumed with yourself, you are always going to be filled with worry and anxiety. But you get consumed with God, enjoy peace, have a great day. You're not worried and you're not anxious.

You're not sticking your head in the sand and acting like it's not happening. You're not denying reality. You're living like God wants you to, so you can be a positive witness. You need to be a positive witness to the people around you. And the nail in the coffin with this Covid thing, let's take a look at **II Timothy**.

II Timothy 1:7: "For God did not give us a spirit of timidity, but a spirit of power, of love and of self-discipline.

That was about as blunt as you can get it. Is that really true? Can I really live as a Christian without worry and fear and anxiety? Even in the midst of Covid? Yeah! So, when you find yourself in a state of fear, that's not from God. That's not His spirit. If you find that in your mind, in your life, in your day, you are off balance Biblically. And dare I say there are many Christians who are freaked out. They don't have their minds renewed by the Word of God and they are listening to the words of man, who is pushing a narrative, as we will see, that is a lie. And it is deliberately putting them into a state of fear that God has not given us to manipulate them.

So, to help alleviate that fear even more so, even though biblically it doesn't matter, even if Covid-19 was as bad and as horrible as they say it is, we still don't need to be afraid as Christians. But let's take a look at the facts. We have two different video clips. The first one is going to deal with the current information. We'll let the so-called experts speak for themselves. This is the current information from the CDC, The Journal of American Medical Association, Johns Hopkins University, and we are just going to deal with stats. Is this really a pandemic? And should people be in such a state of fear as we are seeing even in the church? Absolutely not!

John MacArthur: *"Before we actually launch into questions and I don't want to take a lot of time with this, I am constantly being asked questions about what's going on in the country about Covid, about lockdowns, about all those kinds of things. I want you to know that I don't have any secret inside information, but I do my very best to examine what's available so that I can help people to understand what we are facing. Rather than try to answer these things one piece at a time, let me just share with you some information that I think will be of some help to you, I trust it will be.*

This approach to the virus which has had a devastating impact on many people. In Japan, in one month, there were as many suicides as there have been Covid deaths in almost the entire year long siege. We know about that. There are people who are missing their normal medical care and consequentially they are having some very serious medical complications. In some states as many as a third of the small businesses have closed and are unlikely to open. I read that as many as half of the businesses owned by black people will not be able to open with devastating financial results.

A fascinating article that I read recently is that the expectation that there will be 300,000 to 500,000 fewer babies born next year. That's a remarkable statement made by the Wall Street Journal at the end of November2020. Births were down about 50,000 last year and this year compare that to 300,000 to 500,000. People have such an exponential fear that they are less likely to want to bring children into the world.

We all know the nursing home saga and the sadness of that. There's a new death cause on certificates and its failure to thrive. It's used with those who die in those kinds of facilities. Because nobody can visit them the care descends, and I won't even describe the horrors of how those people are living when they are cut off completely from family. We all know that the price being paid by children is immense. The Journal of American Medicine, probably the premier medical journal in this country, put out a study on November 12, 2020, and the study shows the educational obtainment effect in years of life lost with young children because they are not in school. 44 million children, ages 5 to 11, have been out of school.

They have models that translate that into years. Your length of education and quality of education is the determiner of your length of life. The Journal of American Medicine estimates that we have lost about 5.53 million years in the lives of 5- to 11-year-old children in the future. The single greatest indicator for high school graduation is 4th grade reading skill. And as that plummets because only 60 percent of the kids who are supposed to be doing online learning are actually doing it, and only 1/3 of them are doing it every day. Their ability to read sinks and their ability to get out of high school sinks and there are all kinds of effects of that, that show up in an increased mortality rate.

The Journal of American Medical Association is saying that we are sacrificing our young ostensibly to save the adults that are not vulnerable. CDC survival rate, if you are up to 70 you have a 99.998 percent chance to survive Covid. In California, the courts in our case, it was presented to the courts that you have one chance in 19.1 million to die of Covid. You say it's a serious thing if somebody catches it. It can be. It would be like any kind of flu or virus, and it can very serious if there are comorbidities and that's an important thing to keep in mind. There are some people that should be protected, and we've always been careful to do that, and we should be doing that again. If you're over 70 you have a 95 percent chance to survive and that's with 15 percent of the population in that age group with comorbidities.

Some medical experts are calling for us to stop calling this a pandemic. Essentially, they are wanting us to call it a Syndemic. Pan means "all" by virtue of these statistics from the CDC, if 99.998 people survive, that is not all. Even if they do have some symptoms. What it really is, is a Syndemic that synthesizes with other factors of obesity and heart disease and things like that. In that combination it becomes much more potentially significant.

The Washington Post came out with an article that said everyone wore masks during the 1918 flu pandemic and they were useless. At least 50 million died in that pandemic. There was really no way to resolve it medically. The latest I read, out of the 50 million, 30 million died of pneumonia which is sort of that Syndemic notion. Masks became symbolic. People were told to wear it once and then wash it, sterilize it and once you put it on, don't ever touch it, if you expect it to work.

I received a report from UCLA, an internal report that in their entire system they have tested about 140,000 people for Covid and out of that only 27 people are in the hospital with some Covid complications. 27 out of close to 150,000.

There is one other thing I'd like to mention to you. Johns Hopkins, one of the great medical schools in our country, did a study of Covid-19. They released the study on the 22nd of November, 2020. It is titled, "Relatively no effect in deaths in the U.S." The question that keeps coming up is 'are more people dying now than died in other years?' That is what this study intended to find out. The study declares that the number of deaths is not alarming, in fact it has no effect on the number of deaths in the United States.

Retrieving data from the CDC website revealed that deaths of older people stayed the same before and after Covid. Since it mainly effects older people, experts expected an increase in the percent of deaths in the older group. Data says that didn't happen. The percentage of deaths among all age groups remain relatively the same as from 2014 to 2020. So, if Covid-19 has no significant effect on the total number of U.S. deaths, why does it appear so?

This report says that deaths from 2014 to 2020 were examined. There was a sudden increase in Covid deaths in the year 2020. An analysis of cause of deaths in 2018 show the pattern of seasonal increases in deaths for all causes during the flu season. The leading cause of death was heart disease. In 2020 during that same period, Covid-19 related deaths exceeded heart disease deaths. Unusual because heart disease prevails as the number one cause of death. Looking closer at the number, it is clear that comparing 2018 to 2020 numbers show drastic increase across all causes, rather there was a dramatic decrease in deaths due to heart disease. The total decrease in deaths by all other causes almost exactly equal the increase of deaths from Covid-19. They just assigned a different cause.

There is a declaration called The Great Barrington Declaration signed by 10,000 medical doctors and epidemiologists, experts and public health scientists. The Great Barrington Declaration has great concerns on how Covid-19 is being dealt with. That document says that lockdowns are producing devastating results on short- and long-term public health. This is not the right approach. These 10,000 experts recommend that we allow those with minimal risks to live life normally and build up natural immunity.

Now those are just some things that I wanted to give you, to ease some of the fears that you might have that I said long ago when we first got into this. We are the people of the truth, and we will always do the very best we can to tell you the truth. You don't need to be a victim of lies and deception, but when you see the people who are your leaders sitting around a table for hours and hours together, health officials with the governor, with no masks and no social distancing, having a party, you might wonder if they actually believe what they are asking you to do. I'm not saying that this doesn't exist, it does. I'm not saying that it can't be serious, it can be. It can be anything from the flu to very serious for those who have other prevailing illnesses. But to completely destroy businesses, schools, children, young people, education, churches, and everything else in our society, every normal course in life, is an overreaction. That is not my conclusion, that is the conclusion of 10,000 experts and scientists. That's a fair number.

I'm saying this to you because I don't want to be accused of putting you in jeopardy. People have said about me that I am mocking Covid and people on the internet are saying all kinds of things about me in regard to the fact that I am going to be killing people because we are meeting as a church. We are not naïve about the reality that everyone here is going to die and there are lots of ways that can happen. But at the same time, we have believed from the very beginning that the truth is, this is not a disease that kills everyone, and the statistics are in, 99.998 percent of people survive it. We have simply tried to follow what has become apparent week in and week out, and it started pretty early when it became clear that it was being misrepresented.

The question comes up, why are they doing this? I'm not sure that everybody has the same motive. It can be about fear, it can be about power, it can be about control, largely political, people trying to completely tear down the existing system that we are used to. Power has always been that which maddens people to do the most damage of anything that exists in human ambition. Power is a brutal master. Why they seek power and why they want to overturn things, that's for every person's motive, perhaps nuance a different way than the rest of them, but it comes down to power and control. Changing the world to fit them. This is a collective group, some known and some unknown. And they have done something that has never been done in human history, they have made this global. That in itself is very interesting, because now we are a global world and that is a set up that we have been waiting for through history since the Lord promised us would come in the future, an antichrist, who would have a global government. This is the first time in my lifetime that they literally have such power over people globally that we can shut them down. So, they can't function. That is so culture can come to you. This suits the world of antichrist.

If you look at the book of ***Revelation****, there is the mark of the beast number and if you don't have that you can't buy or sell, you don't exist. Everything about you, they know. People who have access to all your data. They know all of it. You can go out of existence virtually any moment that someone decides that. This is the kind of world that appears to be perfectly suited for the antichrist to come to bring a certain amount of peace. The world falls at his feet. He is the instrument of satan and of course all hell breaks loose.*

And at the time of the great tribulation, God's judgment comes at which time Jesus Christ returns. I don't want to say the Lord is coming soon, but I will say He is coming sooner than He ever has before. The Bible says at the end times there will be lawlessness, and there is lawlessness, an escalating lawlessness and an effort to create more lawlessness by taking restraints away. This is a world that could find itself in such absolute chaos, that the right satanic leader who promises to fix everything could be given the title of King of the World, the antichrist aided by the false prophet by what we see in the book of Revelation.

Many years ago, I thought there were signs of the return of Christ being imminent, and there always have been. We know He could come at any time or any day or any hour, but it seems that this is the world that we never knew could exist. We have the kind of weaponry that could destroy a third of the population, as seen in the ***Book of Revelation****. We have the kind of technology that can literally erase people out of existence. So, it's just up to us to be sure that we are looking at the signs of the times, but I think we have to be aware of the fact that we aren't being told the truth. And that's not surprising, is it? Satan is a liar, and he establishes his kingdom on a lie.*

So be discerning. The Lord has been very gracious to us here. We have been meeting together like this for months and months. The Health Department was here a couple weeks ago to say there is no outbreak here at Grace Church. How is that possible if what they say is so? We are a microcosm of the world. The Lord has even given us protection from the Supreme Court, twice. One case in New York and now Thursday, another case in California. Whatever this virus is, it does not override 1st Amendment rights.

So, we are meeting, but not in a foolish or irresponsible way. With as much knowledge and thoughtfulness as we can have. So, I want to encourage you that spiritually speaking, this is the best place you can be. And physically I don't think we are a threat. We've all been together for weeks and weeks and weeks. I think I had this before Shepherd's Conference. A couple weeks before Shepherd's Conference I didn't feel well at all. I took the normal things that the doctor would give me, and it was over in a few days. You say, well that was way back in March, so you got it early. But you may think it started in January, that's what you read, but do you understand what recently happened?

A serological study was done with the Red Cross. They went back to the blood bank to look at blood that was taken from people in 2019, from October to December, and 2% of that blood they found the antibodies from Covid. It's been around relatively speaking for a long time, and it will run its course like any other bug does. A letter that I got from a Stanford doctor said that 90 percent of the tests are invalid. I asked a football coach what he did to protect his team. He said we swab their nose with bleach. I'm not recommending that.

I'm just very grateful for your faithfulness, very grateful for your trust and confidence in me, and the Lord, and the church, with the wisdom of our elders and for bringing us into contact with people who understand the truth. We don't want anybody to be unprotected. We don't want anybody to be unsafe, but life is a terminal illness. It's far better to be with Christ, so that's the best that can happen to us. But the statistic is so overwhelming, 99.998 percent of people will have no lasting effect from this. How can we literally tear the world to shreds over that? Other forces are at work. We're just glad to be here proclaiming the truth. Worshiping the Lord. Thank you for your faithfulness."

So, based on the facts and based on the truth, and we are people of the truth, and the truth will set you free, is there anything to be afraid of? Not even close! So that brings up the obvious question, why? I agree with John MacArthur, with power and control we will certainly see a global lead up to the antichrist. But two things; I think the reason why is because it's another prophecy related issue, deceit. When you get closer to the 7-year Tribulation, there is going to be some of the biggest deceit you have ever seen in your life.

Look at **Matthew 24,** and then I am going to see if I can answer the why question. Because it's not just happening, there is an agenda. In the context, Jesus is talking about the 7-year Tribulation, signs that it's getting close. Notice what He says right out of the gate, the very first thing. Unfortunately, we usually just skip right over it. Before we get into the wars and rumors of wars, famines, pestilences, and at the midway point with the Abomination of Desolation, it's getting close. But what is the first thing that He says out of His mouth speaking about the 7-year Tribulation?

Matthew 24:3-5 "As Jesus was sitting on the Mount of Olives, the disciples came to Him privately. 'Tell us,' They said, 'when will this happen, and what will be the sign of your coming and of the end of the age?' Jesus answered: 'Watch out that no one deceives you. For many will come in My name, claiming, 'I am the Christ,' and will deceive many.'"

Who are they going to deceive? No one, because they all know the Bible, they are faithful to the scripture, and they are surrounded by churches that preach the truth? No, <u>many</u> will be deceived. And then He goes on to the rest of the list. But what is the first thing out of His mouth? He goes on to talk about false Christs, false messiahs, false teachers. He goes on to say that it will be so powerful that there will be such a strong deception, that if it were even possible even the elect would be deceived, if you're not careful. Well, that's what's going on. It isn't just that they are purposely lying to us, they're trying to get us into a state of fear. And it's not just the state of fear. The premise with the state of fear, as we have seen before in other studies, is to create a crisis so you can manage the outcome.

And there is an outcome. This is not a conspiracy theory, you can check it out for yourself, it's in print. They admit it, it's on tape and it's in video. They are being extremely bold about why they are doing this, because I think this time, they think they are going to pull it off. It's been a long-staged plan, for decades. The Bible tells us where all this is headed. It's the antichrist kingdom, but it's split up into a One World Economy, One World Government, it's a cashless society and it will go into a mark of the beast system. They want to micro-manage the planet in the 7-year Tribulation.

Now the term that they have for why they are purposely dismantling society, destroying people, getting them into a state of fear, and if you get into a state of fear, they know you are more apt to surrender your freedoms than in a time of peace. So, you have to get everybody not only fearful, but you have to let it go on for a long time to get them used to submitting to their solution and then literally, slowly over time, crushing them, their lives, their lively hood, because it's "create a crisis, manage the outcome." You develop a problem, to generate a reaction, and then you come in with a solution. It's a set-up. Now they don't call it "The Great Set-up" but they do call it "The Great Reset." Now, this is not a conspiracy theory. I'm going to just give you an overview. And then we are going to see how they are going to tie every individual on the planet into "The Great Reset."

If you want more on this, I just finished an interview yesterday with Jan Markell and Pastor Brandon Holthaus, from Rock Harbor Church. He and I worked with her for two hours and aired on her website. Tune in, it's a massive amount of detail and we go down deep on this. Now this is what is coming out of "The Great Reset", their words not mine, WEF, the World Economic Forum. It is headed up by a guy named

Klaus Schwab, and with him are the Global Elite. Sounds like a conspiracy theory, but it's all out there. They're not even hiding it anymore.

Bill Gates, of course, is another one, with population control, and of course he is involved with the vaccines. As we saw before, he wants to do wireless birth control that can control whether ladies can have children up to 16 years. We went through that in our AI study. That's nothing new for him. You also have world leaders like Prince Charles. He's still out there behind the scenes in this globalist agenda. But basically, it's a global elite club. You have to be able to join the club with anywhere from $60,000 to $600,000 required to join. The average joe doesn't have that kind of money, so we'll never be a part of it. And even then, they have a tier system in the World Economic Forum. They meet every year in Davos, Switzerland. Just to get into the conference each year, after paying what you had to pay to join, you still have to pay $27,000 to attend.

In the conference, the elite, get what's called a white pass. The white pass people can attend all the meetings including the ones that are secret and will never be televised. So, who knows what goes on in those meetings! What I am talking about is the ones that they do televise, they're still out there, they're on YouTube and they're in print. Basically, they admit that you can't let a good crisis go to waste. Now what crisis do you think it is? They admit Covid-19 is that crisis. And here's what is weird. It's not a conspiracy theory. They met and did a dry run on Covid-19 in October of 2019. As John MacArthur said, when did they find Covid in the blood samples? It was the same time that they met. October 2019 was a dry run, Event 201, it's online, you can check it out, it's not a conspiracy theory. These same elites did a dry run of what's been happening since the beginning. Even as sick as this is, in their laughter and glee, they want to dismantle the world and reset it to their new great plan, "The Great Reset." They even gave each other these little stuffed Covid-19 toys. It's crazy. It's all out there. They're not hiding it.

So, you ask what is "The Great Reset?" They have the problem they created, Covid-19, a global problem. Why? Because they want to literally destroy capitalism, the United States of America is in their way, because we are America first. We honor our sovereignty, and we don't want to go along with globalism. And we had a president, President Trump, who didn't want to go along with that. If you want to do some more research, I was told that he was approached by this same group and he did attend Davos, it's on tape. You can see the speech he gave, as other people said, that they approached him to get him to go along with it. That was when he came out with the speech that really made them mad. He said America first and we are not going along with globalism.

They approached him to sell out, but Trump wouldn't sell out. So that was back then and now the war was on. Because who was the one holding up their Great Reset? Trump. And it has everything to do with the election experience. It wasn't just about getting Trump out of office. When you look at the bigger global plan, Trump was the one messing with The Great Reset. Again, what is the Great Reset? Destroy capitalism, bring in basically in a nutshell, communism on a technological level to the whole planet, including the United States of America.

They had some slogans and one of them is "You'll own nothing and be happy." It's out there. What do you mean, you'll own nothing? What they want to do is replace our way of life, our system, with basically a global government that will dictate everything about your life. Your livelihood, what you eat, what you get to do, if you even get to travel, how you get to live. They want you to live in these micromanaged, little, teeny tiny places and that's even if you get to live. Everything in your life will be micromanaged and basically the Green New Deal, that's not by chance, that's their way of life. They are going to micromanage power; they are going to control everything because "they are doing it for us."

This Great Reset will bring in a utopia. Now what does that sound like? The antichrist kingdom. They call it The Great Reset, but I'm convinced it's the great antichrist kingdom of the 7-year Tribulation. That's how close we are. We can't set a date but man this is crazy and it's all out there. So that's basically what they want to do. Oh, that will never happen! They created the problem, Covid-19, and they have invaded our country for decades. They have taken over the media. We saw that with the election, didn't we?

They have taken over a lot of the government, not all, but a lot of it though. Certainly, the Democrat party, and we have all kinds of RINOs in the Republican party who sold out. I believe that they think they got Trump out of their way, and there is nothing now officially stopping them from pulling off The Great Reset. Because they created the problem and here is the solution. We are going to come in, and we are going to take over the globe, and we are going to micromanage your life.

You would think that there is no way that is ever going to happen, because I'm going to resist. Well, here is the elephant in the room. They didn't just create the problem, Covid-19, to break everybody down, to make them cry out for basically their plan, the solution, the Great Reset, it's also all about the vaccine. You ask, "Why the vaccine?" Because the vaccine is not like any other vaccine in the history of mankind. I don't have time to get into the baby part issue, if you want more on that, get our study on Abortion, the Mass Murder of Children. We go down deep and expose what is really going on with the vaccines.

What I am about to show you on tape is another doctor. We are going to listen to the experts and their take to expose what is in these vaccines, and whether we should be concerned about it. If you want more on this, please get our documentary, Hybrids Super Soldiers and the Coming Genetic Apocalypse. We go deep on this and talk about the sovereignty of God. We released that just before this whole Covid baloney blew up and we didn't even know it. What God put on our hearts to do in the ministry, and it exposes this whole thing. Perfect timing.

Basically, and it may sound crazy, but that vaccine is what they are going to use to connect every individual to The Great Reset. Because in that vaccine, it will literally change your DNA. That's the other thing that is huge, modify your DNA, that's number one. Number two, what also comes with it, it's packed with something that is called Luciferase. Lucifer means light bearer, and this has bio luminescent qualities, and they will know whether or not you have been vaccinated. You can't lie. Number three, it comes with something that was developed by DARPA, and we exposed this in our Hybrids documentary. It's called hydrogel. Hydrogel is the fancy name for nanotechnology.

This nanotechnology is in the vaccine as well and basically what this will do is, it gives you a number and it gives them the ability to wirelessly know what is going on inside your body at all times, 24 hours a day, 7 days a week. It not only transmits that information but also receives information, and people are concerned. First of all, who is all this information going to? Who's in charge of all this? Who's going to receive information? What are you going to do to my body, with nanobots in me now? It sounds crazy but let's take a look at that.

Dr. Carrie Madej: *"So, what do you think about going from a 1.0 to a 2.0 human? What does that mean? Well, going from humans 1.0 as we know as ourselves. A human 2.0 has something to do with transhumanism. If you are not familiar with that term, it's about taking humans as we know ourselves, and melding with Artificial Intelligence. Kind of like being in the Matrix, if you have seen that movie. It may seem rather cool to you. You might have some superhuman abilities, maybe you could think of something and then it happened. Maybe have some physical abilities that are almost superhuman like.*

That's the idea we see in Sci-fi movies. And for myself, thinking about this topic, well I have some time, I think that is many years in the future. However, this question, this idea is right now in this moment. We need to make a decision. And I found out that we need to make a decision about this because I investigated the proposed Covid-19 vaccine, and this is my alarm call to the world. I looked at the pros and cons and it frightened me. I want you to know about this because you need to be very well informed because this new vaccine is not like your normal flu vaccine. This is something very different. This is something brand new, this is completely experimental to the human race.

It's not just about being a different vaccine, there are technologies that are being introduced with this vaccine that can change the way we live, who we are, and what we are. And very quickly. I think that some people that you might know, like Elon Musk, who is the founder of Space X and Tesla Automotive, as well as Ray Kurzweil, who is one of the big wigs of Google. These are self-proclaimed transhumanists who believe that we should go to human 2.0 and they are very big proponents of this.

There are a lot of other people that you might know their names who are also involved, you should look that up. I think the easiest way to explain this to you is to go with one of the front runners of the vaccine. And go into a little bit of the history and how they want to make the vaccine. I think that will speak volumes. So, for instance, Moderna, is one of the front runners for the Covid-19 vaccine.

You should know that Moderna was founded by a person from Harvard, Derrick Rossi. This researcher was successful in taking some modified RNA and being able to reprogram stem cells in the body and change the function of the stem cell. He actually made it genetically modified. It has been proved that you can genetically modify something by using modified RNA. So, they founded the company Moderna on this concept. It's sort of the new kid on the block. It hasn't been around that long. In fact, it hasn't even met any vaccine criteria before, it's made no medicine for a human before, this will be their first run.

You must know that Moderna was in the news recently because it's been fast-tracking the vaccine going from phase one to phase two very, very quickly. In fact, it has gone from phase one to phase three in its experiments, from March of this year until currently. That is unbelievable because it usually takes from 5 to 6 years. How are they able to do this with the safety efficacy data that we need? I want you to know that in phase two we are only using between 30 and 45 humans. In Moderna's past study they only used 45 humans, and with the high dose vaccine, group A, 100 percent of those people got systemic side effects. That's 100 percent. That's only in the short-term side effects profile. In the low-dose vaccine 80 percent got systemic side effects.

Now we don't even know the long-term side effects of that. We would need a lot longer time, right? Maybe years, but we do know based on previous animal studies using this technology, that you can possibly expect an increase in cancer rates, create mutant genes, mutant genesis, also increased auto immune reaction. For instance, in some of the ferret studies they saw that when the ferret was introduced to the virus, that they were trying to protect the ferret, after the ferret got the vaccine, they actually had an exaggerated immune response. They actually hurt the ferret. They had more lung inflammation, more lung fluid and some problems with their livers. It actually hurt them. They had a poorer response. Now those were the long-term reaction that could be seen with the vaccine, but we don't know the data yet. It's not without risks.

Now how are they doing this? They are actually suggesting a platform to explain how they would administer the vaccine. There is a platform called the Microneedle platform developed by MIT. They said it could be very easily mass produced, that is why they are proposing this technology, producing many millions of vaccines quickly. They could also be administered by yourself. So, the idea is to get a Band-Aid, like the one you buy at the drug store.

It would be shipped to you via Amazon, UPS or some other shipping service. You take it out of the package, you put it on your hand, then you take the sticker off and you have been vaccinated. So how is that possible? Well, in the band aid there are little, tiny spicules, little, tiny needles, and this was designed after a snake viper fang bite, a little snake bite. They claim you won't hardly feel these little, tiny spicules. There are little hydrogels inside the needles and inside the hydrogel there is a Luciferase enzyme, as well as the vaccine itself.

So, what does this all mean? First of all, you are getting the vaccine with a modified RNA or modified DNA. So, in that modified RNA, the idea is that the micro-needles would puncture into your cell membrane, and this synthetic piece of RNA is a code for the parts of the virus where it would use the synthetic DNA code, for the parts of the virus to go into your nucleus, and your body would start transcribing it, or reading it, and making more of that part of the virus. So why would you want to make more of the virus? The idea is that your body would get used to seeing it and would know how to make antibodies and would improve T-cell response. The idea is then when you are in the future, your body would already know how to fight it and there would be a better response.

The problem with that is that they are using something that is called Transfection. Transfection is a way that we make genetically modified organisms, like with fruits and vegetables. They are not as healthy as the normal wild type fruits and vegetables. So possibly you could translate that to humans. If we become genetically modified, we would not be as healthy. And we don't have long term studies on this anyway. It's unbelievable.

The vaccine manufacturers have made the statement that this will not alter our DNA, as you know. I say, that is not true, because if we use this process to make a genetically modified organism, why would it not do the same thing to a human? I don't know why they are saying that. If you look at the definition of the word Transfection, it would probably tell you that it could be a temporary change to the cell, and I think that is what the vaccine manufacturers are basing it on, it is temporary, or it's a possibility to become stable, to be taken up into the genome and become so stable that it will start replicating when the genome replicates, meaning it is now a permanent part of your genome. That's the chance we are taking. So, it could be temporary, or it could be permanent. And we would never know that for years down the road.

So, here we go. We have something that could alter our genome. It's a possibility. And another thing on that, if they alter the genome, what would be the effect? I told you previously what some of the side effects would be but also, we need to know that this is a synthetic piece of DNA or RNA, and if it is taken up into the genome of the human, it's synthetic, it's not from nature. If you look at the Supreme Court's ruling on synthetic DNA or gene, it can be patented, and patents have owners. So, what does that mean for us? Does that mean Moderna, or the Bill and Melinda Gates Foundation, or the Department of Defense, all of these people who are involved in the patent, are they going to somehow own parts of our genome? It's a possibility, you need to know that. Now, that is one part of the delivery system. Just one.

Now let me go to the next. The next part of the delivery system is the Luciferase enzyme. They named it and patented it Luciferase. Luciferase because it has bio-luminescent qualities that can produce a light source. All of this would be under your skin, and you wouldn't be able to see it. Now the Luciferase is an idea because they want to make sure you are vaccinated. They don't trust medical records; they don't trust you to say you have been vaccinated. They want to make sure it was successful, a successful transfection or a successful gene modification.

So, when you get the Luciferase vaccination, you have an I-Phone or a special identification, so you can scan over that area and it will give a digital code, a digital imprint, a digital pattern, something that will identify that you were vaccinated. It holds your vaccination record. It also gives you an ID, a number, a bar code, a branding, whatever you want to call it, a tattoo, it's all the same thing. You have now become like a product.

Now the third thing I mentioned is Hydrogel. Hydrogel is actually an invention from DARPA. The Department of Advanced Research Project Agency. This is sort of a Sci-fi group from the Department of Defense Pentagon of the US government. They make these fantastic inventions and one of them is Hydrogel. To find out about Hydrogel you can go on Google, YouTube, and look at Profusa, which is one of the companies at DARPA, as well as Hydrogel, and you will find a little two-minute flick where they describe that Hydrogel is Nanotechnology, microscopic little robots. The little robots, and I know it sounds crazy, they can disassemble or reassemble and make different things.

So, with this Hydrogel, it has this Nanotechnology, so that is something that is robotic or artificial intelligence or has the ability to connect with artificial intelligence. So, this means a human can now connect directly, gather information from your body and connect with your smart phone with the cloud or some other smart device. And once this is done this is 24 hours a day, seven days a week, 365 days a year. Think about that. Think about how immediately that could affect our privacy. It can immediately change our autonomy, immediately change our freedom.

These can gather information like your blood sugar, oxygen level, blood pressure, those sound great. But it can gather many other things. It can gather, they say, your emotions, or your menstrual cycle, your activity, if you fall, the nutrients in your body, if you take medicines, if you take illicit drugs, anything that goes on in your body. And all of this information is going where? That has not been addressed. Who's protecting this information? What are they using it for? This is really serious stuff. This is all to be unveiled in the next vaccine.

Another thing to know about this Nanotechnology, the Hydrogel, Artificial Intelligence hook-up, just like your cell phone, you can send a text message or send an email and you can also receive them back. So that means we can receive information and what kind of information will be coming back into us? Would it affect our mood? Our behavior? Would it affect how we think or our memories? If you haven't watched the movie 'The Matrix' I think you should because there is some truth to that movie. I see so many wrong things with this vaccine. And I see we are not talking about it in media. I feel that these companies are out right lying to us when they say it cannot affect our DNA. Because by all definitions they are using, it can affect our DNA.

I wanted to make this video short, but I really wanted you to do your own research. There are many risks here that we are seeing, and we really need to decide if we want to go from human 1.0 to human 2.0. And let me also tell you that there are some major names behind these vaccines. You are always going to see the Department of Defense of the US government, DARPA, why is our military involved with our vaccine? The Bill & Melinda Gates Foundation is everywhere with this. If you look you will find that name almost always. Look at their track record, what the man stands for. His family comes from a family of Eugenics. What does Eugenics mean? Population control. Meaning there are too many people on the planet. That's important to know. He's been on video stating that he thinks a very good vaccine could decrease the earth's population by 10-15 percent. Well, who is going to stay and who is going to go? And who is he to decide? He doesn't have a medical background, no epidemiology background, no science background, he's not a doctor. He is a software tech. That is what he has.

I would also like for you to realize that I like to look at who has a vested interest, what is their motivation, what is his motivation? We already know his family background. Well, what is very concerning to me is that DARPA as well as the Bill & Melinda Gates Foundation is very interested in what they call 'Gene Drive' Technology, but it is 'Gene Extinction' Technology, and it is exactly what it sounds like. By using genetic mutations, by use of Transfection, for instance, you can exterminate the entire species from the planet.

They are proposing to use the form of mosquitoes in Africa. Our world is a delicate eco system. Who can say one species goes? When you exterminate an entire species, you can affect the whole eco system. Who's going to say who's staying and who's going to go? Why aren't we talking about this? If we can do this through an insect, we can do it to an animal, we can do it to humans. I'm bringing this up because if these agencies that are behind the vaccines, also stand for that, do you trust them with your health, do you trust them with your family, do you trust them with our children?

Another thing is that we are rushing this to production. What is the motivation behind that? We need to really think about this. I have also stated in the past, that here in the United States there have been mandates passed that make the vaccine manufacturers have no liability, zero liability, for any harm done to any human. If people are killed, if they are hurt, paralyzed, maimed for life, it doesn't matter. You have no recourse, and they still make all their profits. So, there is no incentive to make it safe anyway.

I also want you to know that one of the mandates in the Emergency Preparedness Act, they cannot force the vaccine if there is a viable treatment for Covid-19. I want you to know that doctors around the world are being censored about treatment options for Covid-19 or prevention for Covid-19, because if there is a true treatment or prevention, then they can't force the vaccine on us.

I want to bring this up because what in the world is the motivation for doing this. Is it really in the health for all of us? As a doctor, I can't see how this is in the true health of the entire world. I think there is another motive, another agenda going on. The more I look at this the more it comes up. So, I leave you with this. I wanted to make it short and sweet so you can digest it and think about it. Do you really want to go to human 2.0? Don't think it's a fantasy in the movies.

We need to come together and unify our voices because people in the positions of power of taking care of our health, are not in our best interest. But together we have power. Together our voice is strong. So, I encourage you to do your critical thinking, do your own research, form groups in your state, go to your state legislature and you tell them NO! No to these experiments on humans, no to invasion of privacy, no to censorship. We are sovereign human souls, and we need to take our rights back. Thank you for listening and as you know my video are made in the greatest of love and the greatest of peace. Thank you."

The Stew Peters show – Dr. Carrie Madej: 1st US Lab Examines Vaccine Vials Horrific Findings Revealed 9/29/21 (bitchute.com)

Stew Peters: *"Shinning a big bright light into the crevices of darkness, exposing the cockroaches and watching them scatter every day. Welcome to the Stew Peters show, my name is Stew Peters. Well, to prove that there is nothing to fear from the vaccine boosters, resident White House dementia patient, administrator Joe Biden, publicly received a Pfizer booster shot on Monday. At least that is what we are told to believe. Because that is what the media showed us on TV, it has to be legit. One day later the White House announced that the President's trip to Chicago is postponed, supposedly so he can negotiate with lawmakers about the*

Democrats big spending bill, but no you won't see him in public in that span. And why do you ask?

The Biden administration is still pursuing its plan to force the vaccine in the arms of every living and breathing organism that scours, crawls on, or occupies America, regardless of age, health status or religious conviction. But that dictatorial push just isn't enough. So, they are also expanding their push to booster shots. Of course, those will be made mandatory soon as well. Soon everybody will be paying their mandatory tribute to Pfizer, to Moderna, to Johnson and Johnson every six months for the right to travel, go outside, hold a job or have a life. And they are racing forward aggressively.

Even if the CDC's own advisory committee on immunization practices voted against endorsing booster shots for health care workers and teachers, but last Friday, CDC's Rochelle Walensky just overruled them. The Biden administration's political priorities come first. And that means more vaccines being forced into more arms. Dr. Carrie Madej has said she has personally examined multiple vials of the vaccine that are being forced into people's arms, and she said that she was horrified by what she saw. She said she cried harder than she had ever before. She said other American labs have looked at the contents of the vaccine vials, only to shut down shortly after. Dr. Carrie Madej joins us now. Thank you for being with us now."

Dr. Carrie Madej: *"Thank you Stew, it's my pleasure to be here."*

Stew Peters: *"So you sent these images to the show. I've looked at them, and I have to say I was creeped out, but then again, I realized I don't know what I am looking at here, so help me out."*

Dr. Carrie Madej: *"Okay. So, first of all, in July, a local lab in Georgia said they wanted me to examine the contents of a vial that they had just received. This vial was fresh, it had already been injected into at least one patient, because it was at the end of the day, and they were going to discard it. So, they were able to get the vial. This particular vial was*

Moderna. I was there to witness them getting that and putting some of the contents of it on a glass slide, put it under the compound microscope to look at it. Nothing was added to the solution, nothing was diluted, no human tissue was added, only the white lights of the microscope.

But over time it was becoming more room temperature from the refrigeration. First it was just translucent, and then as time went on, about 2 hours, colors appeared. I had never seen anything like this. There was a chemical reaction happening. It was a brilliant blue and royal purple and yellow, sometimes green. So, these colors appeared, and I didn't know what that was. After investigating, more super conducting materials can do that with white light being admitted to it. Super conducting materials can be an injectable computing system. Anyhow, these fibers were appearing more and more.

Some of the fibers had a little fuse structure on them, I'm not sure what that was. And also, metallic fragments were in there. They were not metallic fragments that I am used to seeing. They were exotic radio paste as well as you see on the cover slide, the cover slip. You put a glass partition on top of the glass slide and there are edges. All these colors started to move to the edge. There was some self-assembling going on, things were growing. They were synthetic and then there was one particular, I'd say object or organism, I'm not sure what you call it, that had tentacles coming from it and it was able to lift itself up off of the glass slide."

Stew Peters: *"It was alive? The thing was alive?"*

Dr. Carrie Madej: *"Yes, it appeared to be self-aware or be able to grow or move in space. All I can tell you is this is not something that we were taught in medical school, nothing in my laboratories, nothing I'd seen before and I show this to other people in the field and they don't know what it is either and I thought, when I first saw this, and I kept looking at it over and over again and the colleague with me. And we both thought out loud, like it's self-aware, like it knows we are watching it. It's an intuition, a feeling of mine but it was very upsetting. So, after two or two and a half* *hours it was destroyed. I thought well, maybe it was a fluke in a way. Maybe it was just that one vial.*

So, just recently the lab was able to get more vials in from the same manufacturer, but different batch. Looking at it the same way on a compound microscope, and another one of those tentacle like structures appeared. This was now completely under the cover slip and there was no movement because it wasn't on the edge. But I just couldn't believe I saw another one. It was the same thing. Colors appeared over a matter of time. At this time, I needed to get another video, if they do it again. You could see motion in the video. This is very concerning. I was also able to look at the contents of a vial of vaccine by Johnson and Johnson and there is definitely a substance that looks like graphene. They all have graphene like structures, whether or not they were, I don't have the ability of testing them in this lab but that is what they appear to be. They have fatty substances, like a sticky glue with hydrogel in both of those.

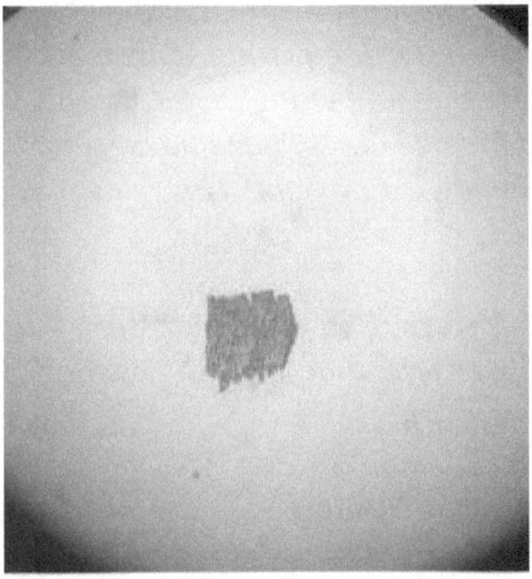

So, that means they are lying to us about the Johnson and Johnson, about not having nano-lipid particles or anything of that substance. In the Johnson and Johnson, they also had colors appear, but their colors were different. Their colors were like a florescent pastel kind of colors. Again, a lot of synthetic structures in there as well. In Johnson and Johnson, the spherical ring structures were there. A lot of sphere structures. These, I'm trying to describe what I am seeing but I have never seen anything like this before. And these are not supposed to be in these injections. These injections, that they are falsely calling vaccines. What are they going to do to somebody? What are they going to do to a child? I started crying when I saw these a second time under the microscope because it was confirmation of what I had seen the first time."

Stew Peters: *"If I looked at a microscope at something that I was told was a vaccine that was supposed to promote health and safety, and some self-aware tentacle equipped creature started moving, I would probably run out of the laboratory. That's just me, I'm not scared of a lot of things but that is scary that that is going into the blood of a lot of global citizens, and you are right. They want to push this into our children."*

Dr. Carrie Madej: *"Yes, this is about 400 times magnification, so we don't have any more information than that. People need to really, really stop and think about what is happening right now, and it doesn't make sense to rush to a decision that you could regret. Something is not right in the world, and I think we all know that right now, and to me it's definitely on the level of a spiritual warfare, looking at it under the microscope, absolutely. And you know this has inspired me to make more of these videos and if we can get the labs to get more of these samples, to do them in real time so you can actually see what we're doing to have proof as, yes this is what is happening. This is what we are seeing. So, you yourself can see what is happening under the microscope. Because I don't think you need to have any science background, when you look at it you will see something is not right. This isn't supposed to be injected into human beings."*

Stew Peters: *"So when you started talking about this self-aware thing, whatever it is, that lifted itself up off the glass, you mentioned something called an injectable computing system. What do you make of that?"*

Dr. Carrie Madej: *"Yes, so when the colors appeared in the solution, and there were no colors, or very little, at the beginning, then all of sudden the most brilliant blue, the most brilliant yellow, the most brilliant purple appeared and more and more over time. I have never seen anything that will do that unless you added another sub-strain for a chemical reaction. You know, it has to react to something. I didn't know it could do that, so I started to talk to some nanotech engineers and genetic engineers, and they told me that the only thing that they knew that could do that is a white light, which a white light did hit it on the microscope. A white light over time will make the reaction on a super conducting material.*

Super conducting is like an injectable computing system, so this is where the electronic components now become visible, under white light, you know where they are. This is proof that they are putting an operating system inside people. This is happened in both the Moderna and the Johnson and Johnson samples that we observed. So, we are getting little pieces of evidence put together one by one by one. But everything is pointing to the very ominous end play, this is the beginning of the advent of transhumanism. This is the beginning of the advent of having surveillance and spying done on people just like Bill Gates said he is doing right now in West Africa.

People need to remember that the Gates Foundation or at least Bill Gates and GAVI, their companies are doing a Mastercard and artificial intelligence program, testing on the people of West Africa with their Covid injection, giving them a digital ID. They can only get their monetary funds through their digital ID, via Mastercard. No other way, no cash, nothing. All their medical information, personal information, all downloaded into this digital format in their bodies. And they said in this research experiment that they are doing on the people, they said, 'If this substance is inside of them, this hydrogel substance, of course, why don't we use it for surveillance, and predictive policing. We are. We are going to start using it for surveillance and predictive policing on the people of West Africa right now'.

They have been doing it since July of 2020. They say that once they have it perfected, they want to unveil it to all the developed nations, and what are they calling it? The Wellness Pass, which is also known as the vaccine passport. So how are they doing that? They have to put something inside your body, to be able to monitor you and know everything that you are doing. So, people need to wake up. What can they put inside your body, and how would they do it? I think Gates is already admitting how he's doing it or how he wants to do it. How much does it take? I don't know. I just am seeing things with my own eyes, things that don't make sense, things that look like they can be used for and have already started doing something with artificial intelligence inside the human body. And we know that the people in charge aren't very trustworthy at all. They lied many times to us. The manufacturers have lied many times to us. So, we don't take this anymore. We don't take this kind of oppression and suppression; we are better than that. We are children of God, we chose to be, right? I for one will not stand for it."

Stew Peters: *"So just to wrap it up here. I know you've got to go but just for responsibility purposes. You've examined things under microscopes before. You know what you are doing with a microscope. These multiple vials that you examined, you have kept track of the chain of custody, nothing was inserted into these things before you were able to look at them. This is all on the up and up, and this is genuinely the contents of what is found in multiple lots now, you have said of Moderna and the J & J vials."*

Dr. Carrie Madej: *"Yes, at least 3 batches."*

Stew Peters: *"This is awful, horrific, I can understand why you cried. Dr. Carrie Madej, thank you so much and when you do have those videos, we trust that you will come back here to share those with the audience. People need to know what it is that is being pushed on them. They need to know that this isn't just an every day run of the mill health and wellness prevention. There is none of that going on here. So, we appreciate it."*

Dr. Carrie Madej: *"Thank you for having me on your show and I'm happy to come on in the future and share more as I get more information."*

Stew Peters: *"Those images that we just looked at together and then hearing the way that Dr. Madej just described and the way that she felt viewing those images through a microscope, horrific, alarming, very concerning and we have to be worried about being around people when we talk about things like transmission and shedding for people who have already gotten this thing, you have to stay healthy."*

Video transcript number two from the Stew Peters Show with Stew Peters as the host.

Stew Peters: *"The freshwater hydra is a pretty incredible organism. It's named after a creature from Greek mythology, if at any time one of its heads was cut off it would grow back two or more in its place. Scientists chose that name well. The freshwater hydra is biologically immortal. It's cells never age as far as we can tell they never die of old age, only from predators or environmental factors. If you cut off a piece of the hydra it will grow back. If you cut the hydra into many pieces all of them will grow into a new hydra. And how about if you stick the hydra in a blender, literally chopping it up into thousands of pieces until it's just a messy soup? Well, if you ball all of the pieces back together, they will merge and become a hydra again. Not surprisingly scientists are very interested in the hydra.*

Our government spends millions of dollars a year researching them for possible findings in biology, genetics and medicine. But is it only research that is happening or is something more going on? We had Dr. Carrie Madej on our show several weeks ago and she told us about the horrifying things she saw when she put vials of the Johnson and Johnson and Moderna, Covid-19 shot vaccines under the microscope. Now she is giving us a look at the Pfizer vial, and she wants to tell us the things that she has seen. Dr. Carrie Madej joins us now. You sent us some horrific slides and videos; I don't know what any of this is, so I am going to rely on your expertise to tell us."

Dr. Carrie Madej: *"Thanks Stew, I'm happy to help. I have worked with Project Veritas, the amazing team there, and they were able to work with the whistle blower from Pfizer and through chain of custody they have brought forth some of the vials. I have some of my own images, but Project Veritas will be coming out, giving their story very soon, which will add so much detail and so much data, so look for that. Anyhow, I also wanted to show a short video from one of the Johnson & Johnson vials that I was able to examine. What I am seeing in all of these manufacturers are synthetic substances, graphene like, also these nano carbon tubes with the metallic flecks, etc. But what I was seeing in this particular Johnson & Johnson was these round spears, they are not air bubbles, there was no way that they were, and many of these rings, as time went on, they would* *get thinner and thinner, and expand out and finally extrude out some gelatinous material. I'm not sure what it was but different things inside these spears, almost like a delivery structure. That is what they are doing.*

On one of these spears or this ring, there was an organism it looked like, a translucent organism that spun around, back and forth. At first, I thought it was another water parasite, another kind, and then I started looking at its movements and I thought that maybe it was moving in a more robotic way. We do have the ability for nanobots. Very much so. I don't know if I gave you a reference for that, but they can put 1 million nanobots inside one syringe needle, not the syringe itself, the needle, one million.

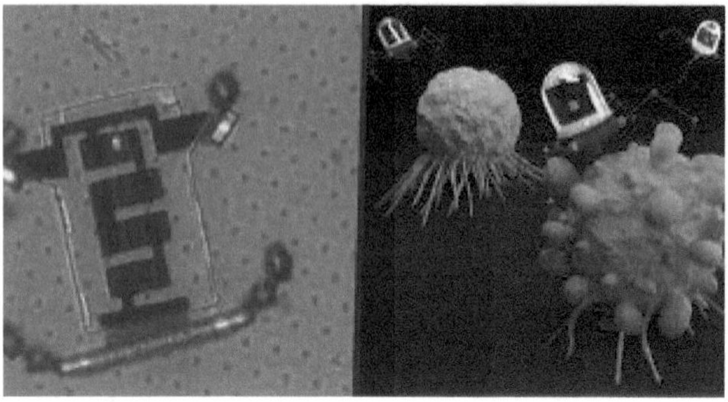

So, this is a possibility, and we need to examine this to see what this is exactly or is it part organic and part synthetic. It's frightening to know that these are being put inside a human being. Now they want to put them inside little children.

We have to stop this right now! These are extreme experimentations. The future of us is in peril. The danger of doing something like this. This is not informed consent by any means. They are trying to use wordplay and going around our human rights, the Nuremberg Code and definitely extending out this emergency use authorization in the worst way ever. So, it's very important to see that video and then looking at the slides from Pfizer, you can see the same kinds of synthetic things in there. Also, something called, or similar to teslaphoresis, that's when these little graphite black metallic particles start to coalesce and to stream like a spider web.

They do that through any external force. It could be light, it could be a magnetic force, it could be an impulse, like a frequency impulse, all these little particles will then coalesce and form their own neuro network, or their own fibers or wires."

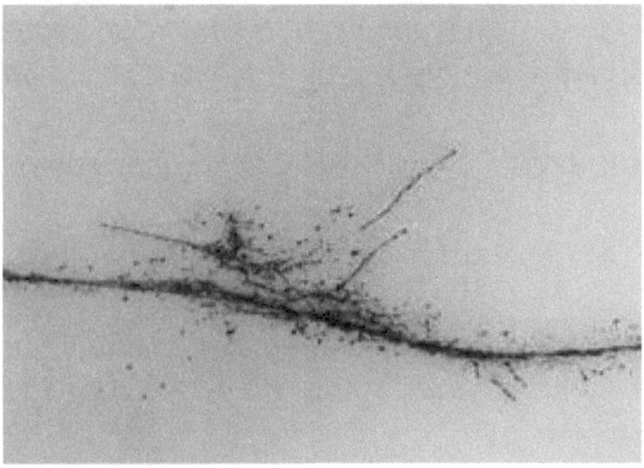

Stew Peters: *"So, like they are building infrastructure."*

Dr. Carrie Madej: *"Yes, like they are taking Lincoln Logs and putting them together and making their own new computer or mother board or wires. You can see that happening in real time."*

Stew Peters: *"This is absolutely mind blowing. I'm sitting here looking at you and you are telling me this and it's like I'm watching a seriously bad "B" movie., a horror thriller. These images are real, I mean there is no way to... And this is almost like a, what do you call it? It's a replication almost, I guess, I don't know if that's a scientific word we can use, but me, as a lay guy, would say we have one scientist in my group that could be the expert and bring us 'this' and we don't really know what 'this' is. And then Dr. Botha brought these discs and she said I need to get somebody to tell me what this is because I don't really know what this is. These things just keep on getting substantiated. And this verification that is going on. These things are alive?"*

Dr. Carrie Madej: *"Yes, we're confirming it. I am confirming it, I don't want it to be right. I'm upset, I'm angry, I'm frightened about what would happen. These are parasitic agents that are being injected into people. I've seen it from multiple different states, multiple different batches, multiple different manufacturers, multiple different times. How much more* *evidence does anyone need to know that something terribly wrong is going on. And now we are seeing it from other countries."*

Stew Peters: *"Okay, so 100 percent? From other countries?"*

Dr. Carrie Madej: *"Yes, Spain, Poland, you've seen Dr. Zelensky. Yes."*

Stew Peters: *"You're saying unequivocally, 100 percent, as a doctor, you're putting your reputation on the line, that there are parasites in these shots."*

Dr. Carrie Madej: *"They appear to be parasites to me, and I don't see anything or in the ingredient list for any kind of structure that would look like a water parasite by these manufacturers. That is correct."*

Stew Peters: *"Okay, so what else, as if we need anything else here, but what from your perspective are you seeing with these things, why are they there? What is really going on? Is there a health benefit to these?"*

Dr. Carrie Madej: *"Well, if you look at the organism, hydra vulgaris, it is one of the model organisms that many of the Transhumanist like to*

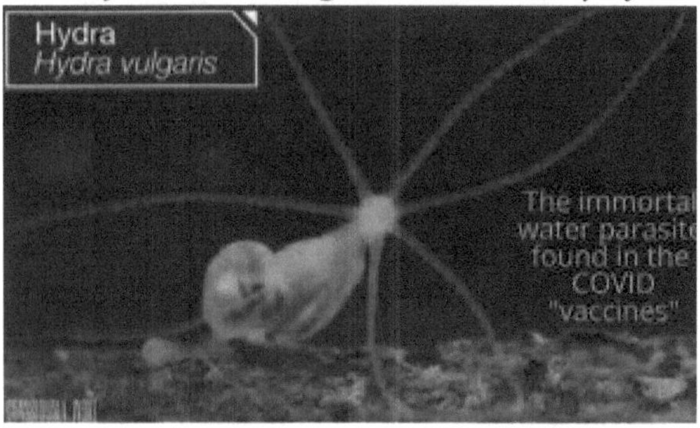
Hydra
Hydra vulgaris
The immorta
water parasit
found in the
COVID
"vaccines"

study and look at. They feel that this is an amazing organism for humanity because (a) it's immortal in the lab, it continuously produces its own stem cells, it never stops. It can make itself innumerable times, you can chop it up into little bits in a petri dish, it forms itself again, and again, and again. You can chop one of its tentacles off and it makes a new one, over and over. So, they think wouldn't it be great if we could put this inside of a human body's genome and then if your hand was chopped off by a trauma, you could grow a new hand. A new hand, right? Be careful about you wish for though. Maybe you couldn't die, and you think that's a great thing. It could be a nightmare too. And what if you grew three hands instead of one. This is a Frankenstein kind of experiment. Is anyone getting permission to do this to us? No, we don't know what they are doing. We do know that they are interested in doing that kind of thing to humanity at some point.

The other thing that they are interested in is that this organism has its own neuro network, its tentacles that go out has no brain but its own network so it's still a thinking kind of organism but in a different way. These neuro networks look like our human neuron, our human nerve, it looks just like it. So, if there's more than one, one here, one here, one here, they can form a mesh network. They can actually communicate between each other almost like you have your own internet inside your body. So, if these organisms are able to keep growing, because they are obviously in the vials and they can keep growing in the body, just surmise that they can make their own neural network, their own outside of yours. This is not good. It means they have their own communication system.

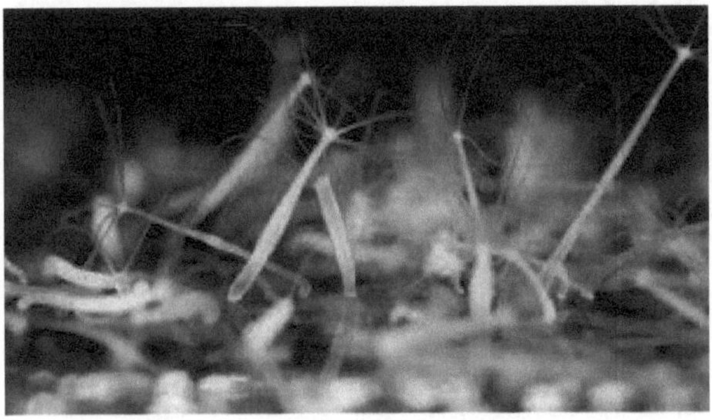

So, let's say, if it has its own communication system, something outward could affect it. Like an impulse, a frequency, something from 5G, a light, a magnet. What if something influenced that communication network but not yours? Would you start thinking things that aren't really your thoughts? How would you know if it was your thoughts? What if you started to get really angry and you didn't know why? What if you had this impulse to do something, like get a shot. What would happen, I'm just giving a hypothesis out here because I'm looking at what I am seeing in a microscope, and I think, why would I see it if it's not in the manufacturer's ingredients list.

Do the research on the people behind it. Like the Transhumanist movement and I see why they are interested. They are interested because of this continuous renewal of cells. They are also interested because of its ability to have its own neural network and to be influenced by magnets and other outside forces. So, you have to look at the people behind this. What are they doing? They lied to us from the very beginning, why would they be telling us the truth now? What would this do to a tiny baby? Or a child that they want to start introducing this to? You know they don't change the amount they give from a baby to an adult, usually it's the same amount. And then what are these delivery rings? What do they really have inside of them? Why are we seeing the phenomenon of teslaphoresis happen? That's some synthetic kind of wires and tubes happening. What that means is that they really are trying to put an artificial intelligence network inside of a human being.

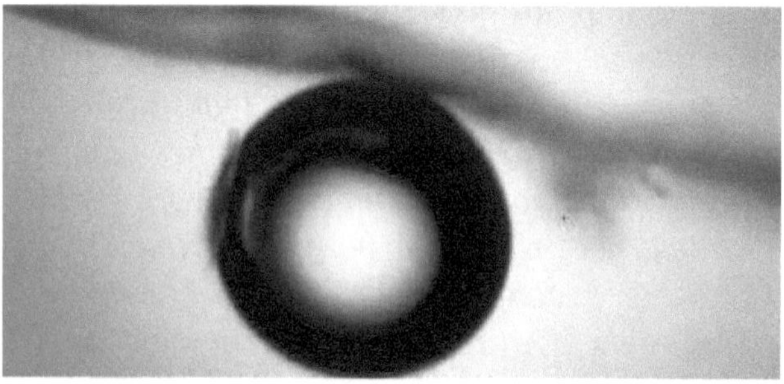

Did we consent to that? No! Again, if you want to be like that, that is your choice as an adult, right? But we are not given a choice right now. This is wrong on so many levels. We don't know what is going to happen. This is the grandest of experiments. I'm providing these pictures and this data for everyone to think for themselves. And to know we can disagree on things, but we have to come together on this because we have to protect our human rights, we have to protect our bodily autonomy, because the future of us is at stake."

Stew Peters: *"Maybe they don't want to be human anymore then we don't have certain rights. I mean if we are going to start thinking of stuff like this. So, let me ask you something as an Internal Medicine Specialist, that's your specialty, internal medicine. We have seen a lot of the common adverse effects, side effects of these shots, stroke, myocarditis, tremors,* *magnetism, what you are seeing now in the vials, do these things make sense to you? I can't make any sense of it but I'm not a doctor."*

Dr. Carrie Madej: *"Well, let's just take the parasites. We're not even going into the spike proteins right now, that's a whole different story. Dr. Sherri Tenpenny does a wonderful job of how inflammatorily dangerous they are. Let's just look at these water parasites. These things have the potential to grow and be innumerable, right? If you are growing things, it's going to clog your arteries. It can clog capillaries; it can clog lymphatics. So, when we are seeing blood clotting happening and what the body's response is to having an infection or a parasitic invasion, would be an inflammatory response, would be to have inflammation, perhaps clotting in that area. So, they are pulling out clots, sometimes almost as big as my hand, it has finger like extensions, like say coming from the heart. It's crazy. It's young people."*

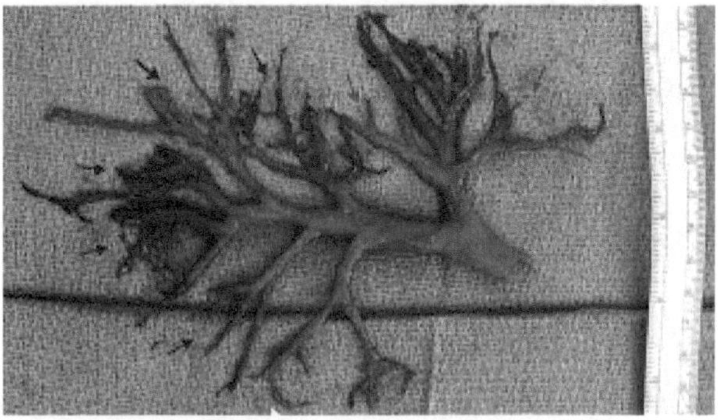

Stew Peters: *"I know, I've seen pictures of what was cut out of somebody that is a personal friend of somebody that I know and trust. It wasn't fake, this thing was huge."*

Dr. Carrie Madej: *"Yeah, I think they need to start examining the clot, taking it straight to a microscope, doing a pathology examination, looking at the tissue and seeing if there is any evidence of an organism, a parasitic organism in there. These things can grow to sontimeters. You know, that's pretty large in a body, right? We don't know what the potential is in the human body. But what we do know is, it should never be injected in us, ever! Under any circumstance."*

Stew Peters: *"If you know this stuff. And you have looked at these. These are images being provided and it's indisputable evidence that these things exist inside of these things, if you know all of this stuff and Project Veritas is going to be doing a big expose' on this, this is obviously not a secret to those people who are making it. Where are all of them? Why aren't those people coming forward and saying, this is what's happening, I mean this is literally, if what you are saying is true, millions of people around the world are in on this plan, know this, what game do they have?"*

Dr. Carrie Madej: *"Well, just like with doctors, if you speak up you lose your job, you lose your profession and people will cave for money. Most, 99 percent, cave for money which is a sad fact but that's true. They are looking for self-preservation, they don't understand that in doing that they won't have any self-preservation because we are all at risk here. No one is going to be exempt from this kind of experimentation. I mean, humanity of course. You have to speak up, it's so foolish to think that you can be exempt from this kind of experimentation. I don't understand why more people aren't speaking up. They don't get the gravity of what is happening here. They don't truly understand that our lives will never go back to normal. I can't understand how people think it's going to ever be normal again.*

Right now, we have to understand who the real enemy is. It's not one another, it's not blacks and whites, it's not Latinos, whatever, it's not left and right, it's humankind against a bigger threat. There are other people, I don't know if you can call them people, I don't think they are people because they are psychopathic. They don't have a conscience, they don't have empathy, they don't care about us, they don't care how many are killed in their experimentation. That's who really, we need to be uniting and fighting against because this is not human kind of medicine. This is not human kind of technology; this is something inhuman. And when I look at it, I know it didn't come from us or God our Father in Heaven and we are in a Spiritual war, so we need to unite and be one with God again. To be close to our Father God in Heaven."

Stew Peters: *"This is really nerve-wracking stuff, but I agree with everything you just said whole-heartedly. That is exactly right, this is good versus evil, get right with God and do it right now. You know how that book ends, so I'm comfortable there. Dr. Carrie Madej thank you so much for your bravery. I don't know why more people are not coming forward either. So, it's really a blessing to have you and I commend you for your courage. I appreciate it. Thank you.*

Dr. Carrie Madej: *"Thank you too, my pleasure."*

Stew Peters: *"We just need to boldly pray. Out in the wide open, fervently pray, please God, don't let our kids be the price that we pay, this has to be stopped. There has to be a worldwide call to stop this, right now! Those images, those things that Dr. Carrie Madej just said, I'm at a loss for words."*

So, do you sit around and get all fearful and freak out? No, you make your own intelligent decision. And what do you need to do? You need to speak up! And we have the right to speak up. We can say no, and while we have the freedoms, we need to exercise those freedoms. But again, as you see, what's important to me is the "why" factor. For something that has a 99.98 percent survival rate, why are they doing this? They already told us why. It's the Great Reset. They created the problem, Covid-19, admittedly, so they could generate the response, reaction, fear and over time dismantle everything in our way of life, economy, everything, to get us to submit to their solution. And they want to use the vaccine to connect us to their global reset, the Great Reset.

Oh, guess what? There are two other slogans; "You'll own nothing and be happy." This is in print. Another two slogans they have had for quite some time is "We're heading for a dark winter", and therefore due to The Great Reset, we need to "Build Back Better." So, who do you think would go along with this? And they sold out on a multitude of levels, but the big elephant in the room, what about Trump. Reports are saying that he resisted their offer, and you see that in the speech he gave after he was there in Davos.

Then the war was on. We have to get rid of this guy!! So, a lot of people believe that was when this plan was put into place. Amongst The Great Reset and Covid-19, this is also going to become the excuse with the Democrat Party and the RINOs in our government and other foreign entities, China, who is on board with The Great Reset, of course because they are a communist country and basically that is what they want to bring to the whole planet. So, they are going to use that as an excuse to one, destroy the economy, but it also makes Trump look bad in the next election cycle.

Number two, it also begins to give the excuse for what they did, and that was to stack the vote with all the mail in ballots. They couldn't have done that before, everything was fine, a so-called pandemic, right? So, it wasn't just to do that, but they killed two birds with one stone. And Trump was one of those birds. And get their guy and the people who have already sold out, and go along with this. And I think that is the reason they are being so bold about this now, in print and video. They think they did it. But have they?

Or is God going to be gracious to us, and do we have a little bit more time left? We know it's not going to last forever but is there a little window of opportunity?

But either way, I don't know about you, but we are living in some really exciting times. Things are ramping up like never before. Even now, God has not given us the spirit of fear, but the power of love and a sound mind. I know I am not to be afraid of this bug called Covid-19. I know it's a scam.

You can call it a Pandemic or a Plandemic or a Scamdemic, whatever you want to say. It's your decision what you want to do with the vaccine. I'm not a doctor and I don't play one on TV. I'm not giving you medical advice. But as a Pastor, I'm telling you, we need to speak up. Because if we roll over and play dead now, and we take the easy way out we keep our mouths shut, The Great Reset will happen. And that is the beginning of the end. I don't know if we are going to leave in the Rapture before that gets completely solved, I don't know. I know we aren't going into the 7-year Tribulation.

My personal prayer is this: "God, please give us more time. I know you have it all mapped out. The 7-year Tribulation and the Rapture is going to happen exactly when you want it to. We're not going to stop that. But please give us more time here in America because we are living in some special days. We can share the gospel with a click of a mouse, 7 days a week, so inexpensively. Never before in the history of the church have we had this opportunity. God, please give us more time. I know it's not going to be forever. Please give us more time so we can bear more fruit for you." That is my prayer and that should be your prayer as well.

Chapter Two

The Motives of Covid

Did anybody ever have a dream that when they grew up you were going to be a clown? Some will say, "Well Pastor Billy you're a clown." Well, I get that, but whether you ever wanted to be a clown or not, did you know that you have been turned into one? In fact, let me tell you the process of how they turned us into a bunch of clowns. Let's see if this sounds familiar to you. 15 days to flatten the curve, remember that? And then they said, "Oh no, two-week lockdown. Now that's how it's going to fix the situation, isn't it? Oh, wait, we all need the vaccine, here comes the wig. Now, what are they saying? Even if you get the vaccine, you still need to wear a mask. Do you feel like a clown yet? You've got to be kidding me,

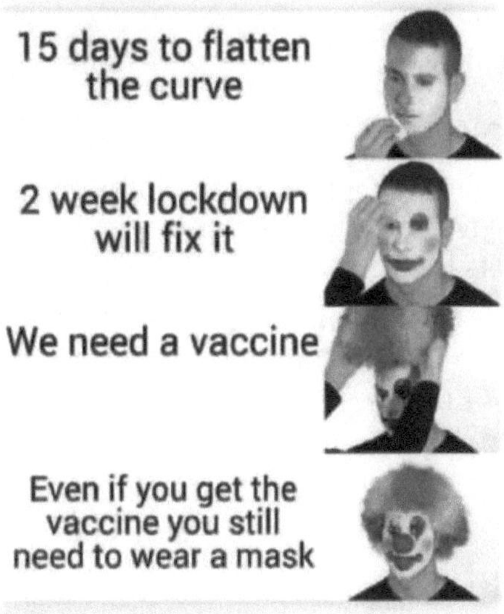

right? They think we are a bunch of fools. The reason why I say that is because we are being deceived on a massive scale.

They are ramping it up again, and the latest thing they are talking about with this Covid, is the new Delta Variant. I don't know if you have paid attention there, but they are following the Greek alphabet. The next one they are already talking about is Lambda. Have you seen that one? They are just going down the list. Are you going to just drag this on? What is going on? We are being deceived! We are being treated like a bunch of fools, a bunch of clowns.

The reason I discovered another layer of deceit about this issue, that I think begins to answer this latest behavior of "Delta Variant", once you understand that layer of deceit, it all makes sense. Really, what they are doing now makes no sense. But when you understand their motives, then it makes sense. So, why are they doing this? For a couple of reasons that I think we can agree. Number one, why did they release Covid? Because it makes President Trump look bad, while he was still in office. I think that was a given. Number two was so that they would have an excuse to bring in the mail-in ballots, to help steal the election. That was an obvious reason as well. Number three, as to why they brought in the Covid issue, is because they wanted to be a part of launching The Great Reset.

The Great Reset is from the World Economic Forum, the global elitists that want to usher in the excuse for the global crisis called Covid, a cashless society, where they will own everything. Remember the slogan, "You'll own nothing, and you will be happy", remember that? It's a direct quote. That's what they want to do. And I believe that is leading up to, what the Bible calls the Antichrist Kingdom, the 7-year Tribulation, the cashless society, the Mark of the Beast system.

But I discovered another layer of deceit that I think has everything to do with this latest round, Delta, basically Covid fear factor, Part 2. On the one hand, we shouldn't be surprised by it, because, the Bible says the closer we get to the 7-year Tribulation, the more you are going to see deceit, deceit, deceit, like never before. That's how the antichrist, the false prophet and satan operate. So, as we get closer to that you can see it ramp up. But don't take my word for it, let's listen to God's. The first thing that Jesus warned us about, that the sign of His coming was getting close, now watch what Jesus says, it's not by chance. He's going to talk about the signs of His coming. Now, He's not talking about the Rapture. It's the second coming at the end of the 7-year Tribulation. So, He basically goes through a literal chronological order of the events of the 7-year Tribulation, and then all the way to the end until He comes back. Notice, before He ever talks about the wars and rumors of wars, famines, pestilence, earthquakes, all those things are on the rise, right? Notice the first thing He warns about, that will be characteristic of that time frame.

Matthew 24:1-5 Jesus left the temple and was walking away when his disciples came up to Him, to call his attention to its buildings. 'Do you see all these things?' he asked, 'I tell you the truth, not one stone here will be left on another, everyone will be thrown down'. As Jesus was sitting on the Mount of Olives the disciples came to him privately, 'Tell us', they said, 'when will this happen, and what will be the sign of Your coming and of the end of the age?' Jesus answered, 'Watch out that no one deceives you. For many will come in My Name, claiming, 'I am the Christ,' and will deceive many."

The prophecy from Jesus came true that in 70 AD, the Romans came in and invaded Jerusalem. If you have ever been to Jerusalem, the Mount of Olives is literally right across the street from the Temple Mount. You go down and then right back up onto the Mount of Olives and you could see the Temple right there. Now, you will notice when asked about the end of the age, the very first thing out of Jesus' mouth is what? Let no man deceive you! No one will be deceived because everyone is sticking to the Bible, because they know the Bible is the only book on the planet that keeps them from being brainwashed from the lies of the evil one. Oh, I'm sorry wrong translation.

But we shouldn't be surprised by the increased level of deceit, even on this issue happening on a global basis as well. I'm not condoning it, but on the other hand I'm not surprised. The closer it gets to the 7-year Tribulation, that is what you would expect. And this shouldn't come as a surprise because this is how the antichrist, the false prophet, and satan, who inspires the antichrist and the false prophet, this is how they operate. It's all lies and deceit. Which makes sense because we have God's what? The Scripture which is God's truth! God doesn't lie. God is Holy, He can't lie. Jesus is the Way, the Truth and the Life. Nobody comes to the Father except through Him.

So, the enemy, what does he do? The exact opposite. God tells the truth, what is satan going to do? He's going to lie. So, let me just refresh that for you. This is why there is going to be so much mass deceit in the last days. Jesus warned about it but that is how they are going to operate. This is the antichrist.

2 Thessalonians 2:9-10 "The coming of the lawless one will be in accordance with the work of Satan displayed in all kinds of counterfeit miracles, signs and wonders, and in every sort of evil that deceives those who are perishing. They perish because they refused to love the truth and so be saved."

They don't want to hear it! You bunch of Christian wackos! You hear all this Jesus stuff; I don't need to get saved. I'm going to listen to this global agenda! The global agenda, these guys are my savior. They are going to bring peace to the planet, and then perish along the way. Then He goes on to say this:

Revelation 13:11-17 "Then I saw another beast, coming out of the earth. He had two horns like a lamb, but he spoke like a dragon. He exercised all the authority of the first beast on his behalf and made the earth and its inhabitants worship the first beast, whose fatal wound had been healed. And he performed great and miraculous signs, even causing fire to come down from heaven to earth in full view of men. Because of the signs he was given power to do on behalf of the first beast, he deceived the inhabitants of the earth. He ordered them to set up an image in honor of the beast who was wounded by the sword and yet lived. He was given power to give breath to the image of the first beast, so that it could speak and cause all who refused to worship the image to be killed. He also forced everyone, small and great, rich and poor, free and slave, to receive a mark on his right hand or on his forehead, so that no one could buy or sell unless he had the mark, which is the name of the beast or the number of his name."

Revelation 12 defines the dragon as satan, so this guy too, the false prophet who works with the antichrist, is also inspired by satan. And again, who are they following? Satan. Jesus tells us, this is what satan does. If these guys work for satan, what do they do? They act like satan.

John 8:43-44 "Why is my language not clear to you? Because you are unable to hear what I say. You belong to your father, the devil, and you want to carry out your father's desire. He was a murderer from the beginning, not holding to the truth, for there is no truth in him. When he lies, he speaks his native language, for he is a liar and the father of lies."

What? These guys, these global elitists who want to depopulate the planet by 90 percent, they are the elites and whoever gets to live according to them, the Bill Gates and others like him. Who do you think is inspiring them? The ultimate murderer, the murderous spirit which comes from satan, it's satanic. What these guys are doing right now in the world is satanic. Satan is the one who is inspiring these guys. They are not just off their rocker, it's a spiritual battle that we are in. So, what did Jesus say? Any lie on the planet, including today, ultimately, you may not have been there in that room when they started that lie, but ultimately, who inspired the lie? Satan.

So, we are being lied to about this covid issue and they are lying again about this latest round, the Delta Variant. Who's inspiring it? Satan, he's the father of all lies. That's why what we are in, not just a battle for freedom, not just a battle for Constitutional and Biblical freedoms, it's a spiritual battle, and this is where it's coming from. But again, it shouldn't surprise us because Jesus warned about it, and the Bible says this is how the antichrist, the false prophet and satan are going to operate, the closer we get to the 7-year Tribulation.

Now I want to say that's where it is leading. These entities will be taking over the world, and if you don't worship this guy as your savior, the antichrist, you will be killed during that time, the 7-year Tribulation. And they are going to institute some kind of global economic system, that they will have complete control over, that somehow you are going to have to be marked in order to interact with that system. You worship the antichrist, take the mark, specifically on your body. That is what is called the mark of the beast system. That's what it's leading to. And they are going to use deceit, deceit, deceit to get people to go along with it.

With that said, I'm not saying that the mask is the mark of the beast. I'm not saying that the vaccine is the mark of the beast. In fact, I'll be blunt. It's not! It can't be, because the mark of the beast does not start until the 7-year Tribulation. Typically, people believe, most prophecy teaches the half-way point; therefore, I think we can agree we are not in the 7-year Tribulation. So, it can't be the mark of the beast. However, I do believe, that in my lifetime, and dare I say in the history of the church, this is what they are doing on a global basis, with Covid, with the mask, and with the vaccine. And specifically, you can't buy and sell. This is being done on a global basis.

This is the biggest preparation I have ever seen. To prepare that society for when the mark of the beast will be instituted in the 7-year Tribulation. It is so abundantly clear, it's crazy. On the one hand it's kind of concerning, but on the other hand it should be exciting. Why? Because that's in the Tribulation and we leave prior. So, what do you do three times a day? Rapture practice, right? That's exactly what you do.

Don't get hooked into the narrative of the media. We are getting ready to expose that in this chapter. They are trying to instill fear in you, when actually we should be getting excited. I'm not condoning, what these guys are doing, but you and I should be excited. That means our departure is getting close, and we need to finish strong and faithful as the bride. So, I believe again, that the mask and the vaccine are not the mark of the beast, but preparing people for it. I think it's pretty obvious.

Now, believe it or not, for those of us who are for freedom, natural sovereignty, United States of America, Biblical freedom, religious freedom, we have an icon, a symbol, if you recall, and that was the Maga hat. And the left and the liberals and the globalists, they hated that. Boy, they were just pouncing on that. Now you do realize that they do the same thing? The leftist or the globalists who do not want freedom, who want global tyranny, not just in the United States, but around the globe, that will lead to the antichrist kingdom, did you know that they have their own symbols? We have the Maga hat, but they have the masks. The masks have become their global symbol of identity, that you are going to follow the narrative and you are going to look at them, the government, the global elitists as your savior, even to the point where you give up your freedoms, and you won't own anything, and you will be happy.

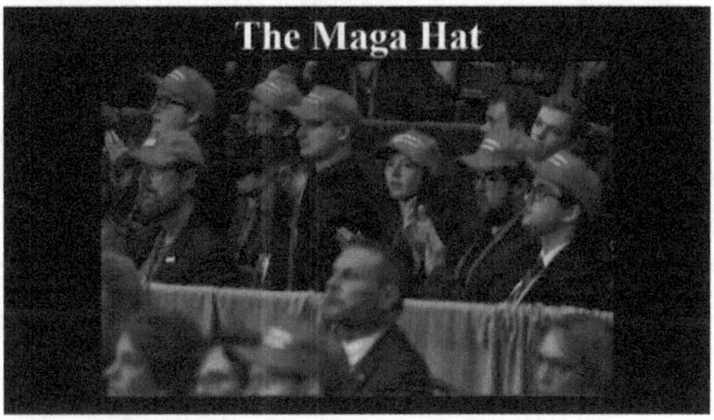

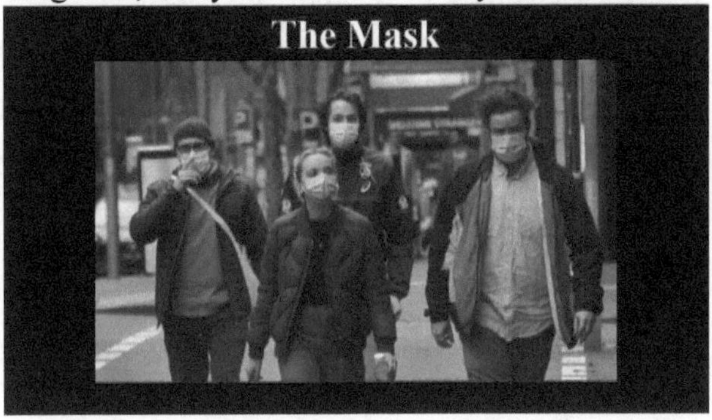

So, again, we are in a spiritual battle. Freedom, not only constitutional freedom and American freedom, but Biblical freedom versus tyranny. Now the sad news is we know, unfortunately, who wins out, and it's going to be tyranny. That is where it is heading, ultimately. Now that doesn't mean we roll over and play dead. I don't know the timing of God. Maybe God will give us another little window of opportunity, I don't know. We need to engage our culture. Basically, that is kind of what is going on.

And again, people will use the phrase, "preparation for the global tyranny, the antichrist system." In the word "mask" all you have to do is remove the "s" and replace it with an "r" for mark because after all, what is the global world considering right now? If you don't have that mask, you can't what? You can't go into a restaurant, you can't go into your workplace, you can't buy or sell. Now they are doing the same thing with the vaccine as well. I'm not saying it's the mark, but I am saying that we are being prepared for that society, where it's global tyranny. You have no freedom, that the antichrist will hijack, and take it to a whole other level, and it's happening right now before our very eyes. Even in the United States of America.

Now let me give you a couple of examples. This was just instituted as of August 3rd, and instituted by New York. It isn't just the mask, now it's the vaccine. They say you will not be able to buy or sell unless you have proof of vaccination. Now let me read this to you. *"New York City will require proof of vaccination from workers and customers at indoor restaurants, gyms, and entertainment venues"*, says Mayor Bill de Blasio. The policy enacted by the mayor, oral, and by executive order, and a Health Department order, will be launched August 16th and phased in, i.e., enforced by September 13th. He says, *"Not everybody is going to agree with this, I understand this, but with so many people, this is going to be a lifesaving act."*

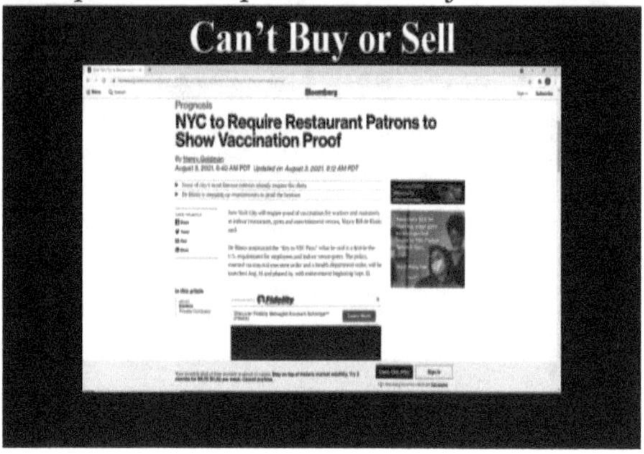

Now again, who do they have their hope in? Wear the mask, take the vaccine, listen to these guys, they are going to bring back normalcy to you, just do what they say, etc. Then what's even more concerning is this. You say, that's too bad for New York. De Blasio continues, *"He hoped that this requirement would be a model for the whole nation."* He was joined by a virtual briefing by National Health Experts including White House Covid-19 advisor Andy Slavitt who said, *"This will be copied around the country."* Not the mask anymore, now we're talking vaccine. Now you are being conditioned against your will.

What is the difference between the mask and the vaccine? The mask is something you can just put on your face, without that you can't buy and sell, it's conditioning you. The vaccine is now not just on your body, but in your body, and where is it ultimately going to go? Into a marking on your hand or on your forehead. It's conditioning. You can't buy or sell. What breaks my heart is that 95% of the American Churches won't even touch prophecy with a ten-foot pole, and this is happening on a massive scale, and they aren't ready, they aren't prepared. They don't know how to deal with it.

And shame on those shepherds, those hirelings, and if you go to one of those churches, I'll just challenge you, you need to run, you need to flee. You need to stop supporting churches who refuse to teach all the scripture, and you need to start supporting the churches that give you the whole council of God and do what God says shepherds are supposed to do. If you are a shepherd and you refuse to teach all of the Bible, you need to quit, or resign, or the church needs to kick you out. You need to go get a different job of picking peaches or changing tires. You have no business handling the Word of God. This is the time to preach God's truth, in all its fullness, because truth is what sets people free. God tells us the truth, including future events, for our benefit. You're not helping people when you are ignoring the truth.

So, what is the mark? Is it a mark of choice? What choice do you have? If you don't do it, you die. If you don't worship this guy you are going to die. If you don't take this, you are going to be shut out of the system. It's not just the mask and the vaccine, preparing for the mark, it's the way they are handling it, it's the term they use. It's a mandate. That's what the mark is. It will be a mandate from the antichrist to follow. And this is happening on a global basis in our lifetime. It's concerning but at the same time, it should be exciting. Because this is going to culminate during the 7-year Tribulation period, we leave prior and it's time to get motivated. But I want to deal with this. Is it really true? Jesus said that many will come in my name and deceive you by saying, "I am the Christ."

What does Christ mean? He is our Savior, and these guys are saying the only way to save our world, to save our planet, to bring back normalcy is what? This savior is the mask, this savior is the vaccine. Our only hope as a people, is that we have to wear masks and we have to take the vaccine. We are being lied to, we are being deceived on a massive scale and I think we all kind of realize this, right? In fact, we realize it and we put memes out there and laugh about it, even though it's not really funny, but it's so obvious. Have you noticed that? Let me review some of those for you.

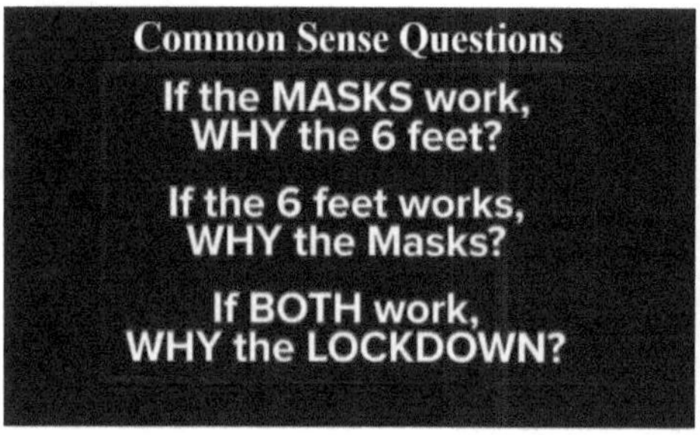

Common Sense Questions
If the MASKS work, WHY the 6 feet?
If the 6 feet works, WHY the Masks?
If BOTH work, WHY the LOCKDOWN?

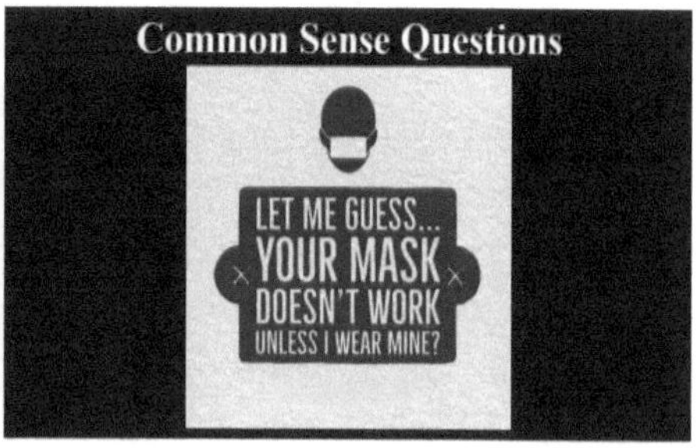

Common Sense Questions
LET ME GUESS...
YOUR MASK
DOESN'T WORK
UNLESS I WEAR MINE?

Have you noticed, they are starting to talk about it again, and that doesn't make sense. If your mask works then what are you worried about? If the vaccine works and I don't choose to get one, as some are choosing not to get, then what are you worried about I'm not a doctor nor do I play one on TV. I'm not giving you medical advice. Some people choose to get the vaccine, and some don't, but that is between you and God. I'm not here to make that decision for you. But can we examine this? If it worked, why are you thinking I have to, if I choose not to? Something's wrong there.

And by the way here is what the virologists wear to protect themselves, but don't worry that bandana is going to work. And when we put it on, we laugh because this is a joke. Oh, and by the way have you ever read the box?

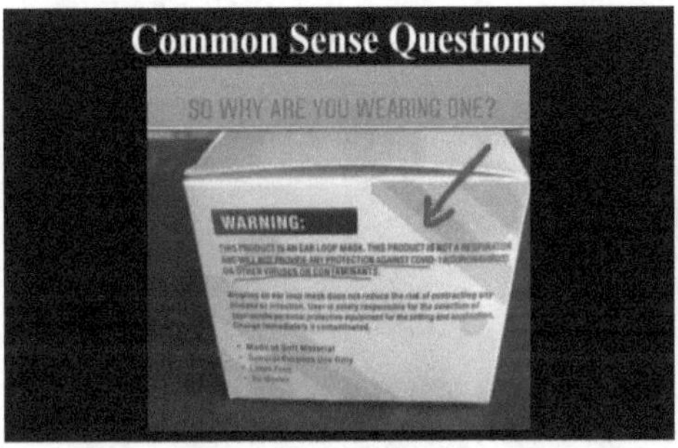
Common Sense Questions
SO WHY ARE YOU WEARING ONE?
WARNING:

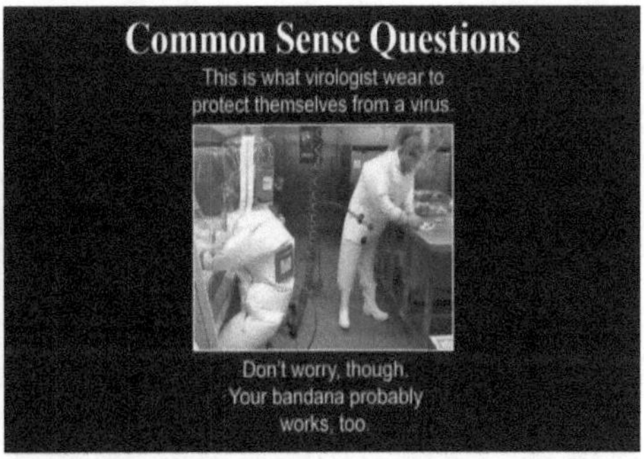
Common Sense Questions
This is what virologist wear to
protect themselves from a virus
Don't worry, though.
Your bandana probably
works, too

Go home and read the box. They admit on the box that these things do not work. They have to because they could be sued. That is a legal disclaimer by the way. And not only does it not help but at the bottom it says cloth masks or medical masks worn longer than 20 minutes actually promote the spread of disease and put you at risk of getting sick. Now it's starting to come out that the longer you wear these things it could actually make you sick and all kinds of other things. So, we know that when they put this out there it doesn't make sense. But haven't you listened to the media? They said … On the way in tonight, on the local broadcast here in Las Vegas, they admitted that the mask doesn't work, the vaccines don't work, but hopefully it will help curb some. And that was the word they used. Curb.

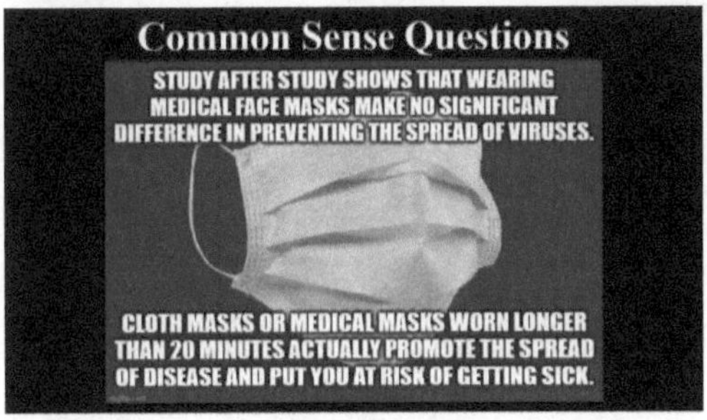

But that's not how it started. They said they did it and fixed it, and now they are saying that the masks don't work and even admitted it on TV tonight. The mask doesn't work! They even showed these little Covid germs flying through the masks. And then the vaccine, the second layer of support, they even showed the germs going through the vaccine. And then they said, "Well hopefully it will catch some of them." But that's not what you have been telling us. You told us a lie, you deceived us. You said if we do it, it will stop it. First the mask and then the vaccine.

Do you think that they know it doesn't work and it's just a bunch of baloney? Let me give you another one. It's all over the news if you pay attention. This is Biden's Covid advisor. Face masks don't help much from Covid-19. This is from a couple of days ago. All of this that I am sharing with you is hot off the press. Let me read what it says here. *"A top Covid advisor, for Joe Biden, has admitted that face masks are not very effective against Covid-19, and said they would only serve as a political purpose."* That is a direct quote. In an interview on Monday, Mike Osterholm said, *"If particles of smoke could get through the mask so could the virus."* And you know what? This one guy said this, *"Yeah, I want a cloth mask to stop the virus, just like I installed a chain link fence to keep out the mosquitos."* We put the memes out there because we know.

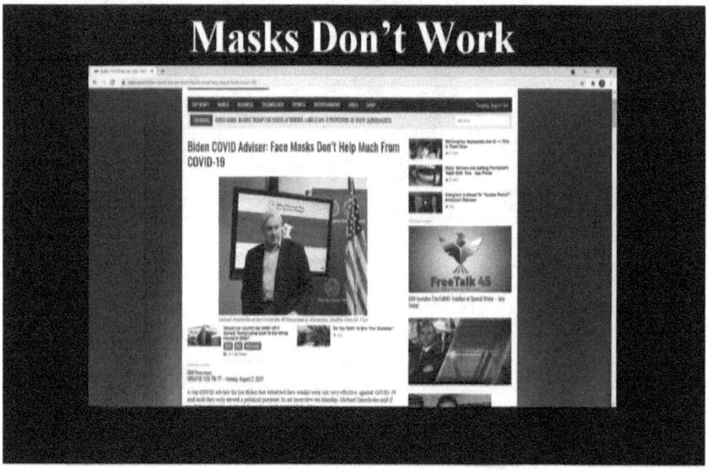
Masks Don't Work
Biden COVID Adviser: Face Masks Don't Help Much From COVID-19
FreeTalk45

We know we are being lied to. Something doesn't add up, it's fishy. In fact, these guy that work with Fauci, if you let them talk long enough, they show their true colors. He admitted in the beginning that masks are important. But then he got caught. He said,

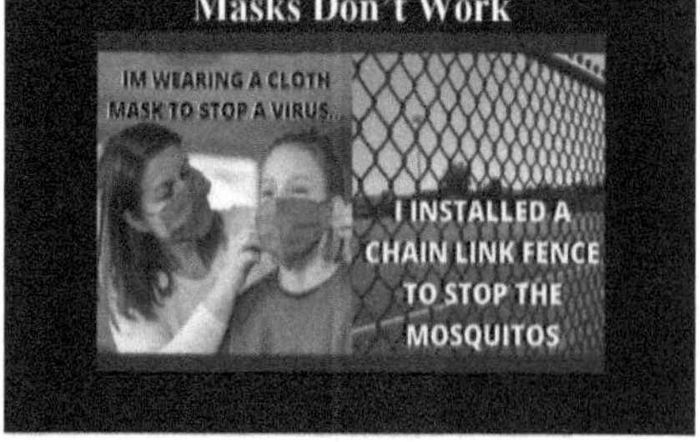
Masks Don't Work
IM WEARING A CLOTH MASK TO STOP A VIRUS...
I INSTALLED A CHAIN LINK FENCE TO STOP THE MOSQUITOS

"There is no reason to be walking around with a mask. Wearing a mask might make people feel better and it might block a droplet, but it's not providing the perfect protection that people think it is. Often there are unattended consequences."

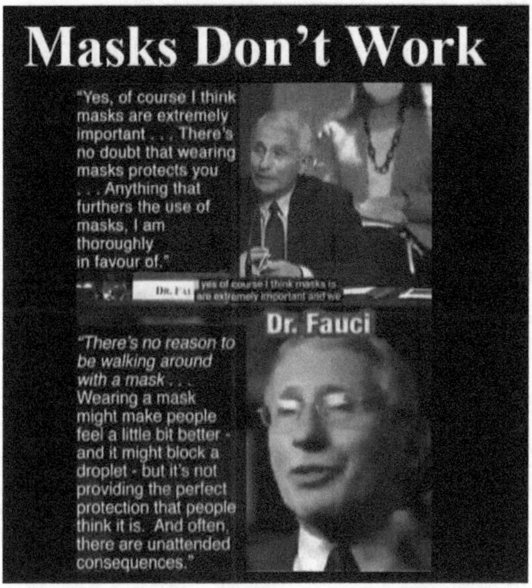

Part of that, they are saying, it will actually make you sick! This is not a conspiracy theory, it's not on Joe Schmo dot com. It's out there and it's legitimate. This is why it went from wear a mask, if you want your life back and you want this tyranny to stop, then you have to wear a mask. Then they said you have to wear two masks. Remember that one that was out there for a while? Then they said, oh, now you can go back to one mask. Then they said, if you get the vaccine you won't have to wear a mask. Now what is it? It doesn't matter if you are vaccinated, you have to wear a mask. And they admitted the masks don't work. It's just for a political purpose.

So again, this tells you that something fishy is going on. Somebody is trying to pull something over on us. We are being, what does the Bible say? Deceived! So, lets recap and look at the trail of deceit that we have been on since they launched Covid. And you tell me if somebody isn't trying to deceive us. Take a look at a transcript of this video clip.

Are you getting the vaccine? *They say the only thing that'll save us is THE VACCINE! The government, media, and celebrities are using fear to force you to do something that you may not be sure about. They expect you to roll up your sleeve and do something to your body that can't be undone. I don't know about you, but I have a few questions. So, we're going to answer them.*

Is the VACCINE safe? *No! According to the FDA, their list of possible adverse event outcomes, AKA side effects, from the VACCINE includes:*

Guillain-Barre Syndrome
Acute Disseminated Encephalomyelitis
Transverse Myelitis
Encephalitis
Myelitis
Encephalomyelitis
Meningoencephalitis
Meningitis
Stroke
Convulsions/seizures
Narcolepsy & Cataplexy
Anaphylaxis
Myocarditis
Autoimmune Disease

Whoa, there are way too many. We don't have time for this. It kind of makes you wonder, these deaths and injuries are already being reported, but rarely by the mainstream media.

Chicago Tribune: *A 'healthy' doctor died two weeks after getting a Covid-19 vaccine; CDC is investigating why.*

Federalist: *Washington Post buries facts about death of volunteer in Covid-19 vaccine trial.*

FOX: *Metro Healthcare worker describes severe allergic reaction to Covid-19 vaccine.*

FOX News: *California resident dies several hours after receiving Covid-19 vaccine; cause of death remains unclear.*

Orange County Register: *Health care worker dies after second dose of Covid vaccine, investigation underway.*

The government's VAERS database is collecting some of the reports. People are having cardiac arrests, respiratory arrests, and other severe reactions. You can look up these reports for yourself. This is just a sampling.

919609-1: Within 15 minutes of receiving the vaccine she developed pain and numbness starting at the injection site traveling down her arm and nausea.

931417-1: Patient began to complain of severe chest pain 3 hours after the vaccine was given ... EKG obtained and revealed ST segment elevation and a "cardiac alter" was called.

934539-1: Patient received Covid-19 (Moderna) vaccine from the Health Department on afternoon of January 8, 2021 and went to sleep approximately 2300 that night. Was found unresponsive in bed the following morning and pronounced dead at 1336 on January 9, 2021.

920545-1: The resident received his vaccine around 11:00 am ... He was found without a pulse, respiration or blood pressure at 1:59 pm.

929341-1: Pt received vaccine and complained of difficulty swallowing and rapid heart rate... Pt then transported to hospital via ambulance.

919087-1: Patient was admitted from 12/27-12/28/2020 at hospital by cardiology team who strongly felt the acute pericarditis was due to the Pfizer vaccine (Doctor was senior cardiologist)

924078-1: Client received vaccine at approximately 3:50 pm, waited in observational area 30 min. Left with husband, stated that she got a few miles down the road and started experiencing tightness in her chest...911 called.

921641-1: Administered first dose of Covid-19 vaccine at 1:29 pm on 1/9/21. At approximately 11:00 pm resident exhibited acute respiratory decompensation.

932145-1: Patient came into the emergency department on 1/8/21 with an acute ischemic stroke with complete occlusion of her left MCA... she received her 1st Covid-19 vaccine dose that morning at 10:31am.

904436-1: The patient was well prior to vaccination... He came to the hospital where he was tachycardia, 200 bpm and hypotensive to SBP10c.

There are already tens of thousands. Other governments are also gathering this information. Like this recent report from Norway:

Norway: 23 deaths associated with Covid-19 vaccination of which 13 have been assessed.

NY Post reports: Swiss nursing home resident reportedly dies after getting Covid-19 vaccine.

Reuters reports: Mexican doctor hospitalized after receiving Covid-19 vaccine.

NY Post reports: Israeli man reportedly dies of heart attack hours after getting Covid-19 vaccine.

Daily Mail reports: Portuguese health worker, 41 dies two days after getting the Pfizer Covid vaccine as her father says he "wants answers."

These are all the immediate side effects. But what happens to the ones that may kick in, in a year? Or 5 years, or 10 years down the road? Or what about long-term effects that are passed from parents to children? No one knows the long-term side effects. Since these injections are making some people sick, it's no wonder that the CEO's making these injections ran to Congress and got a total indemnification of liability from something called the "Prep Act." That means that if you get the shot and that shot injures or kills you, the company that made these injections cannot be held responsible.

So why is the injection making people sick? *Maybe it's because of what is in those syringes. It's experimental and you're the lab rat. You see, nothing like this has ever been used before. This is not a vaccine. A vaccine is where a microorganism, such as a virus, is pumped into the body in a small dose, so your immune system can respond and begin making antibodies. That's the theory anyway. That is not what these shots do! This is an experimental injection and if you get it, congrats, you are part of the biggest mass biological human experiment ever! Because what is in that syringe is not a vaccine any more than a giraffe is a fish!*

So, what is it? *Here's the idea. Your body has DNA in every one of your cells telling your body what to do. mRNA is the messenger that delivers the instructions from your DNA to the rest of your body. What they are going to pump into your arm is a synthetic mRNA. Once the syringe is through squeezing all that experimental juice into you, these tiny nanoparticles will punch holes into your cells and carry into your body the mRNA that was made in the lab. Once in your cells, these nanoparticles will instruct your body to make parts of the Covid-19 virus. It's like hacking a computer but instead of a computer they are hacking your body to make part of a virus.*

The Covid injection bypasses your DNA the same way a hacker bypasses the security firewall of a computer. The computer hacker spreads the virus, and the injection hacker makes part of the virus. But you're not a machine, so how can you be sure that it is safe and that the only code they are uploading into your cells is the code supposedly to fight Covid-19? Next question...

Who loves chemicals? *Well, get ready because they are coming to a syringe near you. Pfizer's version of a Covid injection contains a number of experimental and industrial chemicals including, ALC-0315, a positively charged molecule that helps the nanoparticles form. There's also DSPC & Potassium Chloride, Monobasic Potassium Phosphate,*

Sodium Chloride, and Dibasic Sodium Phosphate Dehydrate. You can find some of ingredients on your favorite bag of fertilizer. Boy! Can't wait to have that in me!

Now let's take a look at the Mode RNA or Moderna injection. Their shot contains similar substances, and they also throw in a drug named Tromethamine, because, why not? And then there is the SM-102 which is proprietary to the company. Proprietary means that this is their super-secret finger licking good family recipe. And they don't have to tell you anything about it. What could big pharma companies be trying to hide? Don't you have the right to know what exactly is being injected into your body? And whether or not it's safe?

Has the experimental injection been thoroughly tested? *No! The FDA's vaccines and related biological products advisory committee decided to approve this experimental injection for emergency use. Arnold Monto presided over the committee. Let's give a listen to see how thorough he was in approving the vaccine for the entire country.*

Member: *"I completely agree with you, but I think ..."*

Arnold Monto: *"Very quickly."*

Member: *"That would be my first question..."*

Arnold Monto: *"I said one part only."*

Member: *"Well, I am just going to put my hand up again then, Arnold."*

Arnold Monto: *"Then you will just go to the bottom of the queue." "We really need to keep this brief..." "Let's keep the answers relatively short." "That's a very big question." "We're not going to worry about adaptive and innate immune responses right now." "We'll take that offline." "I'm going to excuse Dr. Fink from having to answer that part of the question." "I think we want to stay away from discussions about immune response* *and other things that could be taken offline." "And therefore, our work for the day is done."*

Pretty thorough right? Side note. He has received money from Pfizer as recently as December 2018.

"Data from other studies suggest that the vaccine may affect physiological functions (central nervous system, renal, respiratory or cardiovascular system functions) safety pharmacology studies should be incorporated into the toxicity assessment. This does not apply for Covid-19 mRNA vaccine BNT16262."

Those who are supposed to keep you safe felt it unnecessary to see how the injection affects your brain, kidneys, lungs, or heart. ***No*** *studies were done to see how the injections react with other drugs that you may be taking.* ***No*** *toxicity studies were done on a single dose.* ***No*** *toxicokinetic studies were done to see what would happen once these chemicals got into your body.* ***No*** *genotoxicity studies were done to see if these chemicals would damage your DNA.* ***No*** *carcinogenicity studies were done to see if these substances could cause cancer. They have no idea if this is safe for pregnant women.* ***No*** *studies were done on how this experimental injection affects prenatal and postnatal moms or newborns.* ***No*** *studies were done to see what happens when a couple gets the injection and any subsequent children, they may have also received the shot. Look at all those No's!*

Is the experimental injection effective? *Another No! Ask yourself, if the so-called vaccine was effective, why are they still requiring you to wear a mask, after you've been vaccinated? And why have some people gotten Covid after being injected?*

CW Health: Here's why some people test positive after getting a Covid-19 vaccine.

Medpage Today: Vaccinated but sick with Covid-19; reports of post-vax infection a reminder to keep on masking and distancing, experts say.

Healthline: You can still spread, develop Covid-19 after getting a vaccine: What to know...

Have you seen these headlines? Well, the chemical trials for the Pfizer experimental injection did not demonstrate that the shot stopped any of the following:

Still get Covid
Still get sick
Still go to the hospital
Still spread to others

All the clinical trials proved was that the injections reduced the risk of mild Covid-19 symptoms, like coughing or muscle pain. That's it, and how do we know this? Pfizer, the manufacturer tells us:

"Covid-19 was defined according to the food and drug administration (FDA) criteria as the presence of at least one of the following symptoms: fever, new or increased cough, new or increased shortness of breath, chills, new or increased muscle pain, new loss of taste or smell, sore throat, diarrhea or vomiting."

Now for Moderna. According to the FDA, they don't know if the Moderna injection will protect people for more than 2 months. They don't know if it will provide any benefit for people who have already tested positive. They don't know if the injection will stop people from dying of Covid. They don't know if the injection prevents the virus from being transmitted from person to person. They don't know if the injection is safe for a large percentage of the population. They don't know if the injection will make getting the disease even worse. I think the theme here is "They don't know!" And since they are pushing this experimental injection on us as some sort of an emergency...

That must mean that there must be no other safe and effective treatments for Covid-19. Wrong! Doctors have found safe effective and inexpensive treatments that work well in preventing and treating patients with Covid-

19. Like Ivermectin that has been used safely for more than 30 years. But the government is not in support of this effective drug. In fact, there are other therapies including Hydroxychloroquine, vitamin D & C and Zinc that physicians have found to be safe and effective Covid treatments. But the government doesn't want them used either.

Is the Government silencing doctors and ignoring other effective treatments? *Yes! Critical voices from doctors, scientists, nurses and other health care professionals are being censored because if we already have effective therapies against Covid that would make an experimental injection totally unnecessary.*

Don't I have a high chance of dying if I don't get the experimental injection? *No! According to the government's own statistics and good old-fashioned math, your chances of surviving Covid without the experimental injection depends on your age group.*

0 – 14 Survival is 99.9998%
15-44 Survival is 99.9931%
45-64 Survival is 99.9294%
65-85 Survival is 99.6297%
Over 85 Survival is 98.2499%

The numbers don't lie! In fact, the chance of being struck by lightning is about the same as your chance of dying of Covid. Do we need an experimental injection for the potential lightning strike? Oh, by the way, this so-called vaccine wasn't proven to stop anyone from dying of Covid anyway. But your chance of surviving Covid is even better than these statistics. Why? Because the case counts and death counts are inflated since the government's Covid tests, according to the leading scientists are useless. The Covid tests are based on PCR. PCR was invented by a Doctor Kary Mullis who won the Nobel prize for his invention and said on video from his own mouth.

"The PCR Test was never designed to tell you if you are sick. With the PCR, if you do it well, you can find almost anything in anybody. PCR

separate from that is just a process you use to make a whole lot of something out of something. It doesn't tell you that you are sick, and it doesn't tell you that the thing you ended up with really was going to hurt you or anything like that."

In addition, Dr. Anthony Fauci has indicated that most PCR tests are being done wrong and finds dead nucleotides, not infection virus. In other words, the tests are supposedly finding Covid when there really is no Covid. Let's listen:

"If you get a cycle threshold of 35 or more, the chances of it being replication – confident (AKA accurate) are miniscule. We have patients, and it's very frustrating for the patients as well as the physicians. Somebody comes in and they repeat their PCR and it's like a 37-cycle threshold. You almost never can culture a virus from a 37-cycle threshold. I think that if somebody comes in with a 37, 38 or a 36 you have to say, 'You know it's just dead nucleotides, period."

Dead nucleotides, period? Even above 36 cycles, interesting. Guess what the FDA approved? Up to 40-cycles. That means that most of your tests that find Covid are not finding Covid. But in Fauci's words, dead nucleotides. Fragments in the environment.

And finally, the former Vice President of Pfizer, one of the company's making the experimental injections has called the PCR tests useless. So, if someone dies of Covid and the Covid test is useless, what are they really dying from? Probably from one of the other comorbidities. What's that? It means other diseases. According to the CDC. 94 percent of all Covid deaths had an average of 2.9 other comorbidities. In other words, 94 percent of the people who supposedly died of Covid, had on average had about 3 other diseases that could have contributed to their deaths.

Let's recap: *Here's what we know ... Covid vaccine is not a vaccine, it's an experimental mRNA injection that hacks your cells and instructs your body to make parts of the Covid-19 virus. It was rushed through clinical trials, skipped proper safety testing, and is already causing a long list of* *side effects. People are already getting sick and dying from it. The injection was not proven to stop people from contracting Covid, transmitting the virus or preventing people from getting very sick. The list of ingredients are unknown, because the drug company doesn't have to tell us what is in the syringe. Drug companies ran to Congress so they can't be held responsible for when people get sick or die from their so-called vaccine. Ironically, there is an immunity. The injection makers are 100 percent immune from accountability. But safe, effective and proven therapies for Covid exist and they are being ignored and censored. The number of Covid cases and death counts are wildly exaggerated because the test on which they are based is useless. The truth is, none of us really know:*

Why the lockdowns?
Why the inaccurate PCR testing?
Why inflate case & death counts?
What's with the rampant censorship?
What is the real agenda here?

Good question! But I think I found the answer, and I'm going to expose it here in just a second. This is deceit. Stack it all up, this is all verified information. That is why I preach about the interviews, how you can see it's right out of their mouths and you can see what is going on. So, what is the real agenda here? Was it to make President Trump look bad? Yes, that was a given. Was it an excuse to bring in the mail-in ballots to help steal the election? Yes, that was a given. Was it also to begin, on a global basis, to institute the Great Reset, economic cashless society where they are going to own everything, control the buying and selling? Yes, that is a given.

It's also another layer of deceit, and if you read the Bible, it tells you why. Here is the agenda as to why it's so insane and makes no sense, just so you understand why.

1 Timothy 6:10a "For the love of money is a root of all kinds of evil."

Biblical truth, a lot of us know that. In fact, there is an old saying, if you want to find the truth about something, what do you do? Follow the money. I was able to come across the information by, following the money. So, what we are going to see is the proof that we have been deceived. The reason they are pushing vaccines or nothing, and they want to mandate it, is because, just like when Obama first got in office, the first thing he did was bail out the banks, at taxpayer's expense. As we will see it was not just $700 billion, it was close to $13 trillion. The first thing he did was, he came in and bailed out the banks. Now I was like, let them fall, the rest of us have to if we make a bad business decision. Right? Why do taxpayers have to bail these guys out? What we are seeing with this vaccine, it's a bailout for big Pharma. Obama came in and immediately bailed out the banks, Biden came in and he's bailing out big Pharma who were failing and going bankrupt. But not anymore thanks to the vaccine.

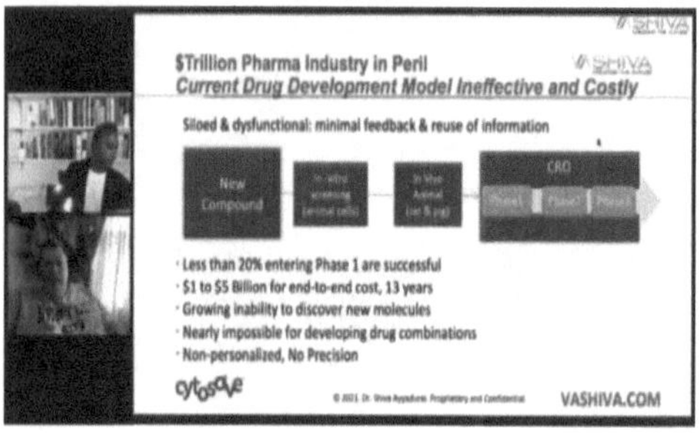

"What you will see here is that the entire Drug Development Model works in the following way: And by the way what is a pharmaceutical? Pharmaceutical is a drug, or a chemical compound, that does not exist in nature. So, a chemical compound that does not exist in nature, would be something like Lipitor or ibuprofen. Something that exists in nature would be something like vitamin C or zinc. These are minerals that exist in nature. When a new compound is created, the drug development industry needs to go through this very, very, long drawn-out process to get that new compound to the market.

Let's say that compound is something like Advil, which, by the way, is a generic drug right now. So, what do they have to do? They have to take that new compound, and the first thing they have to do is file for a patent. The second thing they have to do is they will have to do testing in a test tube. That is called in-vitro testing. In-vitro means in a test tube. In-vitro testing gets done and that will take a couple of years. While in the test tube they have to say this will reduce pain or inflammation. In the test tube they will create the environment where they are creating some cells with inflammatory response. They will drop ibuprofen in and if it makes sense and the data is matching what they predicted, which takes a couple years, then they go into in-vivo testing. Which means they test it on animals. Now you have testing in animals which could take 3 or 4 years, hundreds of millions of dollars, depending on how long you do the testing. So, now you are looking at the synthesis of the product to the in-vivo, that could take about 5 or 6 years.

After that, the Pharmaceutical Company needs to go file for a Clinical testing. Clinical testing means that they have to test on humans. Before they can do that, between the in-vivo and the CRO, they have to go to the FDA and get approval or allowance. Which the FDA looks at their animal data and say, it looks like you're not going to kill human beings. It's not that toxic and you understand the dosages, and that will take a couple of years. Now you are into about 6 or 7 years. Then they start human clinical trials. First trial is called Phase 1, small sets of humans, Phase 2 is larger sets of humans. Phase 3 is many, many, large, hundreds or thousands of humans.

After that they spent close to $5 billion for 13 years. The drug, because patent life is only 7 years, so if it cost them $5 billion and say 100,000 people can take that drug, they have to sell that drug for $50 thousand plus to make back their money. Remember, for pharmaceutical drugs, you can actually sue the pharmaceutical company in court, federal court, state court, if they injure you. So, think about it from the pharmaceutical company's standpoint. It's a lot of money to get this drug out there. And they can be liable. And they can be sued. So, this is the drug development process. Everyone needs to understand this.

It is important to understand this process requires not only money, but it's not working. It is a medieval process, meaning it's an archaic process where it's not even using any real technology. Big Pharma has been spending more and more money in trying to get new drugs through and less and less of the pharmaceutical drugs are actually coming out. Even the FDA is not allowing new drugs to come out, because of the side effects. So, this is where pharmaceutical companies were up until the last ten years. They know they are failing. The R&D process is old, it's not innovative, even big pharma is not allowing those drugs through.

So, this is a reality that pharma has to face every day. They are not making money with this very, very old archaic process. More and more money is put into this old process and less and less drugs are being allowed by the FDA. Now, if you look at the Global Report, this came out at the beginning of last year, when this 'epidemic' was hitting. It says, 'Top 20 Pharma Companies lost $2.6 trillion in Market Cap.' What does that mean? It means, on the stock market, these guys are tanking, $2.6 trillion. By the way, that is the entire size of the weapons industry. One quarter of the pharmaceutical companies lost $2.6 trillion.

Their methodology is old, medieval, they are putting more and more money into it, but they aren't making money back and guess what? Their market value on the stock market is going down. That is what is going on in reality. For every one dollar that the pharmaceutical companies used to spend on R&D they would get ten cents back, a 10.1 percent return. Now it is a 1.8 percent return. Vaccines are growing at a rate of 17 percent per year. If you notice these companies, comparing what they spend on marketing and what they spent on R&D, they are spending double on marketing because the entire drug development process is failing. Pharma spends roughly 30-40 percent on marketing. That is why we are being bombarded on TV with these drug ads all the time.

One of the things to understand, the actual economics of it. How do pharmaceutical companies work? They make money off their patents. So, when they put out a drug, they have twenty years of patent life. When that drug goes off patent, they come crashing and burning. So, it takes them 13 to 15 years to build a drug, and they have a limited amount of time to make money. An example is when Lipitor, which is Pfizer's top drug, in 2010 Lipitor went off the market. Their revenue dropped. So, less and less new drugs are being discovered and more and more of their drugs are coming off patent. This is an industry that is crashing and burning.

Pfizer lost $25 billion in revenue in the last 10 years, from 2011 to 2020. In fact, in the last 4 years, they lost close to $10 billion. You need to understand the background because Pfizer has been tanking and losing money. But the bottom line is that Pfizer has been losing $25 billion in the last 10 years and is a tanking company. Now here is the reality. With the jabs, Bernstein Research, which is one of the most respected research companies on Wall Street, they have predicted that in just one year they are expected to make $15 billion. This prediction was made about a year ago. The recent data is saying that Pfizer will be making about $26 billion this year alone. So, think about that. Pfizer and all of these failing pharma companies are going to make $40 billion in one year.

Now let's look at the Biden administration, just two days ago Biden announced that he's going to buy, with American taxpayers' money, 500 million doses of the Pfizer jab. That will be about $10 billion. Right there Pfizer will be getting $10 billion. Biden was elected in January of this year, and in 6 months he's delivering to them a paycheck of $10 billion. The article says, 'President Biden is slated to announce the plan this week, at the Group of Seven meeting in Britain, where he is expected to be joined by Pfizer CEO Albert Bourla.

Who, by the way, was honored by Israel, just recently, with a Lifetime Achievement Award, and Israel has become the poster child for Pfizer. Meaning that Pfizer did an agreement with Israel back in January, to talk about how everyone should get 'jabinated'. In return, Israel gave Pfizer all that data, essentially making them the poster child. So, what we are seeing is, where does government end and Pfizer begin? Nobody knows. Our American tax dollars, 10 or probably 15 billion in a check to Pfizer, under the guise of helping these countries all over the world. We gotta get them jabbed and America is coming to help them. It's called corruption!

I hope everyone gets this. Your tax dollars are being transferred from American taxpayers, which should be going to infrastructure, building roads, bridges, and water systems, to Pfizer. I hope everyone understands that. Simple stuff and I don't know why the mainstream media and no one else is covering this, because it is in black and white. Now, this just came *out. They created an organization called Covax, which is from the WHO, and guess what they are going to deliver? Two billion doses by the end of this year. Over a month ago I did a deep analysis for everyone, and I shared with you the mathematics of this. Remember I did an excel spreadsheet and I said their goal is to get 2 billion doses out there. Which means 30 percent of the people will be vaccinated, 30 percent of 7.1 billion people, is two billion. The average price that all of the pharmaceutical companies are charging is $40.00, they will get 50 percent, and it will go to all the middlemen, the ad manufacturers will get $20.00. $20.00 time 2 billion is $40 billion. Well, two days ago, the numbers are coming out in black and white. Two billion doses, that is their target.*

This is why they are pushing the 70 percent vaccination, the' jabination'. And the reality is this. Pharmaceutical companies are tanking, they need to be saved. And the way they got saved out of this, is they got 'Operation Warp Speed'. Trump delivered to them 'Operation Warp Speed'. What is 'Operation Warp Speed'? 'Operation Warp Speed' means that 13 years of testing gets eliminated. You don't have 13 years to test anymore. You have nine months of testing, fast tracking. So, Trump did that for pharma. This has nothing to do with Vax or Anti-vax. Forget about the vaccines. Let's assume it is another industry, let's say it was the airplane industry. I'm sure both Biden and Trump gave Boeing the money. Imagine how all of us would feel if they did operation air speed for Boeing. You don't need to do testing; you can put engines on. It takes decades to get airplanes out there on the market.

This reminds me of the Affordable Care Act with Obama, where the insurance companies all got rich off of this, because everybody was a customer. So, in this model, everyone became a customer, because the government and big pharma are working so well together, we are all being forced to become customers. That is what Obama did. So, when you put all of this together, stop creating these fake dialectics. Stop excusing politicians. Recognize that there are two different worlds going on here. One world where the politicians create the dialectic. They can take anything to get you enraged about something. And that is the theater.

Then, over here is the reality. The reality is you have a major industry that has been tanking. Now the jab and the 'jabinations', this product is their life raft. Out of this massively falling industry is falling revenue. So, one guy keyed it up and the other guys are bringing the bacon home. That's all it is."

It answers a lot of questions, doesn't it? Why do they continue with this new false narrative? You have to wear a mask, no masks, two masks, one mask, get the vaccine. Now you don't even have a choice, you have to get the vaccine or they are going to take away your job. All these things are happening. Why? Because they are concerned about your health? No! We are being deceived. The Bible says it will happen in the last days. And it is happening on a global scale. Yes, I believe the Covid virus was released to make President Trump look bad, yes, it was to bring in the mail in ballots to throw the election, yes, the global reset, but like he said, it's an economic bailout as well, at taxpayer's expense.

Again, what's the old phrase? "Those who don't learn their history are doomed to repeat it." Did we forget what Obama did right when he got in office? He was brought in to bail out the banks. This is from PBS, this is their website, so you can't say this is a Christian wacky conspiracy. Even they admit it and I quote:

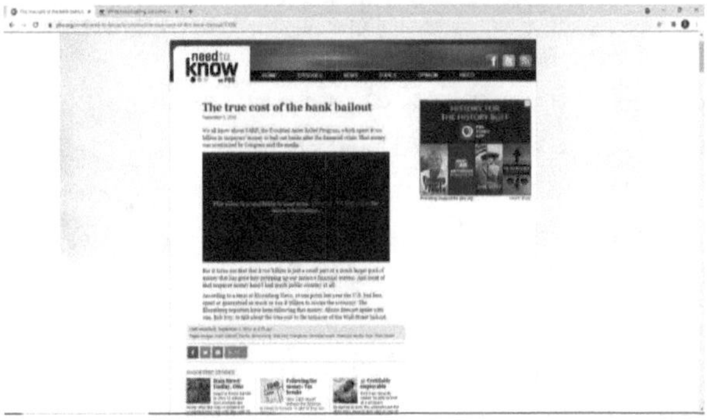

"We all know about the TARP program which sent $700 billion of taxpayer's money. That money was scrutinized by congress and the media, but it turned out that the $700 billion was a small part of a larger pool of money that went into propping up our nation's financial system. And most of that taxpayer money has not had much public scrutiny at all. According to a team at Bloomberg News, the real number is $12.8 trillion."

So, can I translate that for you? We weren't told about this, to bail out the banks. So, Biden comes along, and he bails out Big Pharma.

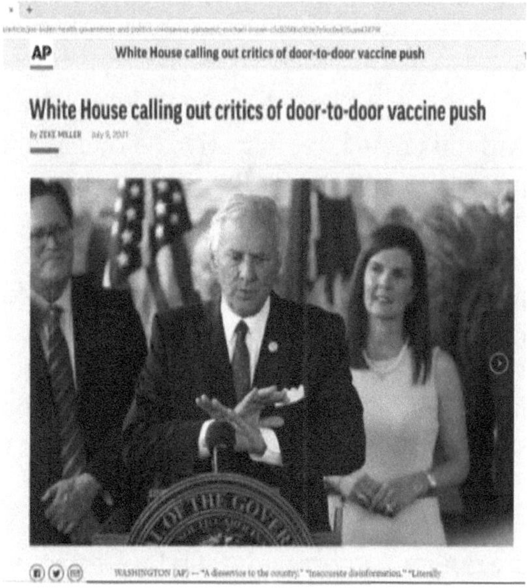

This is why they push it, and it has nothing to do with health. Is Covid real? Of course, it is. I'm not saying it's not. But this insane behavior starts to make sense when you start to understand there is a monetary agenda here. And on the one hand, if we learn our history, they are doing the same thing. Obama bailed out the banks as soon as he got in, Biden is bailing out Big Pharma. This is why they are threatening to go door to door. It's not about your health! Because if they can threaten, and force you, and mandate this, you are a guaranteed customer and the more people they get, the more money they get to bail them out. This is their what? Life raft.

Remember what he said. In ten years, Pfizer lost $25 billion. They are going to make that back and probably a lot more, in one year. And does it show signs of stopping? Unfortunately, no! Again, we know this stuff doesn't make sense. Statistics don't lie. This is from Defending The Republic.org/COVID. This is Sidney Powell's' website, one of the top lawyers in the nation, and they share this, the survival rate is 99.8 percent.

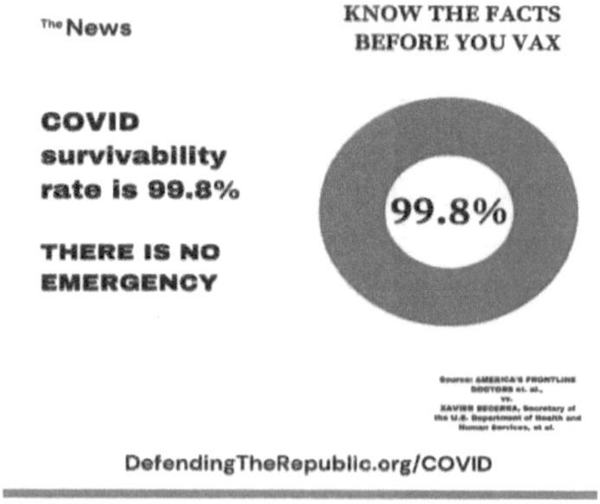

There is no emergency. We say all the time, this is not a pandemic, it's a plandemic. For what? It was a bailout amongst the other issues. It's multi-layered deceit, that's what's going on. One guy says this:

"So let me get this straight in my head, I can have Aids, Chlamydia, Gonorrhea, Ebola, Hepatitis, Meningitis, and Conjunctivitis and I can eat in a restaurant and go to the pub ... but if I haven't had a vaccine for Covid-19 (aka nasty cold virus) ... I'm barred. Seriously?"

Really? It doesn't make sense. Another guy says:

"We went from 'flattening the curve in 14 days' to 'going door-to-door to see your papers' ... Gotta admit, I did N-A-Z-I that one coming."

We know something fishy is going on. This guy says:

"In 6 months, we've gone from the vax ending the pandemic - to you can still get Covid even if vaxxed - to you can pass Covid onto others even if vaxxed – to you can still die of Covid even if vaxxed – to the unvaxxed are killing the vaxxed." When actually the vaxxed are the ones they say are spreading Covid.

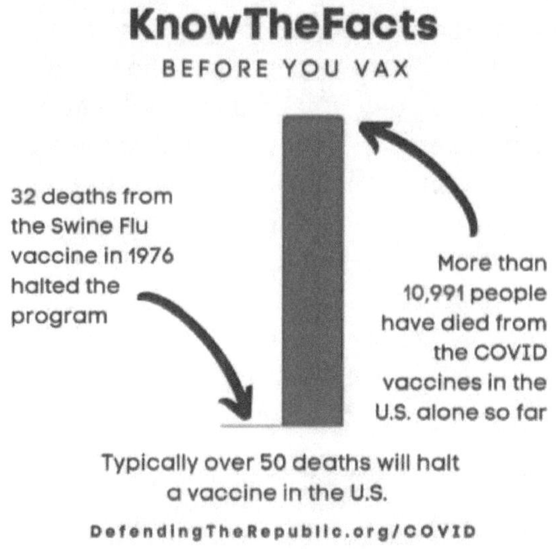

KnowTheFacts
BEFORE YOU VAX
32 deaths from the Swine Flu vaccine in 1976 halted the program
More than 10,991 people have died from the COVID vaccines in the U.S. alone so far
Typically over 50 deaths will halt a vaccine in the U.S.
DefendingTheRepublic.org/COVID

It doesn't make sense, right? And by the way, look at this: Understand it's a bailout. And this is also from Defending the Republic.org/Covid. "Know the Facts before you Vax."

A monetary, evil, sick, twisted, agenda. 32 deaths from the Swine Flu vaccine in 1976 halted that program. That's all it took.

32 deaths and they said, “Get it off the market”. How many have died from the Covid vaccine? 10,991 people and still counting. Some people are saying it’s more like 45,000 or more. But still let’s just take their science and you’re still pushing it? It only took 32 to stop the other one. Why are you letting it go on to 11,000 plus? Or maybe tens of thousands. Why don’t you yank it off the market if you’re so concerned about our health? But that’s not what it is. It’s a bailout! The more people that take this vaccine, the more money they get to put in their pockets. And they call this safe.

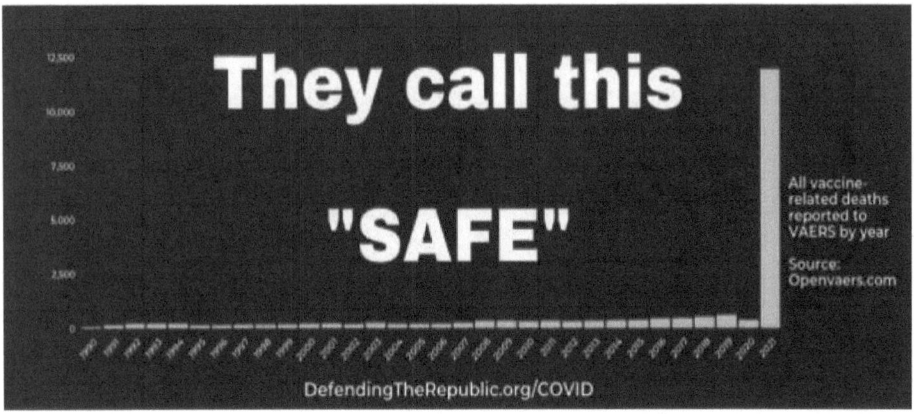
They call this
"SAFE"
All vaccine-related deaths reported to VAERS by year
Source: Openvaers.com
DefendingTheRepublic.org/COVID

These are the vaccine related deaths throughout history. Pretty much stable and then all of a sudden what do you see? If this was about our health, if this was about saving us, and for our good, you should have yanked this baby off the market as fast as you put it on there. But that’s not what is going on. Now here’s my question. How are they doing this? I don’t know about you, but I have my own suspicions. But have you ever tried to talk to somebody, even a family member, about some of these things? It’s like you are talking to a brick wall. Did the peas roll out of your casserole? Did your cheese slide off your cracker? What happened? They have bought into this! It’s because they are using the media to generate the fear, to get people to go along with the program to bail them out. Let’s take a look at part of this video again:

Are you getting the vaccine? *They say the only thing that will save you is the vaccine. The government, celebrities, and the media are using fear to force you into something that you may not be sure about.*

So, what are they using to generate the fear to get people to follow the agenda? Media. And it's working if you look at the latest statistics. Including this latest, Delta Variant. It's working:

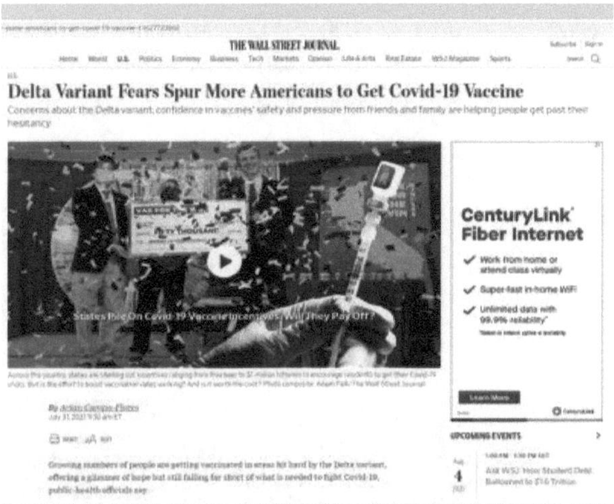
THE WALL STREET JOURNAL.

Delta Variant Fears Spur More Americans to Get Covid-19 Vaccine

Concerns about the Delta variant, confidence in vaccines' safety and pressure from friends and family are helping people get past their hesitancy

Growing numbers of people are getting vaccinated in areas hit hard by the Delta variant, offering a glimmer of hope but still falling far short of what is needed to fight Covid-19, public-health officials say

The Delta Variant fears spur more Americans to get Covid-19 vaccine. People are freaking out. And guess what? It's not about their health, it doesn't cure it, it doesn't even stop it, there's not any good side effects, but what's it really all about? They are scaring people to get more jabs, so they can get more money. It's a bailout. We have been totally deceived. Now, if you don't think the media on a global basis is all interconnected and being used by global elites to produce the narrative, i.e., brainwash people. This is why when we try to talk to people and eek! They are watching social media and the television, and they don't read the scripture, and dare I say even some Christians, and they are freaking out. I'm going to give you a little teaser taste of the proof, that you're not watching the news, you are watching the narrative.

Fox 29 News: "Hi, I'm Jessica Headley." "And I'm Ryan Wolf."
(All saying the same words over each other at the same time)
KATU 2 ABC: "Our responsibility is to serve…."
02 News: "our valley community…"
4 News: "Our Phoenix community…"
Fox 21 News: "Our Eastern Iowa Community…"
Fox 66 News: Our Michigan community…"

4 News: "We are very proud of the quality, balanced journalism we at 4 news produces but..."
All of the stations say these words all at the same time:
"We are concerned about what is plaguing our country."
Eyewitness News: "The sharing and bias of false news has become all to common on social media while alarming some media outlets who report the same fake stories without checking facts first."
Once again, all the stations are speaking on top of one another the same sentence. Like they are all reading the same script. They continue:
"Unfortunately, they push their own personal bias...which is extremely dangerous to our democracy."
Fox 29: "This is extremely dangerous to our democracy."
KATU 2 News: "This is extremely dangerous to our democracy."
Channel 7 news: "This is extremely dangerous to our democracy."
Local 12 News: "This is extremely dangerous to our democracy."
ABC13: "This is extremely dangerous to our democracy."
Fox 11: "This is extremely dangerous to our democracy."
4 News: "This is extremely dangerous to our democracy."

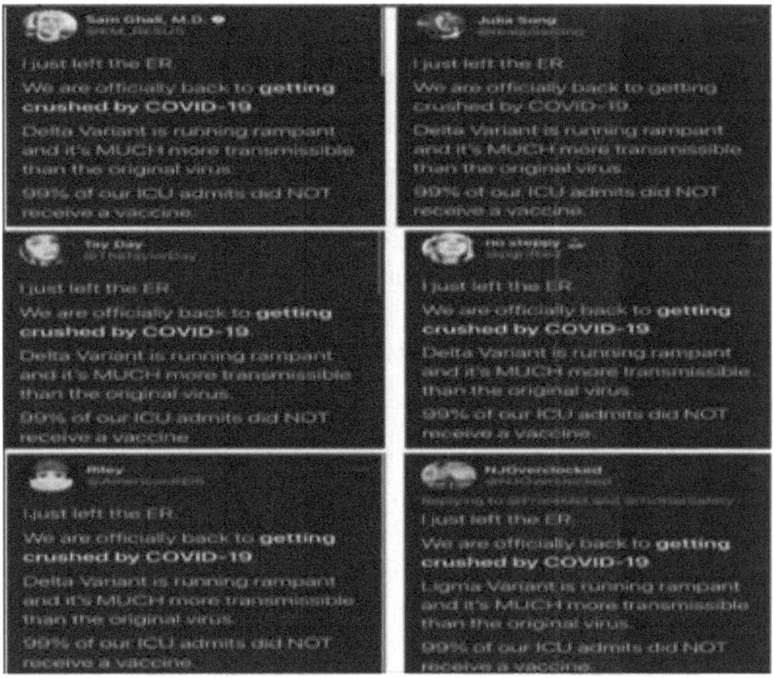

Now, if you don't think this is being done to generate the fear overall about Covid and even this latest Delta Variant, let me just give you one example. This is what's going on in social media. It's all tied together. Pushing the narrative, to get people freaked out to get the jab so they can get their cash. These are posts online, what are the odds, and these are supposed to be individual responses from individuals. But what are the odds that they would say the exact same thing every single time?

I think it is impossible. I think it's AI generating this. These are so-called independent comments. They said the exact same thing, with the exact same caps. We are being lied to. This is generated to generate a fear, with the global elites. And it's not true, that it's with all vaccinated people. I just read an article that Sunrise Hospital here in Las Vegas, eleven nurses came down with Covid after all eleven were vaccinated. So, don't tell me it's just from the vaccinated. But again, it makes no sense unless you understand the motive. What's it about? The bailout.

Now really quick about the bogus media. I don't think it's by chance that two days ago, in God's sovereignty, He had us release our latest documentary called *Subliminal Seduction, How the Mass Media*

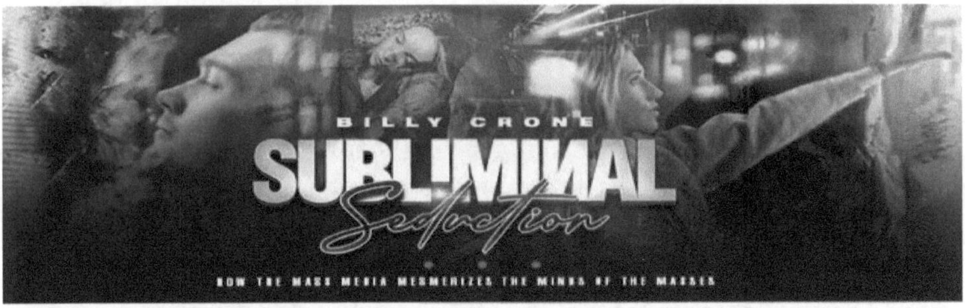

Mesmerizes the Minds of the Masses, as you can see here. We just released this two days ago. We didn't know that they were going to use, once again, the media to generate this Delta Variant, but God did. And it's very interesting for us, as a ministry, and as a church, and me personally, because once again, it's God showing that He is sovereign, and He is in control. Because no way is that by chance. This resource exposes a teaser of what you just saw, how it is all interconnected. And we expose the whole thing on a global basis. All media outlets, and I mean, radio, television, newspapers, books, the educational system and social media are in the hands of a few rich billionaire elites, and they are controlling the narrative on the planet. We exposed the whole thing. That is what it's all about.

And just when Covid was first released, unbeknownst to us, we released *Hybrids Super Soldiers and the Coming Genetic Apocalypse.* And then here comes Covid. This wasn't by chance. Here comes this narrative, and they are using this global media to freak people out. And then we come out with this next one. I'm not saying this to get you to run out and buy the documentary, but I encourage you to do so. But I take that as God saying, "I am in control." He will provide for his people, who want the truth. Remember this, "They perish because they don't want to hear the truth." But if you want the truth, God loves you, He will show you the truth. He'll show you what is going on. This is not a time to be fearful. It is a time to be faithful. In fact, it is a time to get your head out of the news, and get it into the Word of God. Because God says this.

2 Timothy 1:7 "For God has not given us the spirit of fear but of power, and of love, and of a sound mind."

And I will just be blunt in love, as your shepherd, if you are freaking out over Covid, and I'm not saying that it's not real, but if you are freaking out over it and you are literally in a state of panic, that is not from God. I'll guarantee you, it is a media generated fear and they are using you, duping you, deceiving you, to corral you, to go get the jab. That's your choice. I'm not telling you what to do. But to go get it, because they need you to get the jab, to get the cash, to bail them out, we are being deceived. I don't need to be afraid of what's going on, including these global leaders who literally want to take over the world. In fact, it's been a long-standing plan. This is a cartoon from the 1930s. And you tell me if this doesn't sound familiar today. It's a cartoon on how to take over the world.

How to Take Over the World, An Early Warning Cartoon

A black figure is walking down the middle of the street with a gas tank being pulled behind it.

1) *Introduce a Weaponized Influenza*

As the gas tank follows this black figure you can see there are vapors coming out and going into the air.

2) *Flood Newspapers and Radio with Death*

The Radio blasts the news

3) *Shut down shops and churches*

Fences have been put up around the churches to keep people out, boards have been put on the doors of the shops to keep people out.

4) *Use Law Enforcement to Stifle Dissent*

The police are using the sticks to beat a little fellow over the head.

5) *Parade the sick and the dead*

A cart is being pulled down the street by the black figure with a casket in it. The people on the side of the road are very fearful, seeing what could be happening to them next. They all have on their gas masks. All the people in the funeral procession also have on their gas masks.

6) *Inject a "Vaccine" to sterilize the work shy and euthanize the old.*

As each person comes out, they are immediately given the shot. The black figure is issuing the shots.

7) *The people who own banks now own the hospitals; this is their plan to own you! THE END!*

Those who don't know their history are doomed to repeat it. This may be, and I am convinced, especially if you study the global leaders, a lot of them, back in the day knew they weren't going to see the fruition of their globalist behavior in their lifetime. But they continue with this agenda, and now it is coming to fruition. Even though I believe this has been a long-standing plan, I don't have to be afraid. God hasn't given me the spirit of fear. In fact, I need to read **Psalm 2,** and go to sleep. How does God feel about these globalists that are going to take over the world? They say we're going to get rid of God, get rid of Jesus, we're going to get rid of Christianity, we're going to throw off that bondage. We're going to build our own utopia. Look at what God's attitude is on that.

Psalm 2:1-12: "Why do the nations conspire, and the people plot in vain? The kings of the earth take their stand and the rulers gather together against the Lord and against his Anointed One. 'Let us break their chains', they say, 'and throw off their fetters.' The One enthroned in heaven laughs; the Lord scoffs at them. Then he rebukes them in his anger and terrifies them in his wrath, saying, 'I have installed my King on Zion, mu holy hill.' I will proclaim the decree of the Lord. He said to me, 'You are my Son, today I have become your Father, ask of me and I will make the nations your inheritance, the ends of the earth your possession. You will rule them with an iron scepter, you will dash them to pieces like pottery.' Therefore, you kings, be wise; be warned, you rulers of the earth. Serve the Lord with fear and rejoice with trembling. Kiss the Son, lest he be angry and you be destroyed in your way for his wrath can flare up in a moment. Blessed are all who take refuge in him."

Do you really think you are going to overthrow God's agenda? Do you really thing you are going to stop what God has planned for this planet? Do you really thing you are going to stop my Son, Jesus, from coming back and ruling and reigning on this planet? If God is laughing about it. I think we need to lighten up. He does not give us a spirit of fear. We belong to him. Don't you understand that we are going to be with Jesus and ruling and reigning in the Millennial Kingdom? We get Raptured during Hell on earth. Oh, and by the way, all these people that are doing this, with people dying because of this, and this is satanic because he's a murderer and a liar from the beginning, the Bible says that unless they get saved by Jesus Christ, all they are doing is storing up the wrath of God.

You're not going to stop God's plan. He is laughing at these guys. Have you taken refuge in Jesus Christ? God says you are blessed, why? Because we will be with Jesus ruling and reigning on the planet. All this New World Order stuff that is unfolding in front of our very eyes, He is going to come back and fold it right back up. He will rule and reign on this planet with us, His Bride and no man can stop God's plan, no matter how long this has been. We are on the winning team; we won't lose and the only thing we need to do is get excited because the departure is near, and we need to finish strong. You tell people they need to kiss the Son, you need to get saved, or you are going to face the wrath of God. That is how we need to respond to the generated narrative going on.

Chapter Three

The Lies of Covid

How many of you would agree that the days we live in are getting pretty freaky and messed up and weird and wacky out there, especially with all the stuff that's going on? I don't know about you, but what has happened to people? It's like they checked their brains at the door. It's one thing if they want to believe or act that way, but they are trying to get us to go along with their wacky thoughts. Their rationale. Have you noticed that? In fact, tell me if this doesn't sound familiar in the days we live in.

A guy comes walking out to the pool with his towel draped over his shoulder. He looks at the water and gets ready to jump in when a fellow with an orange life jacket, blue baseball cap worn backwards, white sun protection paste covering his nose, black rimmed glasses, that are held together with white tape, jumps in front of him, holds up his hand and asks, "What are you doing?" He is the pool guard.

The prospective swimmer replies, "I'm going to do a little swimming."

Pool guard: "You gotta wear a life jacket or else you can't come in."

Swimmer: "No, I'm good. Thank you though."

Pool guard: “Life jackets are mandatory.”

Swimmer: “Mandatory to wear a life jacket when you swim?”

Pool guard: “Even when you’re not swimming too.”

Swimmer: “Why?”

Pool guard: “Cases of people getting wet are going through the roof. It’s a scary time. Put it on!”

Swimmer: “But that doesn’t mean they are drowning. People get wet every day. It’s part of life.”

Pool guard: “.00001182 percent of all people drown each year. That’s practically everybody. So put on the life jacket!”

Swimmer: “That doesn’t make any logical sense. I’m not putting one on. I know how to swim. I’ve had swimming lessons.”

Pool guard: “Swimming lessons? Do you think those exist? Do you just think your body has this natural ability to traverse through the water in a way that keeps your head up so you can still breathe?”

Swimmer: “Yeah, it’s called swimming.”

Pool guard: “Never heard of it. Flotation devices are backed by science. You don’t believe in science?”

Swimmer: “I do, it’s just that I know how to swim.”

Pool guard: “You are kinda being racist right now.”

Swimmer: “What?!”

There is another guy in the pool waving at the swimmer.

Swimmer: “He’s just standing in the water.”

Pool guard: “Put the life jacket on right now! You are putting everyone at risk of drowning.”

Swimmer: “How am I putting everyone at risk?”

Pool guard: “Their life jackets don’t work unless you have one on.”

Swimmer: “Does his life jacket work?”

Pool guard: “Yes, very well.”

Swimmer: “Then why would he need me to wear a life jacket when his already works?”

Pool guard: “We have to protect the protected swimmers from the unprotected swimmers.”

Swimmer: “But aren’t they already protected?”

Pool guard: “Yes, very well protected.”

Swimmer: “So they should be fine.”

Pool guard: “They would be except they aren’t very well protected because of you! Look, you gotta put one on or you can’t go in.”

Swimmer: “This feels creepy, so where would I get one.”

Pool guard: “Oh, I’m selling them right here.”

Swimmer: “You’re selling life jackets?”

Pool guard: “Yes, of course.”

Swimmer: “You are demanding that everyone wear a life jacket while you are selling life jackets?”

Pool guard: “Yes, for their protection.”

Swimmer: “And they have to buy the life jacket from you?”

Pool guard: “Indeed.”

Swimmer: “Don’t you think that is a conflict of interest?”

Pool guard: “No conflict of interest that I can think of.”

Swimmer: “How much money have you made this year from selling life jackets?”

Pool guard: “Ummm, $27 billion.”

Swimmer: “It seems like you are more interested in making money than keeping people safe from the water.”

Pool guard: “You are an anti-science, anti-life jacket, climate change denier. Cases of people getting wet are going through the roof. I’m getting you to buy a life jacket from me. Put it on, or else you will never have access to swimming pools, showers, rain or drinking water ever again.”

Swimmer: “You are treating me like I am the enemy. If you are concerned with people drowning, shouldn’t you be treating water like it’s the danger, instead of treating me like I’m the danger?”

Pool guard: “Your body is made up of 70 percent water, so you are a ticking time bomb. Put one on!”

Swimmer: “Buddy you are the last person I would want to take directions from. You are so pushy, it’s creeping me out.

Pool guard: "Thank you. Well look, yesterday a guy up the road died from drowning in a head-on collision car accident because he wasn't wearing his life jacket."

Swimmer: "Wouldn't he have died from the car accident?"

Pool guard: "A little water was found in the car, counts as a water death."

Swimmer: "That doesn't make any sense."

Does that sound familiar or what? It doesn't make any sense whatsoever. Of course, what we are really talking about is not life jackets, but what? The vaccine, the Covid narrative, the whole baloney, it's what's going on. By the way, I have to interject this. During this whole time with Covid where are those faith healers?

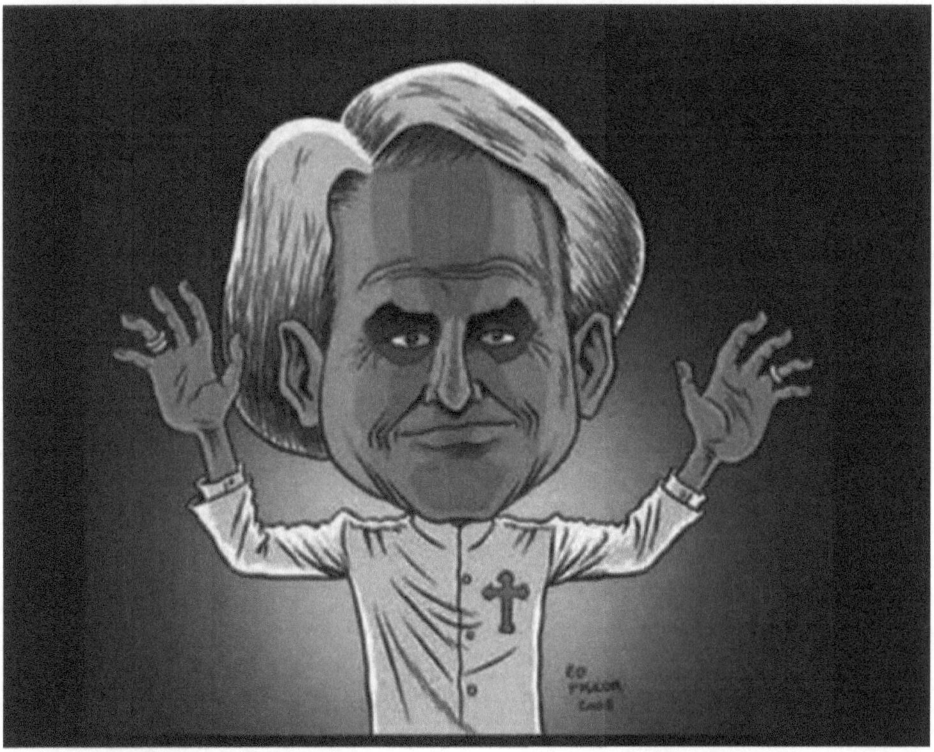

It's your time to shine! But I digress. It's just a little sidetrack issue. But the real issue is that the purpose of this pandemic, or plandemic, was not only to make President Trump look bad while he was in office, to bring in the mail in ballots, to steal the election, to bail out the pharmaceutical companies that were going bankrupt, but also an excuse by the global elites to usher in "The Great Reset." They want to basically take over the planet, bring in the New World Order, basically the rise of the antichrist kingdom. They are using Covid and the whole deception along with it, to get the job done. Take a look at this:

"It's not only a great reset, it's a deception, replacing mom and dad's small businesses and private enterprises, with big tech and big business. Democracy and free enterprise go out the window, totalitarian government control, slides in through the back door. Those behind this scheme are adamant that there can't be, and never will be a return to normal. That life will never again be what it was prior to Covid. That is why they constantly talk about the new normal. The World Economic Forum meets every January in Davos. You may have heard the expression 'Davos Man.' It refers to all those zillionaires, pop stars, popes, princes, and politicians who meet every year to map out our futures. This year's Davos is very, very different from the previous ones.

The World Economic Forum along with the United Nations, the International Monetary Fund, along with any number of prominent globalist organizations and powerful individuals, including Prince Charles. Together they have jointly promised that the 2021 World Economic Forum will be used to introduce via a vast network of connected big tech corporations, online activist movements, and compliant local and national governments, something they call 'The Great Reset.' This isn't just some fantasy conspiracy theory, it's a global commitment they have made to use the panic and fear generated by the Coronavirus as a means to reshape all our economies and laws and move to a new form of capitalism, that focuses on net-zero emissions.

You might think this is a great thing, you might think this is a terrible thing. Even if it is implemented successfully, the Great Reset will undeniably and deliberately, have extreme and possibly have dire repercussions to every single one of your constituents. Already the Great Reset is being widely advertised on posters, and ads, across the UK and Europe, and it will be here before too long. 'You'll own nothing, and you'll be happy'. This is just one of their marketing slogans. The plan involves replacing shareholders of big companies with stakeholders who happen to be left wing bureaucrats and climate change zealots. Replacing mom and dad's small businesses and private enterprises with big tech and big business. Democracy and free enterprise go out the window, and totalitarian government control slides in through the back door.

But remember, it's not only a Great Reset, it's a Great Deception. Because, in order to get everyday people to surrender, many of the rights and freedoms we currently take for granted, the repeatedly stated aim of all of these organizations, is to deliberately use Covid as an excuse to use all the political and authoritarian tools. As Prince Charles puts it, that are currently used around the world to eradicate the virus, such as lockdowns and exclusion zones, forced closure of businesses, heavy fines, making protesting illegal, and so on, and now eradicate carbon emissions.

Those behind this scheme are adamant that there can't be, and never will be, a return to normal. That life will never again be what it was prior to Covid. That's why they constantly talk about the 'New Normal.' This is not me saying this, this is them saying it. The people with the power, and the means, and the obsessional desire to do it. And they keep telling us again and again precisely what they have in store."

Klaus Schwab: *"This is an historical moment in time, not only to fight the virus but to shape the system."*

Prince Charles: *"We have a unique and rapidly shrinking window of opportunity to learn lessons and reset ourselves in a more sustainable path. It's an opportunity we have never had before, and we may never have again, so we must use all the levers we have at our disposal, knowing each and every one of us have a vital role to play."*

Antonio Guterres: *"The Great Reset is a welcome recognition that this human tragedy must be a wake-up call. It is imperative that we reimagine, rebuild, redesign, reinvigorate, and rebalance our world. Rebalancing investments, harnessing science and technology, and advancing the transition to net-zero emissions, all elements of the Great Reset, are fundamental to rebuilding the future we need."*

"And if it's still not clear, get the book written by Klaus Schwab, 'The Fourth Industrial Revolution.' He is setting out precisely how these powerful sources in the world, are lining up to use the Covid-19 crisis as a pretext of introducing a new climate change focus and a One World Economy, that will strip away property rights and basic democratic rights. They are not hiding this stuff; they are shouting it from the rooftops. The World Economic Forum states on its website that the only acceptable response to the Covid crisis is to pursue a Great Reset of our economies, our politics, and our societies."

So, again, that is the bigger issue that's going on. It's a multi-layered level of deception. That's why President Trump had to go, and they used the Covid excuse to get rid of him, and get him out of office with the rigged votes. Why? Because he went to the World Economic Forum, and basically thumbed his nose at them. He told them that America was never going along with this. After he did that, the war was on. That happened in 2018. And this is why they put Biden in.

Biden is all in on this Great Reset. He's all about destroying our country on purpose, because that's what they want to do. He wants to get us to bow our knees to this Great Reset where the globalists take over everything; a One World Government and a One World Economy. Klaus Schwab wants to merge the biological with the digital. He wants to chip everybody, either in the head or in the arm which is not too far from the hand. Why do you think that is? To control everything, to control the economy, what you buy and sell. What does that sound like? And it's on tape. We know where it's headed as Christians, it's headed towards the antichrist kingdom, and will find its fulfillment in the 7-year Tribulation. But as born-again Christians, the good news is we leave prior, so again, it just means for us, it must really be getting close., i.e., the Rapture of the Church, but we need to finish strong.

They got Biden in there because he's going along with that. In fact, his slogan is "Build Back Better".

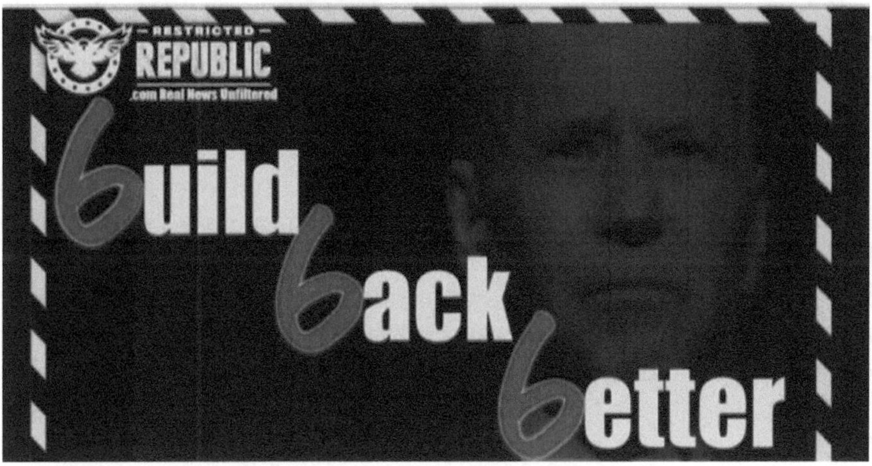

He got that from the Great Reset. He's all in on this. Now I don't know if you noticed, but those "b's" are kind of interesting, in fact not to get too crazy or conspiratorial, it is kind of interesting that a recent video from Biden, talked about getting the job done. And what, of all numbers or miracle phrases he uses to describe how he is going to get the job done, take a look at this.

Joe Biden: "*I'm telling you; we're going to get this done."*

Reporter: *"When?"*

Joe Biden: *"It doesn't matter when. It doesn't matter whether it's in six minutes, six days or six weeks. We're going to get it done."*

Sure thing, Mr. Mark of the Beast. Whatever, not to get too crazy, I just thought that was rather interesting. But again, this is all built on lies and deceit. Now the scripture is very clear. There is no conspiracy. We know, hands down, where this is coming from. Who ultimately is inspiring this? This is leading towards the antichrist kingdom. The antichrist is satan's man on the planet during the 7-year Tribulation. Why? Because any lie comes from Satan and this whole agenda is all built on lies and deception. And that is our opening text:

John 8:31-44 "To the Jews who had believed him, Jesus said, 'If you hold to my teaching, you are really my disciples. Then you will know the truth, and the truth will set you free.' They answered him, 'We are Abraham's descendants and have never been slaves of anyone. How can you say that we shall be set free?' Jesus replied, 'I tell you the truth, everyone who sins is a slave to sin. Now a slave has no permanent place in the family, but a son belongs to it forever. So, if the Son sets you free, you will be free indeed. I know you are Abraham's descendants. Yet you are ready to kill me because you have no room for my word. I am telling you what I have seen in the Father's presence and you do what you have heard from your father.' 'Abraham is our father,' they answered. 'If you were Abraham's children,' said Jesus, 'then you would do the things Abraham did. As it is, you are determined to kill me, a man who has told you the truth that I heard from God. Abraham did not do such things, you are doing the things your own father does.' 'We are not illegitimate children,' they protested. 'The only Father we have is God himself.' Jesus said to them, 'If God were your Father, you would love me, for I came from God and now am here. I have not come on my own; but he sent me. Why is my language not clear to you? Because you are unable to hear what I say. You belong to your father, the devil, and you want to carry out your father's desire. He was a murderer from the beginning, not holding to the truth, for there is no truth in him. When he lies, he speaks his native language, for he is a liar and the father of lies.'"

We have seen this so many times before, but this tells us ultimately who is pulling the strings behind this global movement. Yes, it's the global elites, people in high places and billionaires and tech companies and moguls and all the Transhumanists, but Jesus tells us where it really comes from. So, even though we may not see it, we may not have been in that smoke-filled room. We may not have been there the first day that

Klaus Schwab, the founder of the World Economic Forum, and the other elites were in there smoking their cigars, doing whatever they do and all of a sudden, the idea popped into somebody's head, "Hey, let's do this Great Reset thing! Let's take over the planet and we need a global crisis to get the people to bow a knee and freak out!" We weren't there but we can say positively where it comes from. Satan is the father of all lies. And he is also a murderer.

So anytime you see this sickening desire to mass murder people it is also Satanically inspired. If you don't think that's true when it comes to this Covid narrative, we are going to expose that. Just like the scripture says, we are going to find out where all of this is coming from. These guys aren't just lying a little here and a little there, sprinkling it on a little here and there, they are really laying it on. I can't give you all of them, but I am going to give you sixteen, that's all. How many lies do they have to tell before you just say, "I'm not going to listen to you anymore! You liar! This is Satanic!" It would take three days to go over all of the lies, so I'm just going to give you sixteen. Are these guys really lying like Satan? It's the Satanic agenda because who is the father of all lies? Satan. So, take a look at this Covid narrative. Have we been lied to?

Lie number one was **"Covid is going to kill us all!"** We're all going to die, all over the planet. Remember that? That's not true. As we saw before, Covid has a high survivability rate if you just leave it alone. In fact, you probably have a greater chance of dying from the flu, than this, statistically. We saw this before but let's recap that:

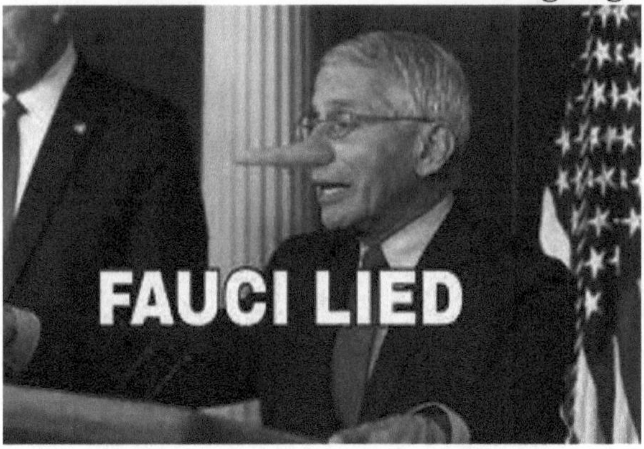

"Don't I have a high chance of dying if I don't get the experimental injection?" The answer is, NO! According to the government's own

statistics and good old-fashioned math, your chances of surviving Covid-19 without the experimental injection depends on your age group:

0 - 14 survival is 99.9998%
15 – 44 survival is 99.9931%
45 – 64 survival is 99.9294%
65 – 85 survival is 99.6297%
Over 85 survival is 98.2499%

The numbers don't lie. In fact, the chance of you getting struck by lightning is about the same as your chance of dying of Covid. Do we need an experimental injection for a potential lightning strike? And, by the way, the so-called vaccine wasn't even proven to stop anyone from dying of Covid anyway."

So, why do we need it? They are lying. We're all going to die!!! No, we are not! Again, you probably have a greater chance of dying from the flu, which we lived with for so long, and we never shut down the country.

Lie number two was **"Only 15 days & a lockdown to flatten the curve."** Well, that wasn't true. Only 15 days, a two-week lockdown and it will flatten the curve. How's that working out for everybody? Last time I checked, for those of you hooked on calendars, how long has it been now? A year and a half. You liar! It just never stops. Then they say, "Well I'll tell you what, this is what is going to prevent it.

Lie number three was **"Wearing masks will stop it."** Now how many times did we get lied to on that one? First it was, wear a mask, then it was don't wear a mask, then it was actually admitted that masks don't work. Let me give you a couple of sources there:

Biden's Covid advisor says, Face masks don't help much from Covid-19." And even Fauci himself, first he said masks and then he said no masks. He admits masks don't work.

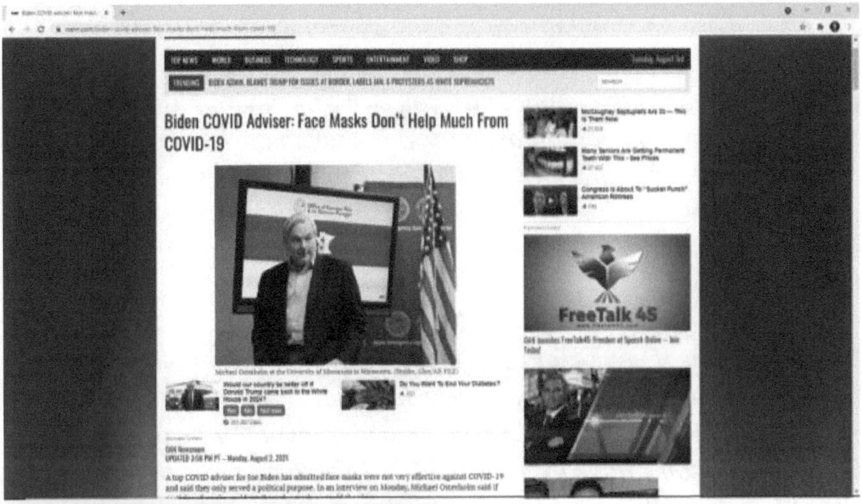

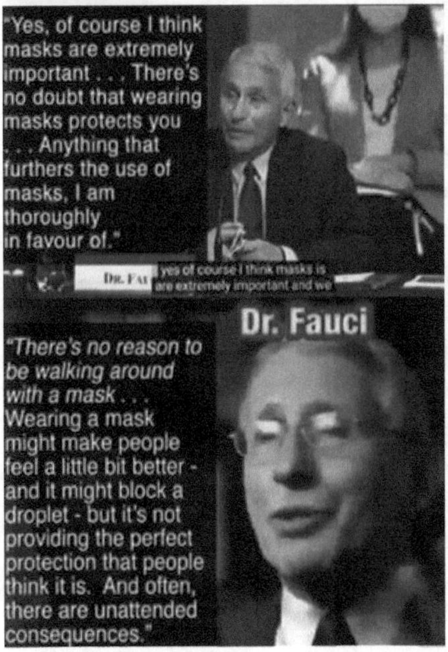

Here's a clip from some interviews where he was speaking about the mask.

"People should not be walking around in masks." "Let me just state for the record that masks are not theater." "Wearing a mask may make people feel a little bit better." "Masks aren't protective." "It's not providing the perfect protection that people think that it is." "There has not been any indication that putting a mask on, or wearing a mask for any certain period of time has any effects…" "There are unintended consequences when people keep fiddling with the mask and they keep touching their faces." "We do not need to wear a mask indoors if in fact you have been vaccinated. If you are vaccinated in a situation where you have people indoors, particularly crowded, you should wear a mask."

"So, even if you are vaccinated you should wear a mask." "If you are fully vaccinated you do not need to wear a mask outdoors or indoors." "When the children go out into the community you want them to continue to wear a mask." "When you look at children outside, particularly when they are with the family, walking down the street, playing a game, what have you, they don't have to wear a mask." "The Academy of Pediatrics, actually makes that recommendation that children should be wearing masks from 2 years on and upward."

"You're asking now if your child is a member of you household can you walk outdoors with your child, without a mask. According to that chart, the answer is yes.' "One mask is better than no masks, but two is better than one, but you don't have to wear two." "It became clear that cloth coverings that you didn't buy in the store, that you can make yourself were adequate." "One of the ways you can make it fit better, if you would like to, put a cloth mask over the first mask, then any leakage from top bottom or sides, is much better contained." He is asked if he is a double masker and we see footage of him sitting in a stadium with no mask on. No answer from Dr. Fauci.

Yeah, you are a double, triple, quadruple liar is what you are. You keep changing your tune over and over again. We have been lied to so much and so often, that you don't get it until you start streaming it together chronologically. And that is just on the mask issue. It's nuts, which leads to the next one. If you are tired of the mask thing, you just get the vaccine, and it will all go away.

Lie number four is **"Just get the vaccine & it will all go away."** How long did that work? Maybe for a little bit for some. But what did he say? Even if you do get the shot, you still have to wear the mask! They lie over and over and over again. Then because there were some fears in the beginning, they were asked if they were going to mandate this stuff or not.

Lie number five is **"Don't worry, we'll never mandate this."** This is America, we would never do that to you. If you don't believe they actually said that, which they did in the beginning just to pacify us, then once Biden got fully into power, they dropped the bomb on us.

Biden: *"I don't think it should be mandatory, I wouldn't demand it to be mandatory, but I will do everything in my power, just like I don't think masks should be made mandatory nationwide.*

Jen Psaki: *"Can we mandate vaccines across the country? No that's not a role that the Federal Government has the power to make."*

Nancy Pelosi: *"We cannot require someone to be vaccinated. That's just not what we can do. It's a matter of privacy to know who is and who isn't."*

Dr. Fauci: *"You don't want to mandate or try and force anyone to take the vaccine. We have never done that. We don't want to be mandating from the Federal Government to the general population. It would be unenforceable, and not appropriate."*

And yet you are doing it! You liar! Again, who is the father of all lies? This is satanic. How many times do you have to get lied to by the same entities before you say, "I'm not listening to anything! I don't care how many science degrees you have; you guys are liars. And I'm not going to trust a liar." Then they not only said, "We are not going to mandate this," and they went ahead and did it anyway, but then they went to the next lie.

Lie number six is **"We didn't purposely make this virus to be released on people."** They said they didn't make this virus, and have it released on the world, so they could manage the outcome. Watch Fauci, once again on tape try to say he didn't manufacture it. And now guess what is now out there in the news, yes, you did in the Wuhan lab.

Fauci: *"I don't know how many times I can say it Madam Chair, we did not fund Gain-of-Function Research being conducted at the Wuhan Institute of Virology."*

CNN: *"In our health lead we now know that a bat Coronavirus was enhanced in a lab."*

Fauci: *"NIH and NIAID categorically has not funded Gain-of-Function Research to be conducted in the Wuhan Institute."*

CNN: *"The National Institute of Health acknowledge that it funded research of a virus that was studied at the Wuhan Institute of Virology. The experiment unexpectedly made the bat coronavirus more contagious than the original naturally occurring one."*

Rand Paul: *"Dr. Fauci, knowing it's a crime to lie to Congress? Do you wish to retract your statement of May 11 where you claimed that the NIH never funded Gain-of-Function Research in Wuhan?"*

Fauci: *"Senator Paul, I have never lied before the Congress, and I do not retract that statement."*

CNN: *"A new letter raising questions about an experiment in the Wuhan lab..."*

Fauci: *"Let me finish."*

Rand Paul: *"You take an animal virus, and you increase it to go to humans and you say that is not Gain-of-Function Research?"*

Fauci: *"That is correct and Senator Paul, you do not know what you are talking about, quite frankly and I want to say that officially. You do not know what you are talking about."*

CNN: *"They used the NIH to provide grant money to Eco Health Alliance who conducted experiments on bat coronaviruses in China."*

Fauci: *"If anybody is lying here Senator, it is you. That's what you are getting, let me finish."*

Rand Paul: *"All the evidence is pointing that it came from the lab. There will be responsibilities for those who funded the lab, including yourself."*

Washington Examiner: *"The National Institute of Health admitted this week that it funded controversial Gain-of-Function Research, researching coronaviruses at a lab in China, at the epicenter of the pandemic, contradicting claims by Dr. Fauci that American taxpayers' dollars never paid for that kind of research."*

Fauci: *"I am not lying before Congress. I have never lied, certainly not before Congress. Case closed!"*

Case closed, you liar! You are lying through your teeth, over and over again. But we are just getting started. They said "Oh no, no need to fear, I know you have heard some things about the vaccine, they could have potential side effects, that they are dangerous, and could cause death.

Lie number 7 is **"No need to fear, the Pfizer Vaccine has FDA approval."** Haven't you heard that the Pfizer vaccine has got FDA approval? That's a lie. Still to this day it has never gotten FDA approval. Let me demonstrate that to you. This is from a Pfizer rep, and he admits that the Covid vaccine is not FDA approved in a recorded call. Let me explain to you what they did. This is from Senator Ron Johnson, he's a Republican from Wisconsin. He made the claim that the US does not have an FDA approved vaccine. Any of them, including the Pfizer, even though the news keeps saying it is. Senator Johnson was criticized, and his claim was buried. Many want to know how the government can say that the vaccine is FDA approved, when it's not.

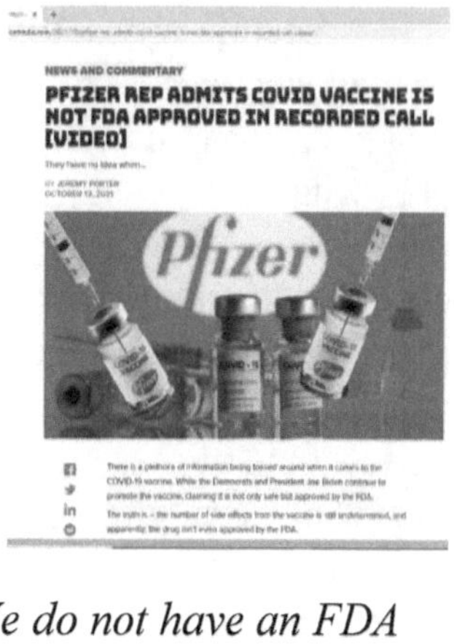
NEWS AND COMMENTARY

PFIZER REP ADMITS COVID VACCINE IS NOT FDA APPROVED IN RECORDED CALL [VIDEO]

Speaking to Fox News Johnson said, *"We do not have an FDA approved vaccine being administered in the US. The FDA played a bait and switch on us."* In other words, they lied. And believe it or not there are still some in Congress that haven't drank the Kool aid on this. "They approved Comirnaty, a version of the Pfizer drug and it's not available in the US. I sent them a letter three days later asking them, *'What are you doing?' What they did was, they extended the emergency use authorization for the Pfizer drug vaccine that is available in the U.S."*

So, the Pfizer vaccine that they are still using, just got the emergency use and still is not FDA approved. They approved something totally different, made by Pfizer, and it still isn't available. And it's still not available in the US. But the media is running with it.

Lie number 8 is **"The vaccine is our only hope."** Don't you want to get back to normal? All we have to do is get this shot. The vaccine is the only thing on the planet that can get rid of Covid. Now Covid is real, and I'm convinced that they developed it in the Wuhan lab, on purpose, with the help of the global elites, to do all kinds of things. Yes, get Trump out (he would never go along with the Great Reset), also to bail out big pharma, but it's being used as an excuse, to usher in all these draconian measures that they want to bring in to frankly, destroy the United States of America.

As we saw in the Great Reset conference, that's part of their plan, and they specifically said, in their eight steps, that America will no longer be called a superpower. This is what is going on. This is why Biden is doing everything he can economically wrong, to destroy our country. And that is what they want to happen. But they said that the vaccine is our only hope. It's true, Covid is real. They released it on us. It's about the same as the flu and you can die from the flu, and you can die from Covid. But the vaccine is not the only hope. In fact, there are other treatments out there that are dirt cheap and that are out there and have been out there for decades. One of these treatments is Ivermectin. But guess what they are doing? They are lying to us. Not only lying, but they are banning effective treatment that can get rid of Covid, just like that. Even the news will admit it once in a while.

Fox News: *"And first this morning, the potentially deadly impact of censorship and media coverups, as evidence mounts, that big tech and corporate media have silenced truthful facts about Covid, to the detriment of the American people. My first guest this morning was studying and questioning potential treatments for Covid-19, throughout the pandemic. Despite evidence of safety and efficacy of early treatment from at least one drug, that has been on the market for treating other sicknesses, any mention of either Ivermectin or to a lesser extent, Hydroxychloroquine, was met with attacks and take downs by political operatives and some media. Such mentions or posts were censored by social media."*

Now why would they do that? If you really care about people and you really want to get rid of this so-called Covid crisis thing, then why aren't you releasing it out on a massive scale? You can still do your vaccines; people have a choice. By the way, I'm not a doctor and I don't play one on TV, and I'm not here to give medical advice. This is not a hospital, I'm just sharing with you what I have come across and you can make your own adult decisions. But again, if it works, why would you hide this? Especially if it's cheaper? Because you can't make money off of that. And you can't keep using this other narrative to get people to say it's the jab or nothing. Oh, and by the way it really does work. It works on a massive scale. We have testimonies of that right here in our own congregation.

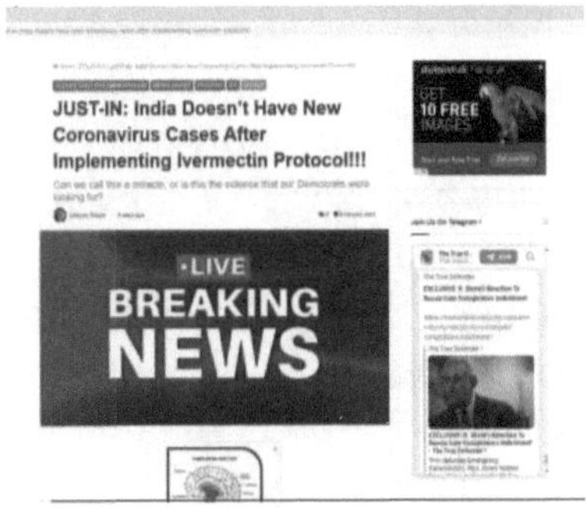
JUST-IN: India Doesn't Have New Coronavirus Cases After Implementing Ivermectin Protocol!!!
GET 10 FREE IMAGES
•LIVE
BREAKING NEWS

India, big news in India. India has not bought into this narrative, by and large, and they are not pro-vaccine. Praise God for their government, and it's not even a Christian nation, but they know better. They have released Ivermectin to their people, and it's wiping it out, completely! No new Covid cases in India after implementing Ivermectin protocol! Across the country it's wiping it out, in the whole country, nationwide. Which tells us, if our leaders would quit bowing the knee to the Great Reset people, and would release this medication, then guess what? This whole thing would be done tonight. But you can't have that, you keep extending it, so you can take our rights away. They say, well you can trust our numbers, because the numbers don't lie.

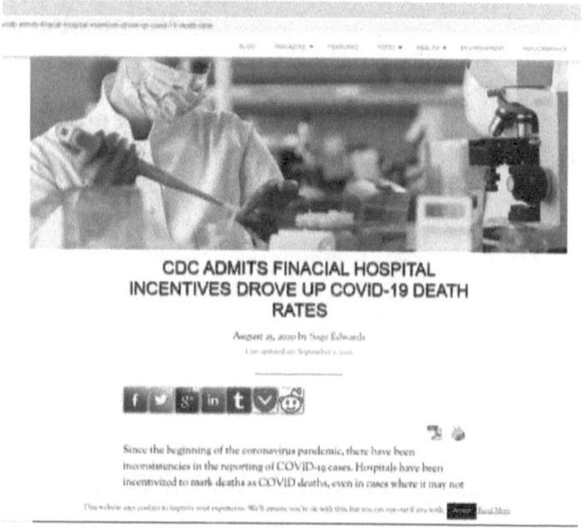
CDC ADMITS FINACIAL HOSPITAL INCENTIVES DROVE UP COVID-19 DEATH RATES

Since the beginning of the coronavirus pandemic, there have been inconsistencies in the reporting of COVID-19 cases. Hospitals have been incentivized to mark deaths as COVID deaths, even in cases where it may not

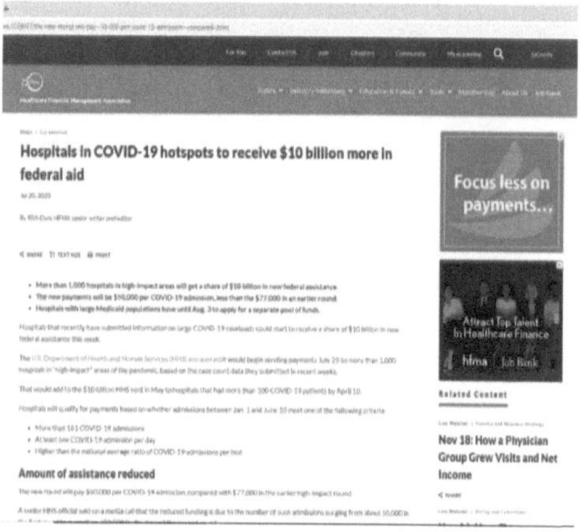
Hospitals in COVID-19 hotspots to receive $10 billion more in federal aid

- More than 1,000 hospitals in high-impact areas will get a share of $10 billion in new federal assistance.
- The new payments will be $50,000 per COVID-19 admission, less than the $77,000 in an earlier round.
- Hospitals with large Medicaid populations have until Aug. 3 to apply for a separate pool of funds.

Hospitals will qualify for payments based on whether admissions between Jan. 1 and June 10 meet one of the following criteria:

- More than 161 COVID-19 admissions
- At least one COVID-19 admission per day
- Higher than the national average ratio of COVID-19 admissions per bed

Amount of assistance reduced

Lie number 9 is **"You can trust our numbers."** Yeah, you liar. You are lying about the numbers. That was part of the initial scare. People are dying like flies. You gotta get the shot! Well, let's take a look at the numbers. Now it's coming out, that the numbers were completely inflated. Key word – Inflated with a capital "I". The reason why, hospitals were paid to inflate the numbers. That's all coming out now. Now hospitals admit that incentives drove up Covid-19 death rates. We're not talking about to the tune of millions, we are talking billions. Billions of dollars were given in Federal aid to those who had Covid patients. Let me break it down for you. And I quote from this article, *"The new payments for hospitals will be $50,000 per Covid-19 admission."* Which is down from the previous round of billions of dollars of aid, to these hospitals of $77,000. "Hospitals will qualify for payment based on whether they meet the following criteria; more than 161 Covid admissions." And if you don't have that what are you going to do? What's that, you stubbed your toe, you've got Covid. You may laugh but we have members here at our church, where family members went into the hospital with one thing, and they had to fight with them, because they didn't go in for Covid. They don't have Covid. And why? Because they are getting billions of dollars to do that. They have to have at least one Covid admission per day, to qualify for billions of dollars. So, you have to make sure that whoever comes through that door, at least one of them, has Covid. Or you have a higher than national average of Covid-19 admissions per bed. You would think this was a big joke.

Here a man is eaten by a shark but dies from Coronavirus and Pelosi blames Trump. We laugh about it because it is so true. We have our own stories. What is going on? But you know why they are inflating the numbers? So they can gain billions of dollars. But they say, don't look at that, we just have to deal with the stats. On this website Worldometer, which is one of the statistical sights. You can check it out. It's a legitimate source. Here is what they say this week. "Right now, in the United States of America, there have been 775,262 people die of Covid." So, you see that's why we have to do all these draconian measures. Well, I don't trust your numbers because you are paying people to inflate them or whatever. Now what has come out from the CDC, is guess what? 94 percent of the reported deaths are not from Covid alone. So, I got hooked on a calculator this week and at 94 percent, only 6 percent have really died of Covid. For those of you who are hooked on math, the real figure is

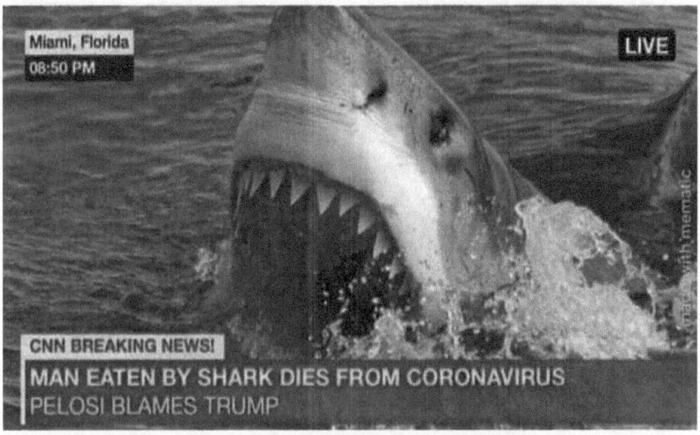
Miami, Florida
08:50 PM
LIVE
CNN BREAKING NEWS!
MAN EATEN BY SHARK DIES FROM CORONAVIRUS
PELOSI BLAMES TRUMP

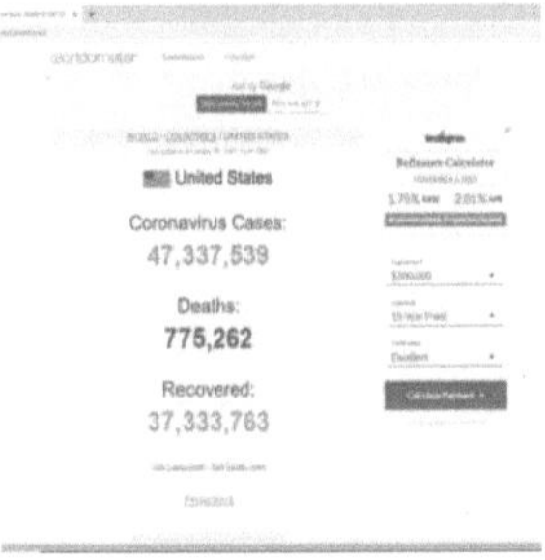
United States
Coronavirus Cases:
47,337,539
Deaths:
775,262
Recovered:
37,333,763

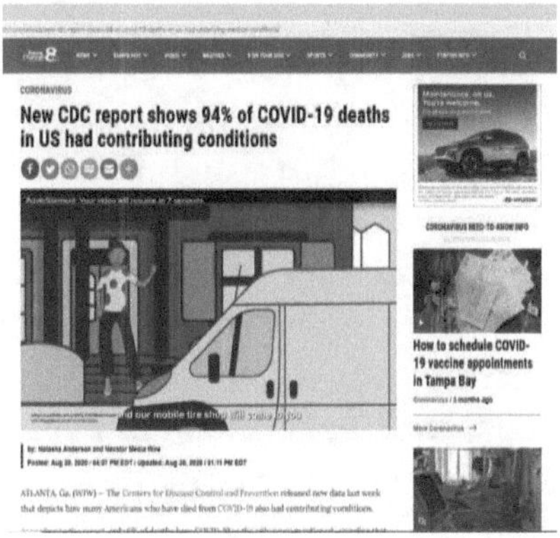
CORONAVIRUS
New CDC report shows 94% of COVID-19 deaths in US had contributing conditions
How to schedule COVID-19 vaccine appointments in Tampa Bay

46,515. I'm just using the math, from the CDC. That is 6 percent of the 775,262. So, they shut the country down for 46,515 people? Granted, that is a lot of people, but you shut the whole country down, and you don't get to reopen it until you comply with the mandates and the vaccine… that's our only hope?

Well, let's compare it with the other causes of death that we deal with every single year. This is the National Center for Health Statistics, it's their own website.

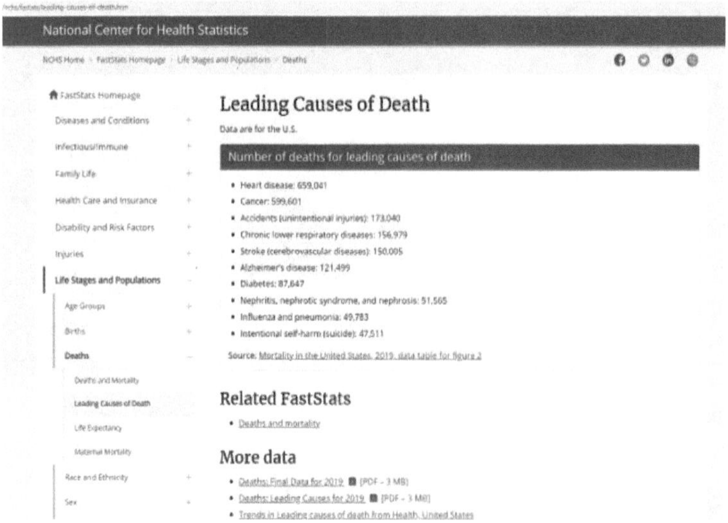
National Center for Health Statistics

NCHS Home > FastStats Homepage > Life Stages and Populations > Deaths

FastStats Homepage
Diseases and Conditions
Infectious/Immune
Family Life
Health Care and Insurance
Disability and Risk Factors
Injuries
Life Stages and Populations
Age Groups
Births
Deaths
Deaths and Mortality
Leading Causes of Death
Life Expectancy
Maternal Mortality
Race and Ethnicity
Sex

Leading Causes of Death

Data are for the U.S.

Number of deaths for leading causes of death

- Heart disease: 659,041
- Cancer: 599,601
- Accidents (unintentional injuries): 173,040
- Chronic lower respiratory diseases: 156,979
- Stroke (cerebrovascular diseases): 150,005
- Alzheimer's disease: 121,499
- Diabetes: 87,647
- Nephritis, nephrotic syndrome, and nephrosis: 51,565
- Influenza and pneumonia: 49,783
- Intentional self-harm (suicide): 47,511

Source: Mortality in the United States, 2019, data table for figure 2

Related FastStats

- Deaths and mortality

More data

- Deaths: Final Data for 2019 [PDF - 3 MB]
- Deaths: Leading Causes for 2019 [PDF - 3 MB]
- Trends in Leading causes of death from Health, United States

The number one killer every year is heart disease, with 659,041, with cancer in second cause of death at 599,601, and then accidents at 173,000. At the bottom of the list is suicides at 47,511 with Covid deaths at 46,515. Covid didn't even make the top 10. In fact, it's below the flu, meaning the flu is more dangerous. I'm not inflating numbers; I'm just using their numbers. And yet they say we have to do what they tell us to do. You liar!

Lie number 10 is **"The vaccines are highly effective."** The vaccines are just so good, and they will get rid of this virus lickety-split. Excuse me? Take a look at Fauci once again. Pay attention to him when they first started releasing these vaccines. I love sharing these clips because it's showing how much we are being lied to. He says, "highly effective, highly effective" and then watch the numbers go down completely into the toilet where they say it is colossally stupid.

Fauci: *"So now we have two vaccines that are really quite effective." "The mRNA vaccine is highly effective." "Extraordinarily efficacious 94 to 95 percent for mild to moderate diseases, virtually 100 percent efficacious." "For the real-world effectiveness is even more impressive than the results of the clinical trials."*

"No hospitalization and no deaths: All three US vaccines 'highly efficacious'", Fauci says. "Vaccines are safe and effective against Delta. You might not know that from the media fearmongering." "Experimental coronavirus vaccine highly effective." "The Pfizer-BioNTech Vaccine is said to be powerfully protective in adolescents."

GOOD JAB: "Coronavirus news UK latest – June 21 lockdown lift 'looking good' as vaccines 'highly effective' against Indian variant."

"Covid vaccine found highly effective in real-world US study."

"The Covid-19 vaccines are highly effective, and the chance of an adverse reaction is rare."

"Covid vaccine found highly effective in real-world study."

"New study finds Covid-19 vaccines are highly effective in preventing hospitalizations among older US adults."

"FDA scientists endorse 'highly effective' Pfizer/BioNTech Covid-19 vaccine ahead of key panel."

"mRNA Covid vaccines highly effective at preventing symptomatic infection in health workers."

"AstraZeneca Covid Vaccine is 100 percent effective preventing severe disease."

"Vaccine was 100 percent effective in preventing severe disease as defined by the U.S. Centers for Disease Control and Prevention and 95.3

percent effective in preventing severe disease as defined by the U.S. Food and Drug Administration. Vaccine was 100 percent effective in preventing Covid-19 cases in South Africa, where the B.1.351 lineage is prevalent."

"Novavax Vaccine 100 percent effective against both moderate and severe Covid-19 and it's easier to distribute than the current vaccines, which require ultra-cold storage."

"Moderna says its Covid vaccine is 100 percent effective in teens, plans to seek FDA OK in early June."

"AstraZeneca Covid-19 vaccine 100 percent effective in preventing death, hospitalization: U.S. Study."

"Covid-19: Novavax jab 100 percent effective in protecting against moderate and severe disease, trial results suggest. President of research and development at Novavax said, 'Our vaccine will be a critical part of the solution to Covid-19.'"

"The Pfizer vaccine is 100 percent effective for people this age, study says, 'Clinical trials found that it fully prevented any covid infections in participants.'"

"J&J asks for booster go-ahead, says second vaccine does provides 100 percent Covid protection."

"Covid-19 vaccine AstraZeneca confirms 100 percent protection against severe disease, hospitalization and death in the primary analysis of Phase III trials."

"Pfizer/BioNTech says its Covid-19 vaccine is 100 percent effective and well tolerated in adolescents."

"Pfizer-BioNTech says Covid vaccine is 100 percent effective in kids ages 12 to 15."

"Moderna says its Covid vaccine is 100 percent effective in teens, plans to seek FDA OK in early June."

"The Johnson & Johnson vaccine is 100 percent effective at this one thing. This is why Dr. Fauci says the new vaccine has shown 'spectacular results.'"

"Moderna's Covid-19 vaccine found to be 100 percent effective in children 12 to 17. Four who received the placebo tested positive for the virus, a result consistent with a vaccine efficacy of 100 percent."

"Real-world vaccine study shows 99 percent effective rate."

"Israeli Health Ministry: Pfizer vaccine close to 99 percent effective. The vaccine will allow us to return to the routine of life we all long for only when those under 16 are also inoculated, says Health Ministry director general."

"Pfizer coronavirus vaccine is 98 percent effective – expert. The actual effectiveness of the Pfizer-BioNTech coronavirus vaccine is 98 percent according to the results of its use."

"Pfizer vaccine 97 percent effective against symptomatic Covid-19, study shows. Pfizer-BioNTech's coronavirus vaccine offers more protection than earlier though, with effectiveness in preventing symptomatic disease reaching 97 percent, according to real-word evidence published Thursday by the pharma companies."

"Pfizer vaccine 96.7 percent effective at preventing Covid deaths, Israeli data shows. Shots also 97.5 percent effective against serious illness and 95.3 percent effective in preventing infection, according to study published in prestigious medical journal."

"Moderna vaccine is more effective against Covid-19 infection at 96 percent compared to Pfizer shot at 89 percent, another study finds."

"One Covid vaccine jab 96.6 percent effective in averting deaths, two 97.5 percent: A Covid vaccine tracker will be launched with details of vaccinations and the number of fatalities among vaccinated people after breakthrough infections, the health ministry said."

"Updated Pfizer data shows vaccine is 95 percent effective."

"The Pfizer and Moderna vaccines are 94 percent effective at preventing hospitalization in older adults, a study finds."

"Moderna's Covid-19 vaccine still 93 percent effective after 6 months, company says."

"Vaccine 92 percent effective against Delta variant: AstraZeneca."

"CDC reports two vaccines 91 percent effective."

"CDC: Pfizer and Moderna vaccines are 90 percent effective in real-world conditions."

"Novavax Covid vaccine is 89 percent effective and could be approved in UK in weeks."

"Study: Pfizer vaccine 88 percent effective against delta variant."

"Getting both Covid-19 vaccine shots has 87 percent efficacy; Japanese university study."

"Pfizer Covid vaccine 86 percent effective after third shot – Maccabi."

"Pfizer Covid-19 vaccine 85 percent effective after single dose, Israeli researchers find."

"Pfizer's CEO says Covid vaccine effectiveness drops to 84 percent after six months."

"Pfizer says immunity can drop to 83 percent within 4 months in people who got its Covid-19 shot, further bolstering the company case for a booster."

"Coronavirus first dose is 82 percent effective in preventing death, second dose 95 percent effective: Study. There has been a big disclosure about the coronavirus vaccine. Research reveals that taking the first dose reduces the risk of death by 82 percent and the second dose by 95 percent."

"Bharat Biotech's Covid-19 vaccine shows interim efficacy of 81 percent."

"One dose of Pfizer or Moderna vaccines was 80 percent effective in preventing Covid in CDC study of health workers."

"AstraZeneca vaccine found to be 79 percent effective in U.S. Trial, no increased risk of blood clots."

"Pfizer Covid vaccine shows 78 percent efficacy in pregnancy."

"Moderna's effectiveness against hospitalization held steady over a four-month period, while Pfizer's fell from 91 to 72 percent. This research is still limited, and more data is needed to fully understand the differences between the two vaccines."

"AstraZeneca says Covid-19 vaccine 76 percent effective in new analysis, to seek US approval."

"FADING HOPE Covid vaccine effectiveness falls as low as 75 percent against Delta, study warns."

"Effectiveness of Pfizer's Covid-19 vaccine drops to 74 percent after five months, study finds, as the U.S. prepares to roll out boosters next month. A new study from the U.K. found that the effectiveness of Pfizer's vaccine drops from 88 to 74 percent after five to six months."

"Researchers determined that individuals fully vaccinated with the Pfizer-BioNTech vaccine had an overall 73 percent effective protection against Covid-19 infection and a 90 percent effective protection against Covid-19 related hospitalization."

"Moderna vaccine 72 percent effective against Covid after just one dose."

"Johnson & Johnson booster waiting on approval, original dose only 71 percent effective."

"Pfizer vaccine 70 percent effective against Delta variant, claims study."

"Full Covid-19 vaccination provides 69 percent protection against infection by Delta variant: Singapore Study."

"Johnson & Johnson is 68 percent effective on Covid-19 strains, seeks FDA approval."

"First DNA Covid vaccine found 67 percent effective in clinical trials."

"CanSinoBio's Covid-19 vaccine 65.7 percent effective in global trials, Pakistan official says."

"Pfizer vaccine protection against infection declines to 64 percent in Israel."

"The WHO's Strategic Advisory Group of Experts on Immunization, known as Sage, has been scrutinizing evidence from vaccine trials. Its interim recommendations say the vaccine is 63 percent effective overall."

"Yes, recent data from the Oxford/AstraZeneca and Moderna vaccine trials suggests their candidates also have high efficacy. Oxford data indicates the vaccine has 62 percent efficacy when one full dose is given followed by another full dose."

"The vaccine developed by Oxford and the pharmaceutical company AstraZeneca in Cambridge, UK was 69 percent effective against a high viral load 14 days after the second dose, falling to 61 percent by 90 days. The drop in effectiveness shouldn't be cause for alarm, says Sarah Walker, a medical statistician at the University of Oxford who led the study. For both of these vaccines, two doses are still doing really well against Delta, she says."

"The study found overall vaccine effectiveness against symptomatic disease in risk groups is approximately 60 percent after one dose of either AstraZeneca or Pfizer-BioNTech, with little variation by age."

"Covid-19: Oxford vaccine could be 59 percent effective against asymptomatic infections, analysis shows."

"Researchers: Best Covid-19 vaccines 58 percent effective at 250 days."

"Johnson & Johnson 1-dose vaccine tests only 57 percent effective against South African Covid-19 variant."

"Meanwhile, a Canadian study that's still awaiting peer review found that a single dose of Pfizer's shot was 56 percent effective at preventing symptomatic infections caused by Delta after two weeks."

"In a smaller trial conducted in South Africa – where volunteers were primarily exposed to another newer, more contagious variant widely circulating there and spreading around the world – the Novavax vaccine was only around 55 percent effective but still fully prevented severe illness and death."

"An Israeli study showed that Pfizer's vaccine was 54 percent effective against Covid-19 from 13 days to 24 days after vaccination, a figure comparable to the late stage trial data presented to the FDA."

"Researchers found the effectiveness of the Pfizer vaccines against delta variant infections was 93 percent a month after the second dose and fell to 53 percent after four months."

"According to Pfizer data published in December 2020, the Pfizer-BioNTech vaccine is roughly 52 percent effective after the first dose. Out of 36,523 participants in the phase three trial – the final stage of testing where people either received two full doses, 21 days apart, or a placebo – who had no evidence of existing infection, 82 people in the placebo group and 39 in the vaccine group developed Covid-19 symptoms."

A Covid-19 vaccine may be only 50 percent effective. Is that good enough?"

"The mRNA Covid-19 vaccine was only 47 percent effective after 5 months."

"A large observational, real-world study from Israel estimates that the Pfizer/BioNTech Covid-19 vaccine is 46 percent effective at preventing infection 14 to 20 days."

"Moderna Covid vaccine 76 percent effective against Delta, Pfizer 42 percent: Study. Covid-19 jabs that were developed by U.S. drug makers Pfizer and Moderna may not be as effective against the Delta variant compared to as they were against the original strain of the virus, says study."

"Pfizer's Covid vaccine is only 42 percent effective against Indian Delta variant while Moderna's jab is 76 percent effective, Mayo Clinic study suggests. The two most commonly used Covid-19 vaccines in the U.S. may not be as effective against the Indian Delta variant, a new study finds."

"Israeli Research claims Pfizer shot now only 41 percent effective against Delta strain. Nathan Jeffay wrote: New data from Israel and the U.K. painted a confusing and contradictory picture on Thursday as to the effectiveness of Pfizer's Covid-19 vaccine in fighting off the Delta variant

of the coronavirus. New Health Ministry statistics indicated that, on average, the Pfizer shot – the vaccine given to nearly all Israelis – is now just 39 percent effective against infection, while being only 41 percent effective in preventing symptomatic Covid. Previously, the Pfizer-BioNTech vaccine was well over 90 percent effective against infection."

"Health Ministry says Covid vaccine is only 40 percent effective at halting transmission."

"Officials say Pfizer vaccine is only 39 percent effective against the Delta variant in Israel. The country's health ministry says the vaccine remains effective at preventing severe illness and hospitalization."

"JAB BLOW One dose of vaccine only 33 percent effective, leaving over-60s vulnerable, Israeli experts claim."

"Pfizer's Covid vaccine efficacy against infection plunges to just 20 percent after six months – but protection against severe illness barely dips, study concludes. Pfizer's Covid jab is only 20 percent effective at stopping people getting infected after six months, real world data revealed today."

"CDC back Pfizer Covid-19 vaccine booster shots for millions of seniors and others at risk."

"For people who got the J&J vaccine, some doctors are advising boosters ASAP."

"Pfizer CEO says third Covid vaccine dose likely needed within 12 months."

"Israeli vaccine passports now expire after six months, boosters required."

"Fauci says, US going in 'wrong direction' may need booster."

"Pfizer, BioNTech to seek authorization for Covid booster as Delta variant spreads."

"Breakthrough data outlines need for booster, Pfizer CEO says. This adds to the literature suggesting waning immunity among initial Covid-19 vaccines."

"Why top FDA official says Covid booster shots may be needed for all adults. A top FDA official is saying that all adults may soon need a booster shot to have a 'harmonized approach' to boosters for all three vaccines."

"Covid: Pfizer and AstraZeneca approved as booster vaccines."

"If you got Pfizer, this is when you'll need a booster, CEO says."

"New Pfizer data makes case for booster shots 6 months after primary doses. It comes days before the FDA's advisory committee will discuss booster shots."

"Third AstraZeneca Covid shot can be effective booster."

"Fauci says quite possible Americans may need Covid-19 vaccine booster in coming months."

Fauci: *"We know that it's highly effective."*

"It never ends: Israel says fourth 'booster' vaccine will be required to keep covid 'green pass' active."

"Iceland halts use of Moderna's Covid vaccine amid concerns over heart-inflammation risk. Iceland's chief epidemiologist decided to suspend the use of Moderna's Covid-19 vaccine citing growing concerns over risks of heart inflammation."

"U.S. halts Johnson & Johnson Covid-19 vaccine shipments: report."

"Hong Kong halts Pfizer/BioNTech Covid vaccine, investigates packaging."

"India halts clinical trial of Oxford-AstraZeneca Covid vaccine."

"Sweden halts use of Moderna vaccine for young adults."

"Japan suspends 1.6 million Moderna Covid vaccine doses over contamination concerns."

"Tennessee no longer encouraging vaccines of any kind for minors. The state Department of Health is stopping all of its vaccine outreach, not just for Covid-19 vaccines, internal documents show, amid pressure from Republican lawmakers. The decision comes directly from Health Commissioner Dr. Lisa Piercey, the internal report states."

"U.K. halts AstraZeneca Covid vaccine trial on kids amid blood-clot concerns."

"Japan halts vaccines after deaths of 4 children."

"Sweden, Denmark, halt Moderna's Covid shot for younger people."

"South Africa halts vaccine rollout."

"How the Covid-19 vaccine injected billions into Big Pharma – and made its executives very rich."

"Covid vaccine profits mint 9 new pharma billionaires."

"From Pfizer to Moderna: who's making billions from Covid-19 vaccines?"

"Vaccine maker earned record profits but delivered disappointment in return. Emergent BioSolutions was awarded a $628 million federal contract with no competitive bidding. Top executives received big bonuses

while factories mostly sat idle, and tens of millions of Covid-19 doses were thrown away."

"Global Billionaire Pandemic Wealth Gains Surge to $5.5 Trillion. As the wealth divide grows deeper, global advocates call for one-time 99 percent emergency tax on billionaires' pandemic windfalls to fund Covid-19 vaccines for entire world."

"Moderna posts profit for first time. Modern recorded a profit for the first time and raised its 2021 sales forecast for its covid-19 shots. Fred Katayama reports."

"Moderna's founders make their debut on the Forbes top 400 richest people in America list after cashing in on the pandemic with Covid vaccine. Moderna co-founders Noubar Afeyan and Robert Langer and early investor Timothy Springer all made Forbes' richest people in America this year."

"As covid vaccines drive record profits, CEOs get ultra-rich off massive pay packages, questionable stock sales."

"Covid-19 vaccine leads to Moderna's first profitable quarter."

"Pfizer's posts $4.9B 1Q profit as vaccine strategy pays off. Selling vaccines during a pandemic has boosted Pfizer's bottom line and proven that a strategy it embarked upon over a decade ago is now paying off handsomely."

"Stunning study reveals how ineffective Pfizer vaccine actually is. Biden official: 'If that's not a wakeup call, I don't know what is.'"

"Past vaccine disasters show why rushing a coronavirus vaccine now would be 'colossally stupid.'"

How many times, do you have to be lied to, to say, "You know what, I'm not going to listen to you again?" And again, you don't get it because we have been lied to so much, so often, until you string it all together and it is colossally stupid. That we would believe anything that these guys are saying. It's not effective. But hey, don't look at that.

Lie number 11 is **"The vaccines produce great immunity."**

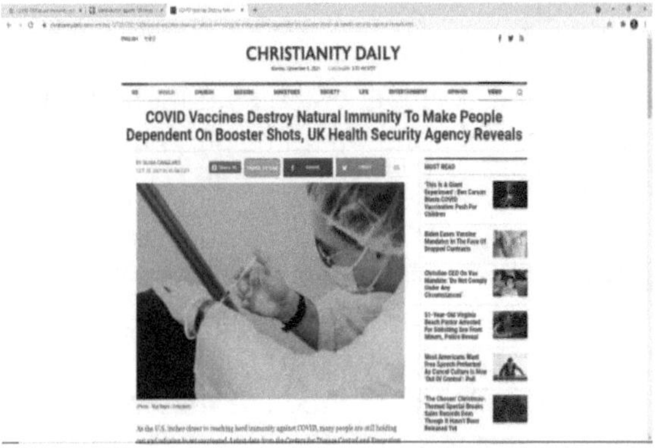

Actually, once again, shocker, they actually destroy your immunity. And I quote: "Covid vaccines destroy natural immunity to make people dependent on booster shots." Again, if it worked, why would I need booster shots? There is a reason why for that and we'll get to that in a second and it rhymes with money again. This is coming from the U.K. Health Security Agency. Now other health industries like the U.K., and also Israel, outside of our country. We are being lied to on a massive scale, by the current administration and others. As crazy as it sounds, in the United States of America, we have to go outside of our own country, to find out what's really going on. It actually destroys your immunity. In fact, so much so, that now they are saying, the ones that have already got the shot, it's not only

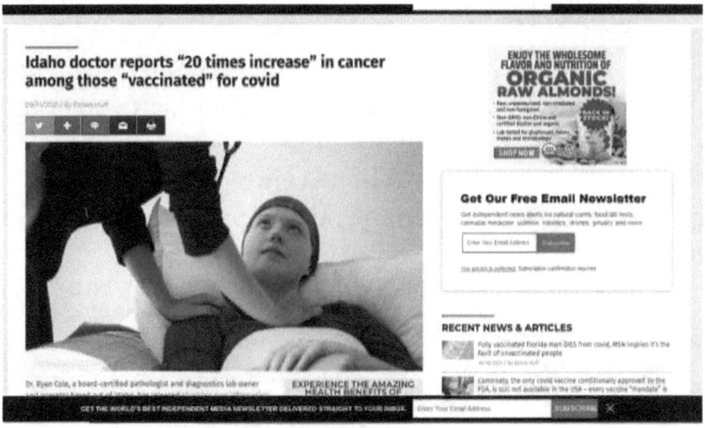

destroying their immunity, but now that your immunity is being destroyed, it makes you susceptible to other things that you can't fight off.

This is an article from the Medicine News, not Joe Shmoe dot com, where an Idaho doctor reports, 20 times increase in cancer among those vaccinated for covid. Because you don't have an immune system anymore. It's destroying your immune system. And what we are going to see in just a little bit, it not only destroys your immune system, what it basically does, is any previous condition that you do have, if you get the shot, it will make it that much worse. So, if you had a little bit of history of cancer, it's going to come back. If you have intestinal problems that is going to come skyrocketing back, if you have diabetes, it's going to go through the roof. Because your immune system is being destroyed.

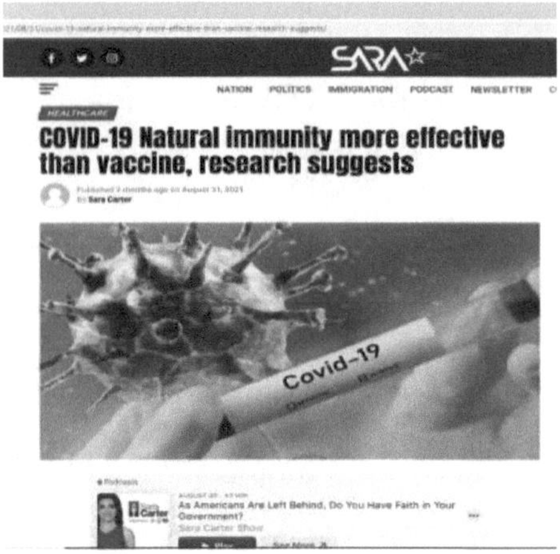
SARA

NATION POLITICS IMMIGRATION PODCAST NEWSLETTER

HEALTHCARE

COVID-19 Natural immunity more effective than vaccine, research suggests

Covid-19

As Americans Are Left Behind, Do You Have Faith in Your Government?

Sara Carter Show

Oh, and by the way, what about your natural immunity? You can still get Covid, many of us here had Covid, did the Ivermectin, or just sweated it out. It's like the flu. It's dangerous and some people die. Some people die of the flu, but your God given natural immunity is tons better, lasts for years, than this thing that does the exact opposite and destroys your immunity.

Natural immunity is more effective than the vaccine. So, why do I need it? It's another lie. They flat out say, "This is going to keep it from ever happening. It prevents Covid."

Lie number 12 is **"The vaccines prevent Covid."** No, actually what we are now discovering is that it produces Covid for those who got the shot.

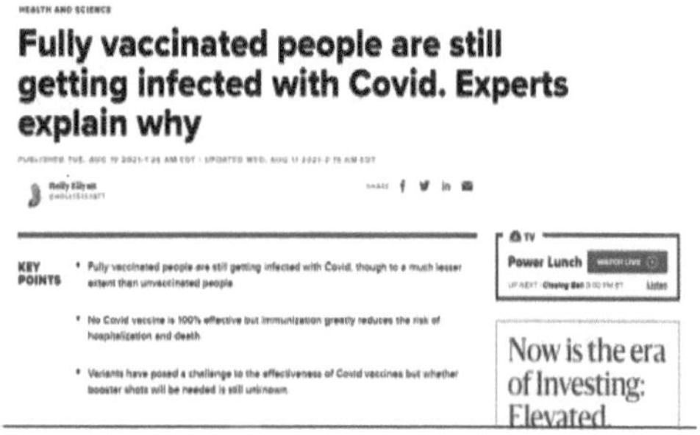
HEALTH AND SCIENCE

Fully vaccinated people are still getting infected with Covid. Experts explain why

KEY POINTS

- Fully vaccinated people are still getting infected with Covid, though to a much lesser extent than unvaccinated people
- No Covid vaccine is 100% effective but immunization greatly reduces the risk of hospitalization and death
- Variants have posed a challenge to the effectiveness of Covid vaccines but whether booster shots will be needed is still unknown

Power Lunch

Now is the era of Investing: Elevated

Vaccinated people are still getting infected with Covid. Now can I translate that for you? It doesn't work! Now you can't say, it doesn't work, so have you noticed the "word speak" they are using? It's called a "breakthrough case".

Doesn't that sound positive? Doesn't that sound fantastic? Something scientific just occurred. It's a breakthrough. No, it doesn't work! But you have to spin it to make it sound wonderful. It's like that goof-ball climate change thing. They used to call it global warming. Well, they had to stop doing that because we demonstrated it wasn't true. So, they had to pick another term, climate change. Well, last time I checked it changes every day. But you can't get them on that. This is the same thing. They can't say the vaccines don't work. No, it's a breakthrough case. It's a joke. And let's keep going. What about this? 60 percent of covid hospitalizations in 65 or older are patients that have been fully vaccinated. Now what's the news out there, you hear it on the radio, you hear it on the news. 95 percent of all hospitalizations are all caused by the unvaccinated. That's a lie. They are making those that have chosen not to be vaccinated out to be the bad guys. Covid case rates among the fully vaccinated are now higher than the non-vaccinated.

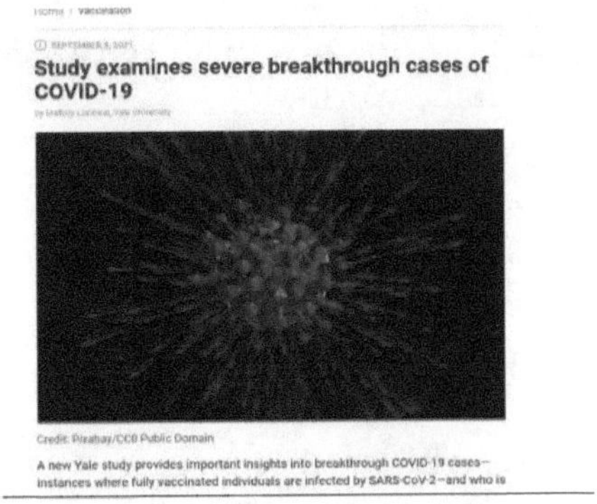

Study examines severe breakthrough cases of COVID-19

Credit: Pixabay/CC0 Public Domain

A new Yale study provides important insights into breakthrough COVID-19 cases—instances where fully vaccinated individuals are infected by SARS-CoV-2—and who is

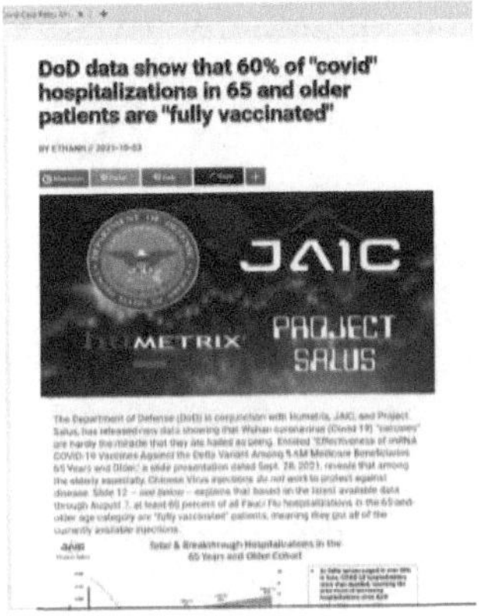

DoD data show that 60% of "covid" hospitalizations in 65 and older patients are "fully vaccinated"

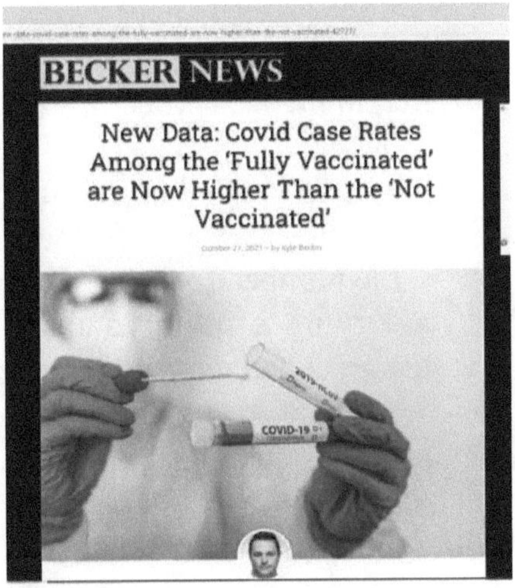

BECKER NEWS

New Data: Covid Case Rates Among the 'Fully Vaccinated' are Now Higher Than the 'Not Vaccinated'

Sounds to me like it's not only not working, but it's also causing Covid. In fact, I have a video clip, showing that if people get the shot, and this is happening all over the world, if you didn't already have Covid, you typically will get Covid. Here is a video clip showing the rise in illnesses around the world.

'"Look vaccines make people sick.' On the graphs in every country, illnesses were leveled out until they started giving out the shots and immediately the needle went straight up showing how many people got sick from the shot. 'Just say NO! Worldwide'"

The spirit of Nancy Regan is all over this. Remember her "Just say NO!" campaign to drugs? Well, just say no to that shot. It actually gives you Covid. Which is what this one lady said. Talk about a patriot with common sense.

This retired California RN is asking the question we all need answered. *"Why do the protected need to be protected from the unprotected by forcing the unprotected to use the protection that didn't protect the protected in the first place?"*

Right? That's just common sense. Which leads to the next lie.

Lie number 13 says, **"Unvaccinated are harming vaccinated."** They are trying to split us and divide us. If you haven't got vaccinated, boy, you are a bad guy. Well, actually that's not true. Here is a video clip from the Senate, with Senator Ron Johnson on the Senate floor. He is demonstrating that when Covid was on its way down, as soon as the vaccines came out and people started getting the vaccines, it caused the Delta spike. You won't see this in the news, and this is our own Congress. He is showing how the vaccine is actually causing the virus to continue.

"We need to recognize people's health autonomy. This is their body. They should be able to make these choices. I want to talk about some of the information that we are not getting from our health care agencies that people who are choosing not to get vaccinated are looking at. And it's not just information, this real information is being withheld from the public by our health care agencies, by the media and the social media. The first thing I want to show, is a chart I put together. This comes from the CDC

in terms of the number of new cases per day, as well as the number of deaths per day. Deaths are on the chart at the bottom in a very thin line. But you can see by this chart, the initial surge of Covid pretty well peaked in late December, early January. The vaccines got the emergency authorization about mid-December. The orange line shows the Americans that were fully vaccinated. You can see the initial pandemic, or surge, was winding down before the vaccines could even take effect.

Now we all hoped and prayed, that the vaccine would be 100 percent effective and 100 percent safe. But when we look at this chart, as the pandemic is winding down, the amount of fully vaccinated individuals is going up, what you would expect to see would be a complete winding down of the pandemic. But that is not what we have seen. We see a new surge, of a variant called Delta. So, what are we to make of this? Let's look at some data. The kind of data that we are not getting from our health care agencies, so we have to look, unfortunately, to England and Israel. They are more transparent. In England, of the 600,000 new cases of Delta of over 2,500 deaths, 63 percent of those deaths, 1,613 people were fully vaccinated. 28 percent were un-vaxxed. Now this is probably information the American people have never heard. It's information, that if I give it, I will be attacked, I will be vilified, I will be censored, I will be suppressed. The reason I came to the floor of the Senate, is to reveal this information because the American people need to know."

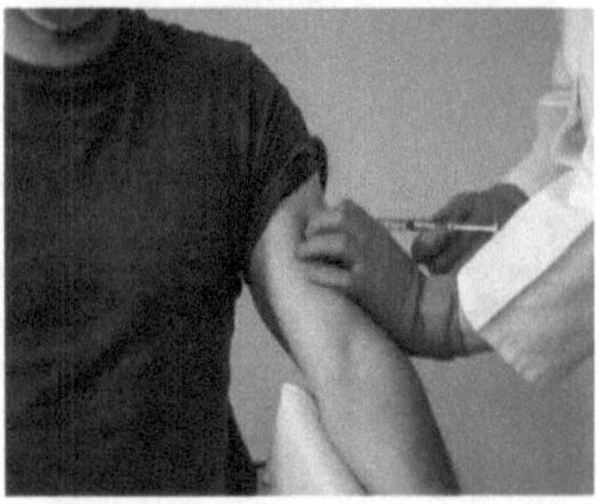

VAERS System Is Only Recording "Fewer than 1%" of Covid-1 Vaccines Side Effects and Deaths

About what? That we are being lied to. Right, but unfortunately, that's not all. Well, maybe it doesn't work so well and actually it may continue on, but what?

Lie number 14 is, **"Hardly any deaths or adverse reactions to vaccines."** What's the phrase? It's safe and effective. You liar! Let's take a look at that and examine some numbers. They are saying it's safe, only a handful of people have died from the vaccines. This is from the CDC reporting system. I don't know if you saw this, but they have finally said that the VAERS system, is only recording fewer than 1 percent of Covid-19 side effects and deaths. It says fewer than 1 percent but let's just go with 1 percent. That means that we are not hearing about the other 99 percent adverse reactions and the deaths. So, let's go to VAERS, this is the latest one this week, they are saying that Covid deaths according to VAERS is over 18,000. They died from the vaccine. Now wait a second.

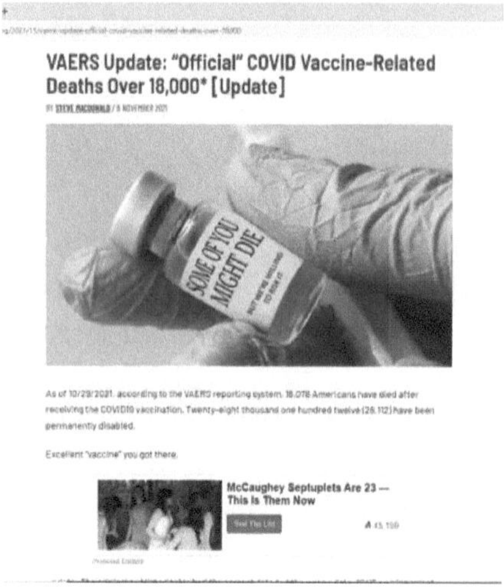
VAERS Update: "Official" COVID Vaccine-Related Deaths Over 18,000* [Update]
SOME OF YOU MIGHT DIE
As of 10/29/2021, according to the VAERS reporting system, 18,078 Americans have died after receiving the COVID19 vaccination. Twenty-eight thousand one hundred twelve (28,112) have been permanently disabled.
Excellent "vaccine" you got there.
McCaughey Septuplets Are 23 — This Is Them Now

With other vaccines, when just a handful of people die, they pull it from the market. That is historically what has gone on. How many more thousands, and it's not just thousands, there's a lot more than that, let's put it to the test. They said 18,000 but 18,000 represents 1 percent. Really, less than 1 percent, but let's play along with them. So, once again, here is the real number. 1,782,000 have died from the Covid shot, just in the United States of America. That's what is really going on. I don't know about you but I'm hearing stories from everybody including here at Sunrise. Everybody knows somebody that has died from the shot, basically. And multitudes of people, but you don't hear about them. This is what is really going on. I'm using their numbers, but according to the numbers, they reported 1 percent and that is 18,000 so times that by 99 and you get 1,782,000. So, there you go. And I'm not the only one who can do math. People are saying you're right. According to the VAERS report, when they only report 1 percent of the recording, of the adverse reactions and death, it's nearly 2 million people.

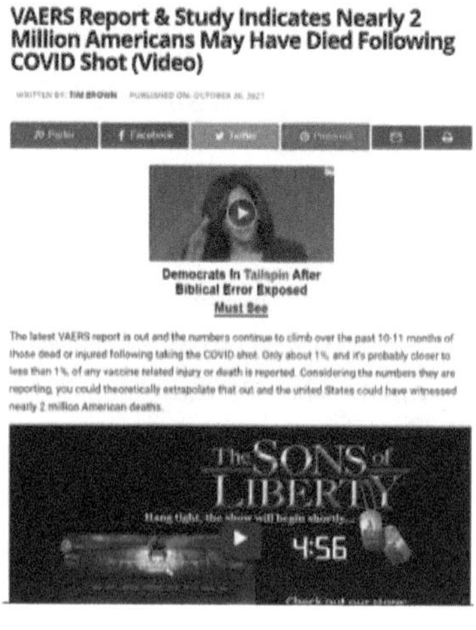

This is gross, this is sick! Can I use the word that has historically been used? The word is "Genocide" and that's just America, what about the rest of the world? Who's not only a liar but the father of all lies and a murderer and has been one from the beginning? This is satanic. A satanic agenda is going on here as well. Which means again, it leads to the next lie.

Lie number 15 is **"We would never lie about deaths or harmful side effects."** Yes, there is a massive, huge cover-up going on. And let me demonstrate that to you. If you are so honest in your reporting and you just want to give us the facts that the vaccines are safe and effective. You say trust the signs, then why is OSHA instructing Federal Agencies not to record Covid vaccine side effects? It's in print. Why would you do that? If it's all about honesty and transparency, and you want to get the truth out there? You're covering up. So really how many more are there, than when we just did the math? If there's a cover-up some of them would never even get reported. So, maybe it's even more than 2 million. And then there is this:

OSHA Instructs Federal Agencies Not to Record COVID Vaccine Side Effects

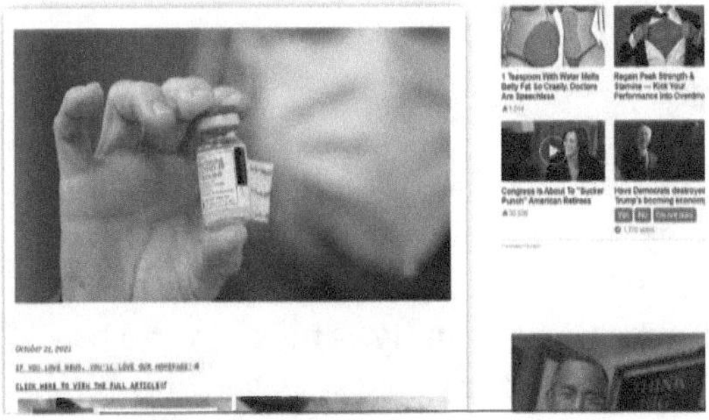

Now the CDC is listing vaccinated deaths as unvaccinated deaths. This came out a couple weeks ago. Let me explain the old switcheroo that they are doing. Like the Pfizer vaccine, that they did the old

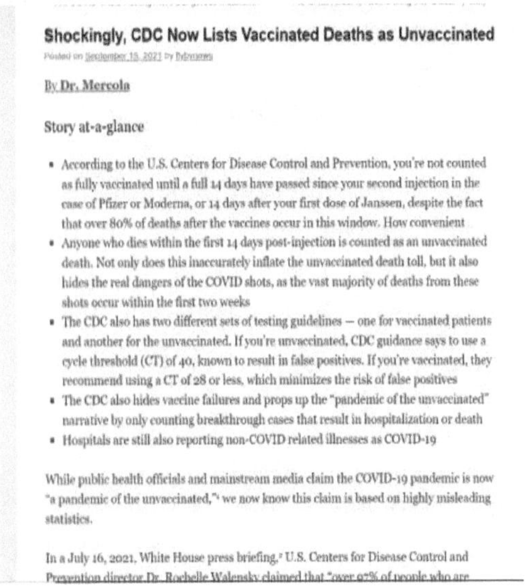
Shockingly, CDC Now Lists Vaccinated Deaths as Unvaccinated

Posted on September 15, 2021 by

By Dr. Mercola

Story at-a-glance

- According to the U.S. Centers for Disease Control and Prevention, you're not counted as fully vaccinated until a full 14 days have passed since your second injection in the case of Pfizer or Moderna, or 14 days after your first dose of Janssen, despite the fact that over 80% of deaths after the vaccines occur in this window. How convenient
- Anyone who dies within the first 14 days post-injection is counted as an unvaccinated death. Not only does this inaccurately inflate the unvaccinated death toll, but it also hides the real dangers of the COVID shots, as the vast majority of deaths from these shots occur within the first two weeks
- The CDC also has two different sets of testing guidelines — one for vaccinated patients and another for the unvaccinated. If you're unvaccinated, CDC guidance says to use a cycle threshold (CT) of 40, known to result in false positives. If you're vaccinated, they recommend using a CT of 28 or less, which minimizes the risk of false positives
- The CDC also hides vaccine failures and props up the "pandemic of the unvaccinated" narrative by only counting breakthrough cases that result in hospitalization or death
- Hospitals are still also reporting non-COVID related illnesses as COVID-19

While public health officials and mainstream media claim the COVID-19 pandemic is now "a pandemic of the unvaccinated,"[1] we now know this claim is based on highly misleading statistics.

In a July 16, 2021, White House press briefing,[2] U.S. Centers for Disease Control and Prevention director Dr. Rochelle Walensky claimed that "over 97% of people who are switcheroo, which isn't a vaccine that was FDA approved, it really wasn't. It was a different one that isn't even here in the US. The news ran with it and lied to us.

Watch this: *"According to the CDC you're not counted as fully vaccinated until a full 14 days have passed since your second injection, in the case of the Pfizer or Moderna vaccine, or 14 days after your first dose of the Johnson & Johnson. Over 80 percent of deaths due to these vaccines of Covid occur within that 14-day period. How convenient. Which means anyone who dies in the first 14 days, after getting the vaccine, is now counted as an unvaccinated death. Not only does this inaccurately inflate the unvaccinated death rate, making us look bad, but it hides the real danger of the Covid shot, and how many people are really dying."*

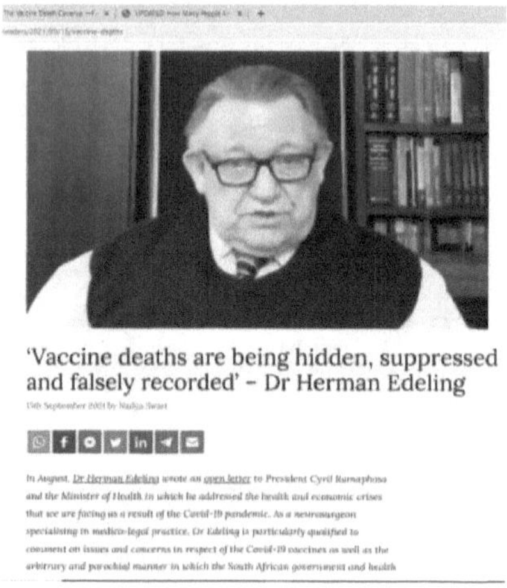

'Vaccine deaths are being hidden, suppressed and falsely recorded' – Dr Herman Edeling

In August, Dr Herman Edeling wrote an open letter to President Cyril Ramaphosa and the Minister of Health in which he addressed the health and economic crises that we are facing as a result of the Covid-19 pandemic. As a neurosurgeon specialising in medico-legal practice, Dr Edeling is particularly qualified to comment on issues and concerns in respect of the Covid-19 vaccines as well as the arbitrary and parochial manner in which the South African government and health

Like flies, you liars! And that is why some people are beginning to blow the whistle. Including some in the medical community. This is from Dr. Herman Edeling. He says vaccine deaths are being hidden, suppressed and falsely recorded.

We are being lied to about this.

Others are saying that there is a suppressing of covid vax info from the public. They are keeping the truth from us. That is really what is happening. It's causing mass adverse reactions, radically destroying people's lives, and killing people all over the world. Here's another one calling it a "vaccine death coverup."

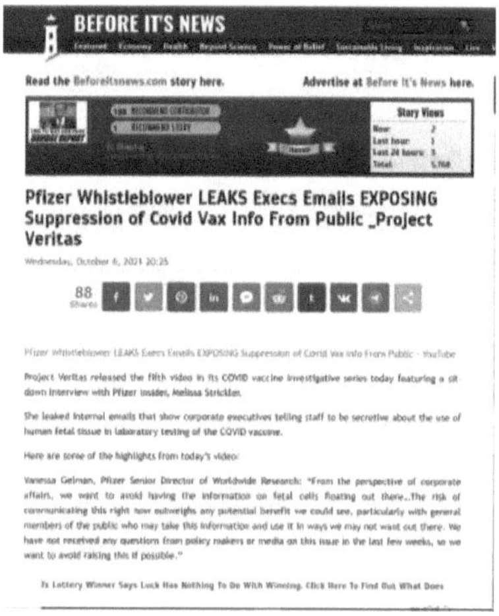

BEFORE IT'S NEWS

Read the Beforeitsnews.com story here. Advertise at Before It's News here.

Story Views
Now: 2
Last hour: 1
Last 24 hours: 1

Pfizer Whistleblower LEAKS Execs Emails EXPOSING Suppression of Covid Vax Info From Public _Project Veritas

Wednesday, October 6, 2021 20:25

88 Shares

Pfizer Whistleblower LEAKS Execs Emails EXPOSING Suppression of Covid Vax Info From Public - YouTube

Project Veritas released the fifth video in its COVID vaccine investigative series today featuring a sit down interview with Pfizer insider, Melissa Strickler.

She leaked internal emails that show corporate executives telling staff to be secretive about the use of human fetal tissue in laboratory testing of the COVID vaccine.

Here are some of the highlights from today's video:

Vanessa Gelman, Pfizer Senior Director of Worldwide Research: "From the perspective of corporate affairs, we want to avoid having the information on fetal cells floating out there...The risk of communicating this right now outweighs any potential benefit we could see, particularly with general members of the public who may take this information and use it in ways we may not want out there. We have not received any questions from policy makers or media on this issue in the last few weeks, so we want to avoid raising this if possible."

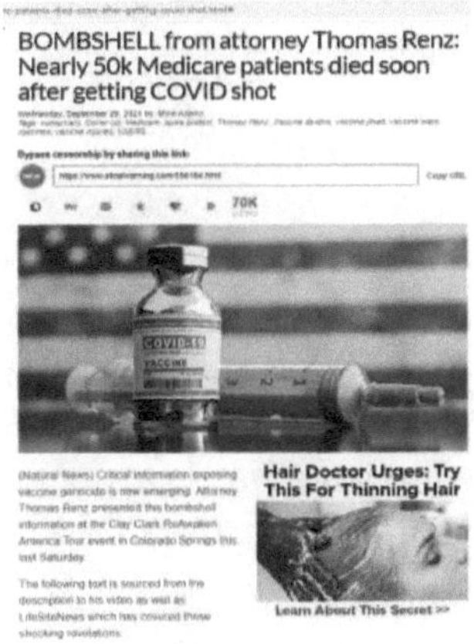

BOMBSHELL from attorney Thomas Renz: Nearly 50k Medicare patients died soon after getting COVID shot

(Natural News) Critical information exposing vaccine genocide is now emerging. Attorney Thomas Renz presented this bombshell information at the Clay Clark ReAwaken America Tour event in Colorado Springs this last Saturday.

The following text is sourced from the description to his video as well as LifeSiteNews which has covered these shocking revelations.

50,000 Medicare patients die after getting the Covid shot. This blew up in their faces. I don't know if you saw this headline. They asked for stories about the unvaxed dying from Covid. They want to put it in the press as to how bad those unvaccinated people are. But it blew up in their face and instead, they got 180K responses of vaccine injured and dead instead, from one city.

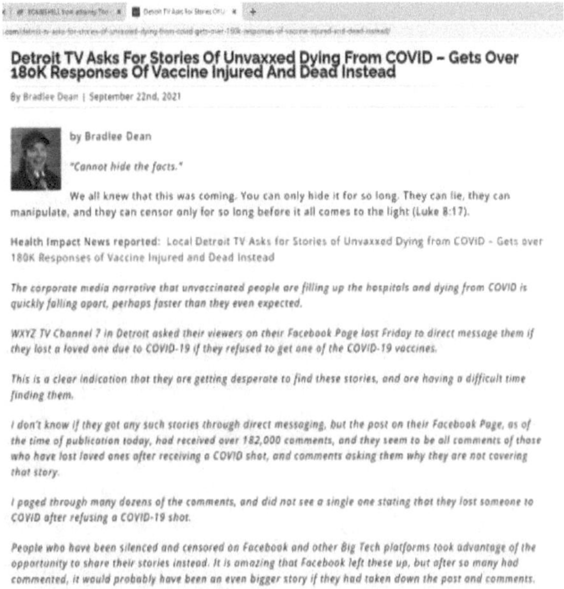

Detroit TV Asks For Stories Of Unvaxxed Dying From COVID – Gets Over 180K Responses Of Vaccine Injured And Dead Instead

By Bradlee Dean | September 22nd, 2021

by Bradlee Dean

"Cannot hide the facts."

We all knew that this was coming. You can only hide it for so long. They can lie, they can manipulate, and they can censor only for so long before it all comes to the light (Luke 8:17).

Health Impact News reported: Local Detroit TV Asks for Stories of Unvaxxed Dying from COVID – Gets over 180K Responses of Vaccine Injured and Dead Instead

The corporate media narrative that unvaccinated people are filling up the hospitals and dying from COVID is quickly falling apart, perhaps faster than they even expected.

WXYZ TV Channel 7 in Detroit asked their viewers on their Facebook Page last Friday to direct message them if they lost a loved one due to COVID-19 if they refused to get one of the COVID-19 vaccines.

This is a clear indication that they are getting desperate to find these stories, and are having a difficult time finding them.

I don't know if they got any such stories through direct messaging, but the post on their Facebook Page, as of the time of publication today, had received over 182,000 comments, and they seem to be all comments of those who have lost loved ones after receiving a COVID shot, and comments asking them why they are not covering that story.

I paged through many dozens of the comments, and did not see a single one stating that they lost someone to COVID after refusing a COVID-19 shot.

People who have been silenced and censored on Facebook and other Big Tech platforms took advantage of the opportunity to share their stories instead. It is amazing that Facebook left these up, but after so many had commented, it would probably have been an even bigger story if they had taken down the post and comments.

Which leads to the next one. Now they say we want to give this to kids. But don't worry, it's safe for the kids.

Lie number 16 is **"Don't worry it's safe for the kids."** Now this is sick! A Pfizer executive admitted that kids are 50 times more likely to die from the Corona vaccines than the virus itself.

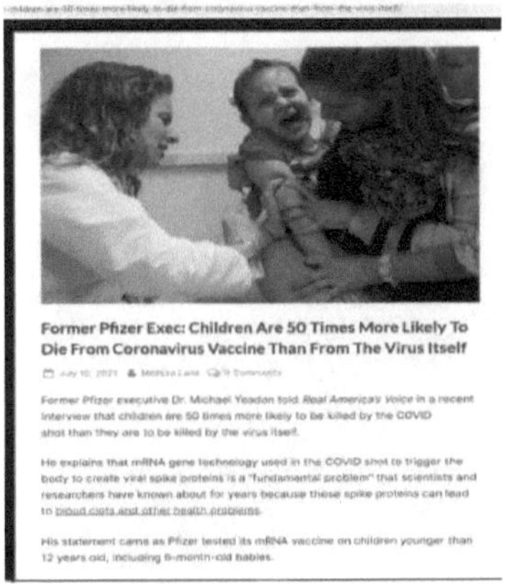

Former Pfizer Exec: Children Are 50 Times More Likely To Die From Coronavirus Vaccine Than From The Virus Itself

Former Pfizer executive Dr. Michael Yeadon told *Real America's Voice* in a recent interview that children are 50 times more likely to be killed by the COVID shot than they are to be killed by the virus itself.

He explains that mRNA gene technology used in the COVID shot to trigger the body to create viral spike proteins is a "fundamental problem" that scientists and researchers have known about for years because these spike proteins can lead to blood clots and other health problems.

His statement came as Pfizer tested its mRNA vaccine on children younger than 12 years old, including 6-month-old babies.

And if you don't believe me, here he is saying it on tape. Here it is:

The Covid Vaccine in Children/Adolescents

Dr. Anthony Fauci: *"High School kids will likely get vaccinated as we get into the full term and children of any age will likely get*

vaccinated by the time we get to the end of the year."

Dr. Soumya Swaminathan: *"Children can get infected with Covid-19 and they can transmit the infection to others. They have a much lower risk of getting the disease compared to older adults."*

Deanna De Paoli, Attorney, America's Front-Line doctors: *"The risk level that they face a fatality from Covid-19 is statistically 0 percent. To force an experimental agent upon children, when you do not have the long-term effects, there are so many unknowns upon children who at effectively 0 risks of fatality from this disease, is a ridiculous proposition and yet they are moving forward. We have to be particularly sensitive and cautious around children, because their bodies are still developing. They are not simply mini adults. There are many other medical factors at play in their growth and development, and we don't know what the effects that these experimental agents are on children."*

Dr. Soumya Swaminathan: *"It's not necessary that children must get the vaccine before they can go back to school. We have seen in many countries that schools have been kept open very successfully."*

Steve Bannon, Americas Voice News: *"According to Dr. Fauci, this is from Fauci's interviews, that they are going to start vaccinating 12- to 15-year-olds, kids in middle school, in high school, as soon as they get back in the fall and, that the school children will be vaccinated by the end of the year. Walk us through your thoughts about this vaccine, particularly for adolescents and school age children and younger."*

Dr. Michael Yeadon, Fmr. Pfizer VP: *"I'm generally pro-vaccine, but I'm for safety and these Covid-19 vaccines are not safe. Young people are not susceptible to Covid-19. If they acquire the virus, they usually have no symptoms and they shrug it off very easily. So, they are not at risk. It's a crazy thing to vaccinate them with something that is actually 50 times more likely to KILL them, than the virus itself."*

What do you call that? Murder. We are going to see another doctor and he simply calls it child sacrifice. That is the only reason you would give a child the vaccine. And this is why we are seeing headlines around the world. Hang with me, we are going to rip through them. But it's pretty easy for you to see these kinds of headlines around the world.

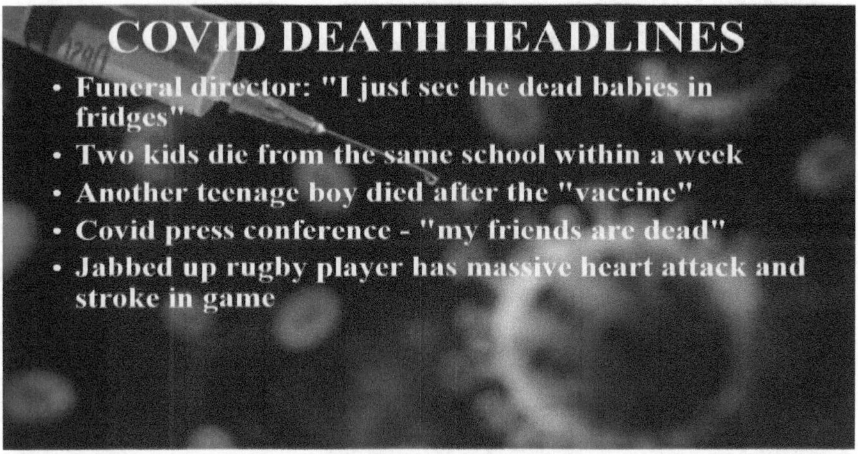
COVID DEATH HEADLINES
• Funeral director: "I just see the dead babies in fridges"
• Two kids die from the same school within a week
• Another teenage boy died after the "vaccine"
• Covid press conference - "my friends are dead"
• Jabbed up rugby player has massive heart attack and stroke in game

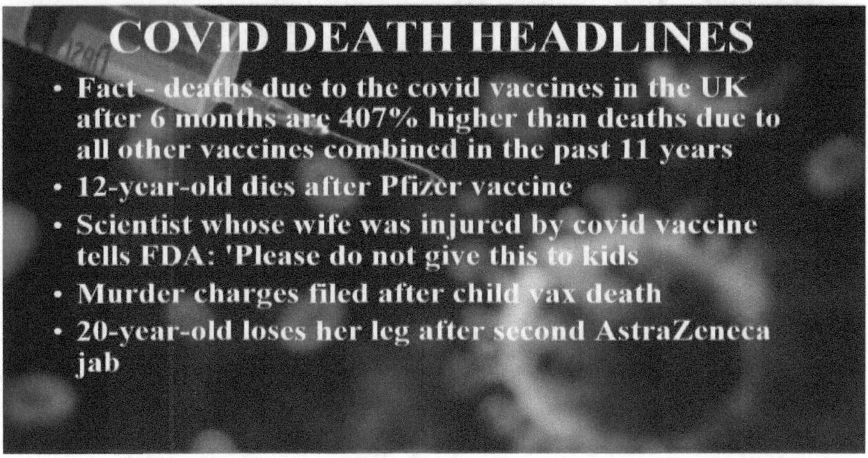
COVID DEATH HEADLINES
• Fact - deaths due to the covid vaccines in the UK after 6 months are 407% higher than deaths due to all other vaccines combined in the past 11 years
• 12-year-old dies after Pfizer vaccine
• Scientist whose wife was injured by covid vaccine tells FDA: 'Please do not give this to kids
• Murder charges filed after child vax death
• 20-year-old loses her leg after second AstraZeneca jab

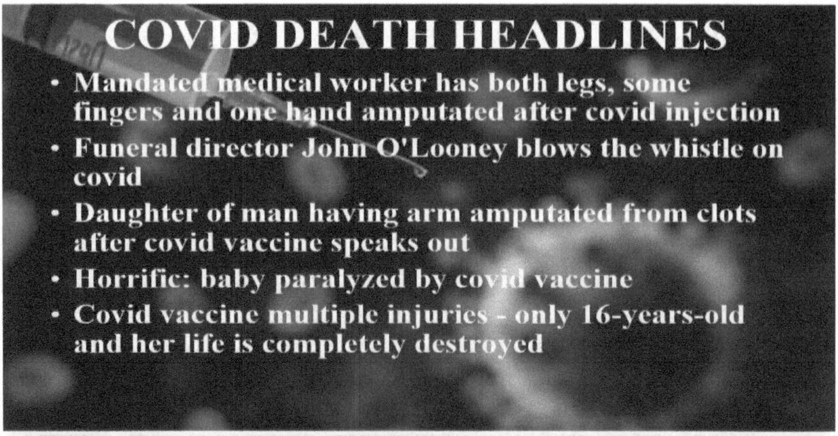
COVID DEATH HEADLINES
• Mandated medical worker has both legs, some fingers and one hand amputated after covid injection
• Funeral director John O'Looney blows the whistle on covid
• Daughter of man having arm amputated from clots after covid vaccine speaks out
• Horrific: baby paralyzed by covid vaccine
• Covid vaccine multiple injuries - only 16-years-old and her life is completely destroyed

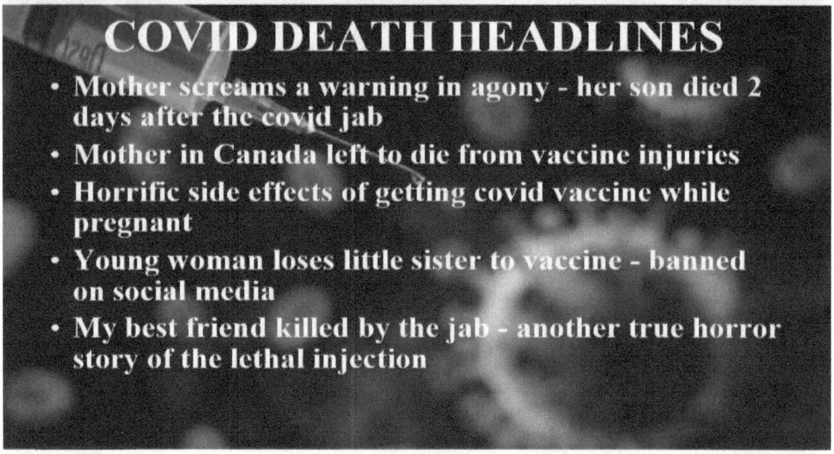
COVID DEATH HEADLINES
• Mother screams a warning in agony - her son died 2 days after the covid jab
• Mother in Canada left to die from vaccine injuries
• Horrific side effects of getting covid vaccine while pregnant
• Young woman loses little sister to vaccine - banned on social media
• My best friend killed by the jab - another true horror story of the lethal injection

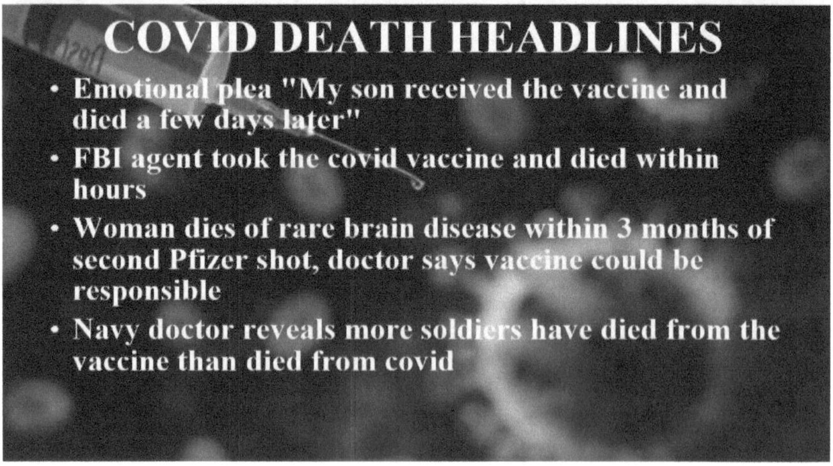
COVID DEATH HEADLINES
• Emotional plea "My son received the vaccine and died a few days later"
• FBI agent took the covid vaccine and died within hours
• Woman dies of rare brain disease within 3 months of second Pfizer shot, doctor says vaccine could be responsible
• Navy doctor reveals more soldiers have died from the vaccine than died from covid

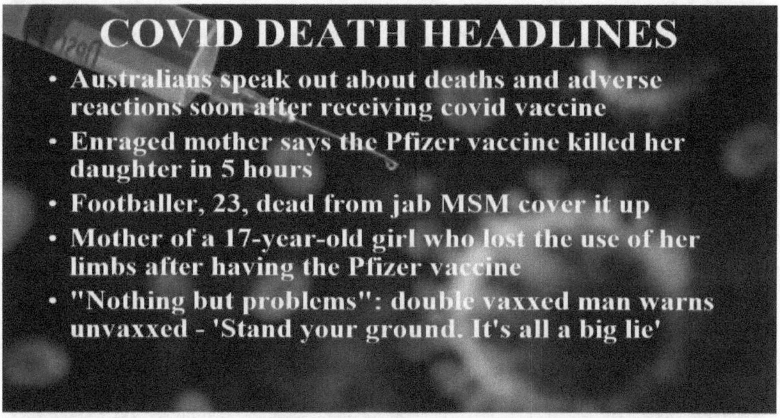
COVID DEATH HEADLINES
• Australians speak out about deaths and adverse reactions soon after receiving covid vaccine
• Enraged mother says the Pfizer vaccine killed her daughter in 5 hours
• Footballer, 23, dead from jab MSM cover it up
• Mother of a 17-year-old girl who lost the use of her limbs after having the Pfizer vaccine
• "Nothing but problems": double vaxxed man warns unvaxxed - 'Stand your ground. It's all a big lie'

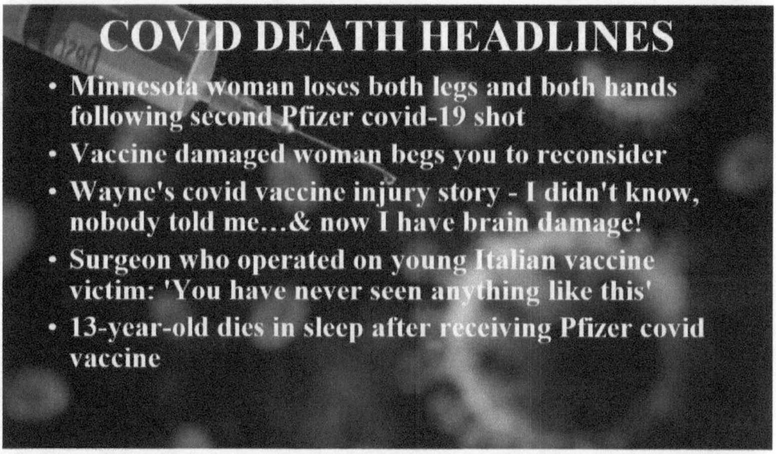
COVID DEATH HEADLINES
• Minnesota woman loses both legs and both hands following second Pfizer covid-19 shot
• Vaccine damaged woman begs you to reconsider
• Wayne's covid vaccine injury story - I didn't know, nobody told me…& now I have brain damage!
• Surgeon who operated on young Italian vaccine victim: 'You have never seen anything like this'
• 13-year-old dies in sleep after receiving Pfizer covid vaccine

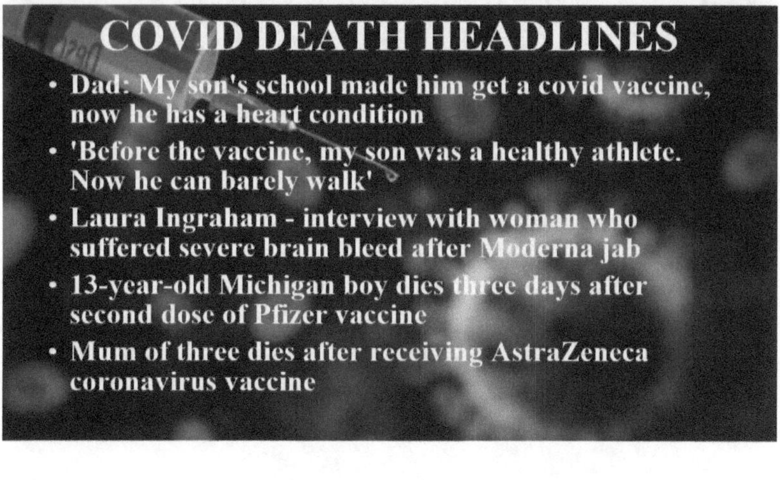
COVID DEATH HEADLINES
• Dad: My son's school made him get a covid vaccine, now he has a heart condition
• 'Before the vaccine, my son was a healthy athlete. Now he can barely walk'
• Laura Ingraham - interview with woman who suffered severe brain bleed after Moderna jab
• 13-year-old Michigan boy dies three days after second dose of Pfizer vaccine
• Mum of three dies after receiving AstraZeneca coronavirus vaccine

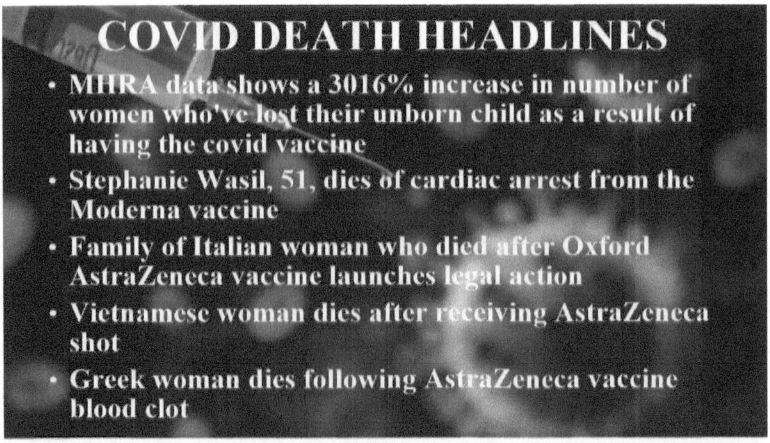
COVID DEATH HEADLINES
• MHRA data shows a 3016% increase in number of women who've lost their unborn child as a result of having the covid vaccine
• Stephanie Wasil, 51, dies of cardiac arrest from the Moderna vaccine
• Family of Italian woman who died after Oxford AstraZeneca vaccine launches legal action
• Vietnamese woman dies after receiving AstraZeneca shot
• Greek woman dies following AstraZeneca vaccine blood clot

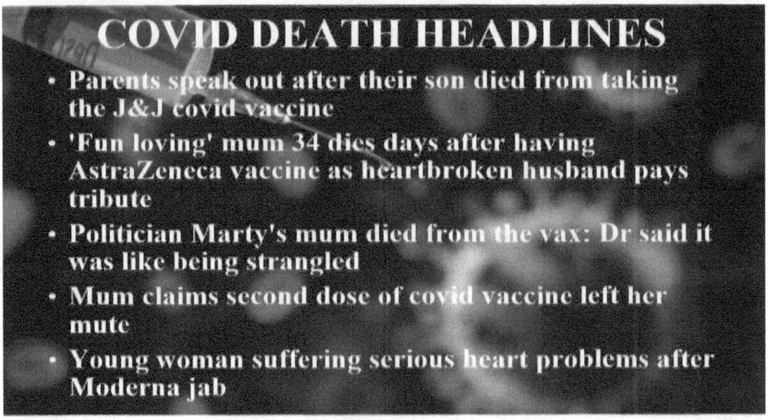
COVID DEATH HEADLINES
• Parents speak out after their son died from taking the J&J covid vaccine
• 'Fun loving' mum 34 dies days after having AstraZeneca vaccine as heartbroken husband pays tribute
• Politician Marty's mum died from the vax: Dr said it was like being strangled
• Mum claims second dose of covid vaccine left her mute
• Young woman suffering serious heart problems after Moderna jab

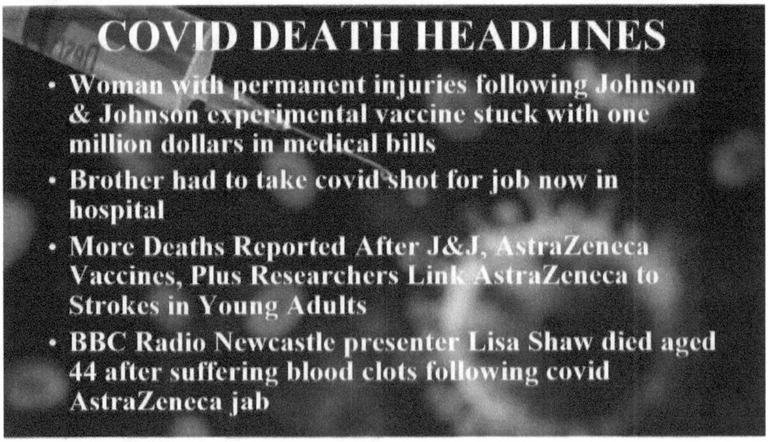
COVID DEATH HEADLINES
• Woman with permanent injuries following Johnson & Johnson experimental vaccine stuck with one million dollars in medical bills
• Brother had to take covid shot for job now in hospital
• More Deaths Reported After J&J, AstraZeneca Vaccines, Plus Researchers Link AstraZeneca to Strokes in Young Adults
• BBC Radio Newcastle presenter Lisa Shaw died aged 44 after suffering blood clots following covid AstraZeneca jab

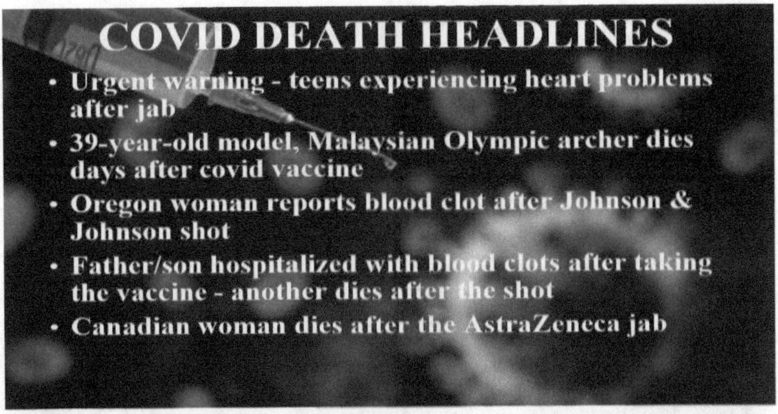
COVID DEATH HEADLINES
• Urgent warning - teens experiencing heart problems after jab
• 39-year-old model, Malaysian Olympic archer dies days after covid vaccine
• Oregon woman reports blood clot after Johnson & Johnson shot
• Father/son hospitalized with blood clots after taking the vaccine - another dies after the shot
• Canadian woman dies after the AstraZeneca jab

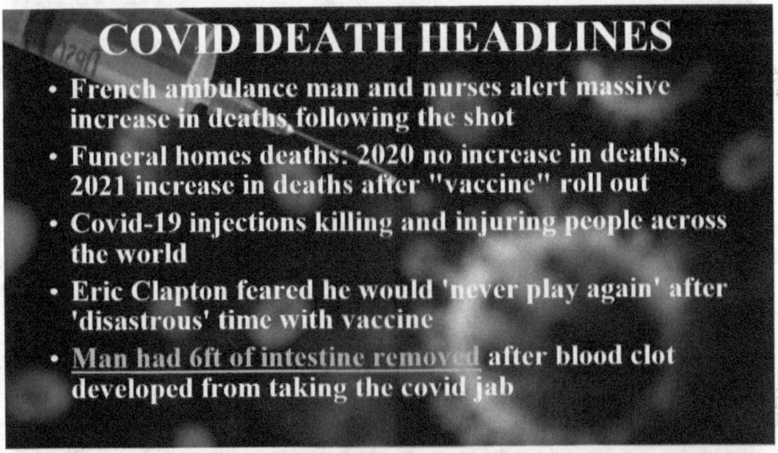
COVID DEATH HEADLINES
• French ambulance man and nurses alert massive increase in deaths following the shot
• Funeral homes deaths: 2020 no increase in deaths, 2021 increase in deaths after "vaccine" roll out
• Covid-19 injections killing and injuring people across the world
• Eric Clapton feared he would 'never play again' after 'disastrous' time with vaccine
• Man had 6ft of intestine removed after blood clot developed from taking the covid jab

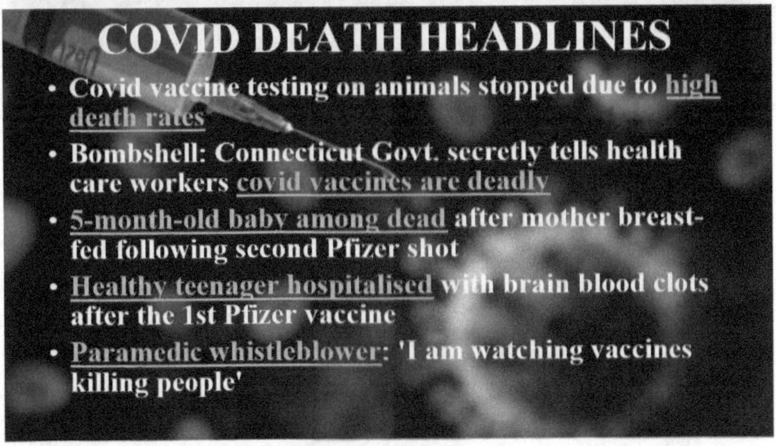
COVID DEATH HEADLINES
• Covid vaccine testing on animals stopped due to high death rates
• Bombshell: Connecticut Govt. secretly tells health care workers covid vaccines are deadly
• 5-month-old baby among dead after mother breast-fed following second Pfizer shot
• Healthy teenager hospitalised with brain blood clots after the 1st Pfizer vaccine
• Paramedic whistleblower: 'I am watching vaccines killing people'

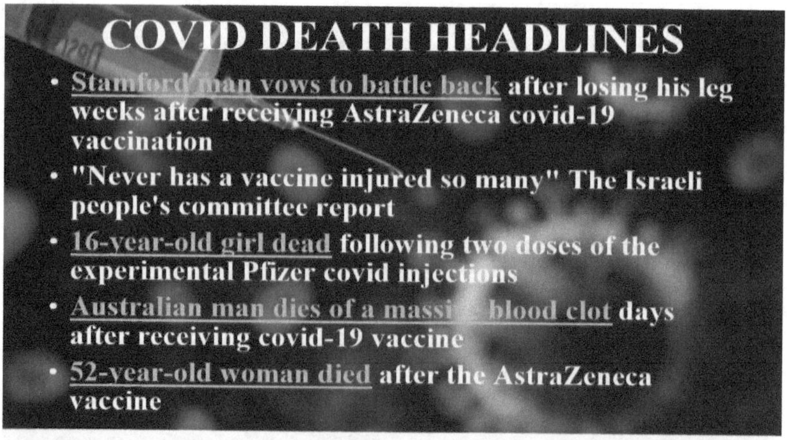
COVID DEATH HEADLINES
• Stamford man vows to battle back after losing his leg weeks after receiving AstraZeneca covid-19 vaccination
• "Never has a vaccine injured so many" The Israeli people's committee report
• 16-year-old girl dead following two doses of the experimental Pfizer covid injections
• Australian man dies of a massive blood clot days after receiving covid-19 vaccine
• 52-year-old woman died after the AstraZeneca vaccine

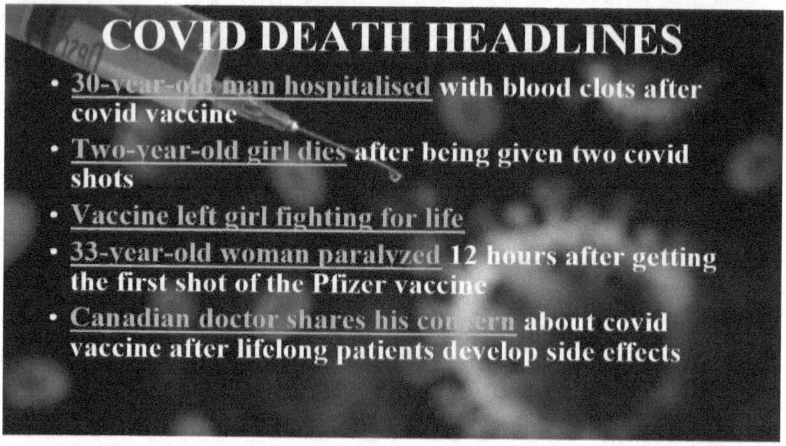
COVID DEATH HEADLINES
• 30-year-old man hospitalised with blood clots after covid vaccine
• Two-year-old girl dies after being given two covid shots
• Vaccine left girl fighting for life
• 33-year-old woman paralyzed 12 hours after getting the first shot of the Pfizer vaccine
• Canadian doctor shares his concern about covid vaccine after lifelong patients develop side effects

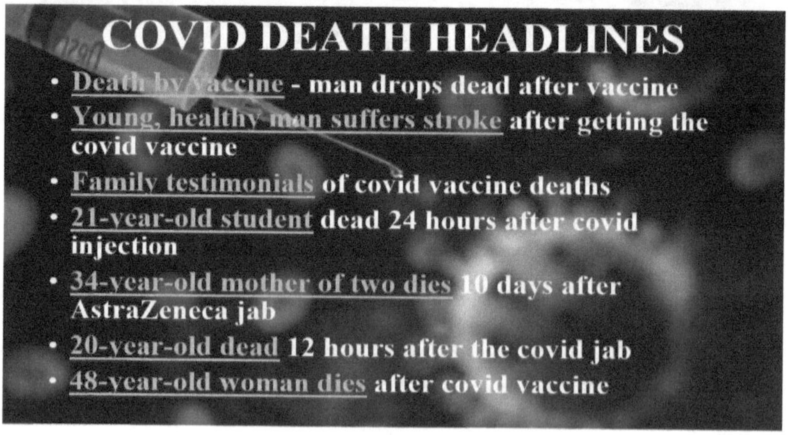
COVID DEATH HEADLINES
• Death by vaccine - man drops dead after vaccine
• Young, healthy man suffers stroke after getting the covid vaccine
• Family testimonials of covid vaccine deaths
• 21-year-old student dead 24 hours after covid injection
• 34-year-old mother of two dies 10 days after AstraZeneca jab
• 20-year-old dead 12 hours after the covid jab
• 48-year-old woman dies after covid vaccine

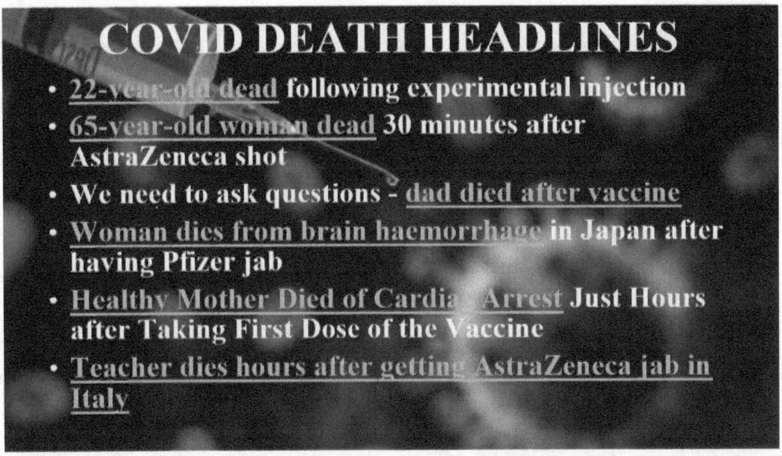
COVID DEATH HEADLINES
• 22-year-old dead following experimental injection
• 65-year-old woman dead 30 minutes after AstraZeneca shot
• We need to ask questions - dad died after vaccine
• Woman dies from brain haemorrhage in Japan after having Pfizer jab
• Healthy Mother Died of Cardiac Arrest Just Hours after Taking First Dose of the Vaccine
• Teacher dies hours after getting AstraZeneca jab in Italy

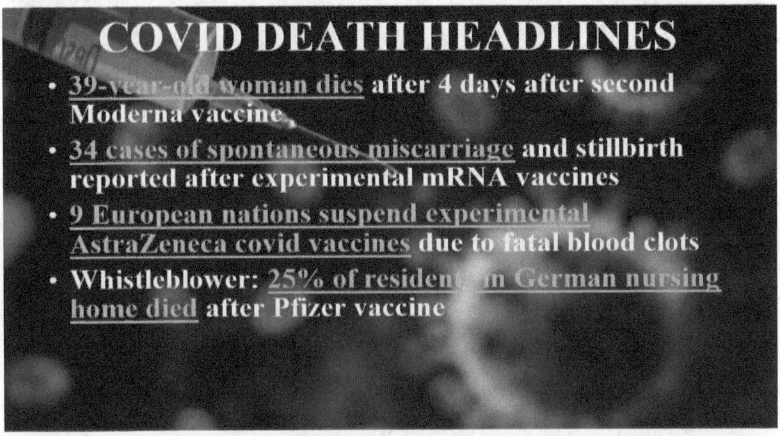
COVID DEATH HEADLINES
• 39-year-old woman dies after 4 days after second Moderna vaccine
• 34 cases of spontaneous miscarriage and stillbirth reported after experimental mRNA vaccines
• 9 European nations suspend experimental AstraZeneca covid vaccines due to fatal blood clots
• Whistleblower: 25% of residents in German nursing home died after Pfizer vaccine

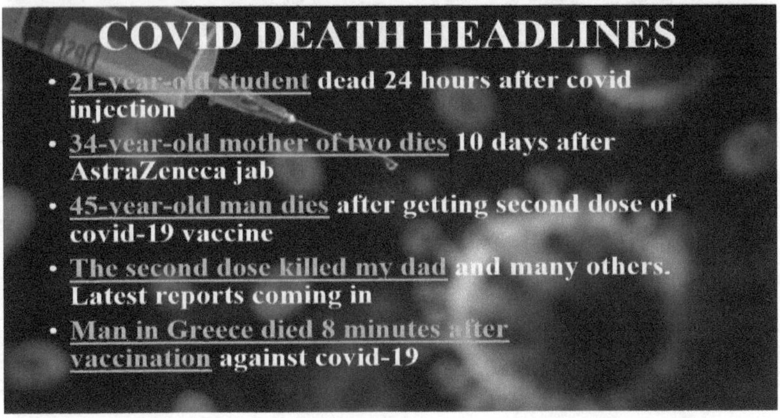
COVID DEATH HEADLINES
• 21-year-old student dead 24 hours after covid injection
• 34-year-old mother of two dies 10 days after AstraZeneca jab
• 45-year-old man dies after getting second dose of covid-19 vaccine
• The second dose killed my dad and many others. Latest reports coming in
• Man in Greece died 8 minutes after vaccination against covid-19

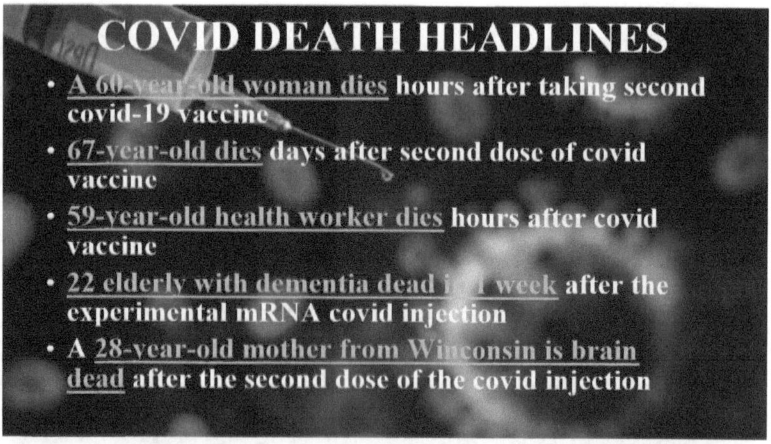
COVID DEATH HEADLINES
• A 60-year-old woman dies hours after taking second covid-19 vaccine
• 67-year-old dies days after second dose of covid vaccine
• 59-year-old health worker dies hours after covid vaccine
• 22 elderly with dementia dead in 1 week after the experimental mRNA covid injection
• A 28-year-old mother from Wisconsin is brain dead after the second dose of the covid injection

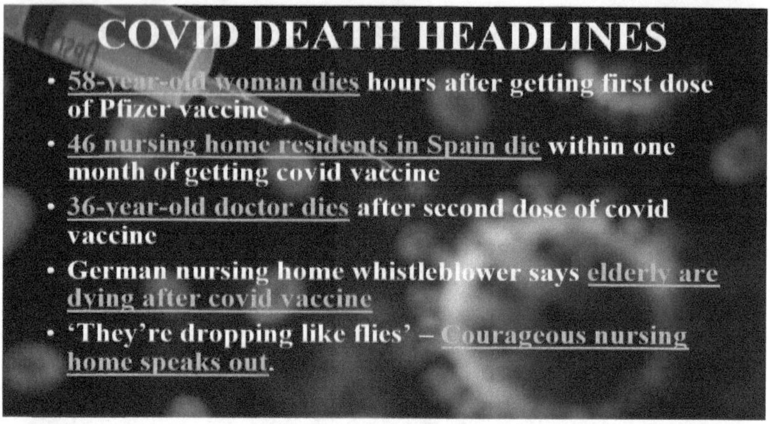
COVID DEATH HEADLINES
• 58-year-old woman dies hours after getting first dose of Pfizer vaccine
• 46 nursing home residents in Spain die within one month of getting covid vaccine
• 36-year-old doctor dies after second dose of covid vaccine
• German nursing home whistleblower says elderly are dying after covid vaccine
• 'They're dropping like flies' – Courageous nursing home speaks out.

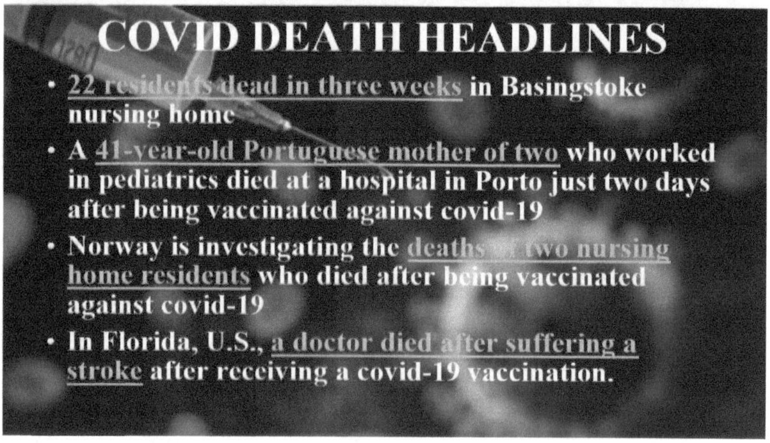
COVID DEATH HEADLINES
• 22 residents dead in three weeks in Basingstoke nursing home
• A 41-year-old Portuguese mother of two who worked in pediatrics died at a hospital in Porto just two days after being vaccinated against covid-19
• Norway is investigating the deaths of two nursing home residents who died after being vaccinated against covid-19
• In Florida, U.S., a doctor died after suffering a stroke after receiving a covid-19 vaccination.

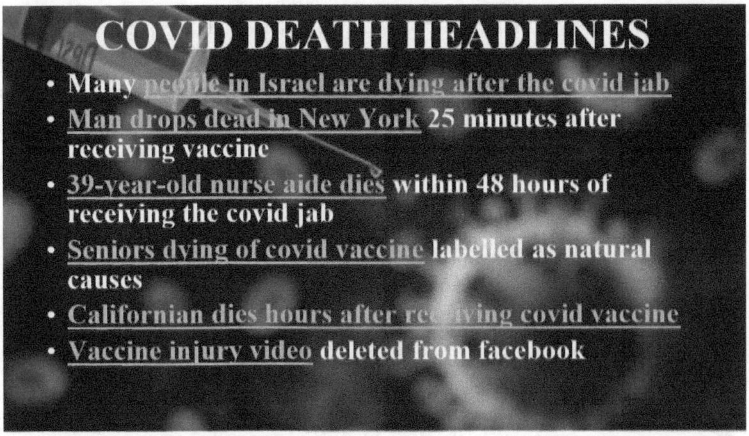
COVID DEATH HEADLINES
• Many people in Israel are dying after the covid jab
• Man drops dead in New York 25 minutes after receiving vaccine
• 39-year-old nurse aide dies within 48 hours of receiving the covid jab
• Seniors dying of covid vaccine labelled as natural causes
• Californian dies hours after receiving covid vaccine
• Vaccine injury video deleted from facebook

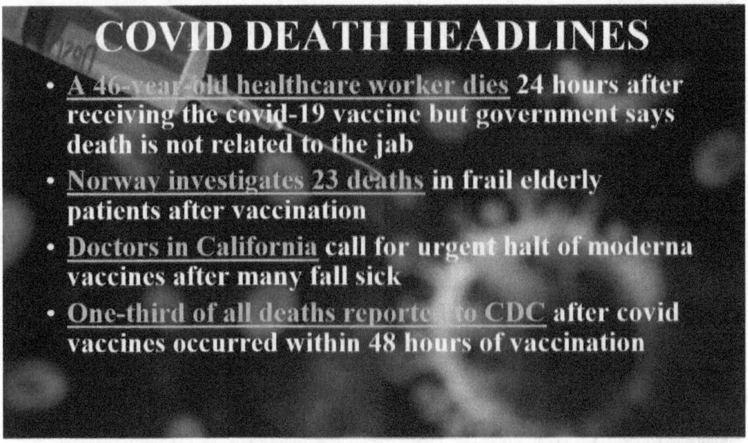
COVID DEATH HEADLINES
• A 46-year-old healthcare worker dies 24 hours after receiving the covid-19 vaccine but government says death is not related to the jab
• Norway investigates 23 deaths in frail elderly patients after vaccination
• Doctors in California call for urgent halt of moderna vaccines after many fall sick
• One-third of all deaths reported to CDC after covid vaccines occurred within 48 hours of vaccination

Looking back at where the school made the father get his son a covid vaccine and now he has a heart condition. I have said it before and I will say it again, get your kids out of public schools and homeschool your kids. If you don't think they are going to start sneaking the vaccine into the schools, let me tell you. Kids can already get contraceptives in school; they don't have to tell parents about it. They are watching pornography, homosexuality, lesbianism, and they don't have to tell you, the parent. If you don't think they are going to do this, give me a break. They can get an abortion at school, and they don't even have to tell a parent. You better wake up!

But don't worry, the vaccine is safe and effective. And we can go on and on and on, but it is effective if you want to murder people. That's why I do not hesitate to say what's going on, it's a satanic agenda. It's not just full of lies, but it is murdering people like flies. That's why some people are speaking up and saying, "You know what, the Covid vaccine is poison." In fact, it's from Johns Hopkins.

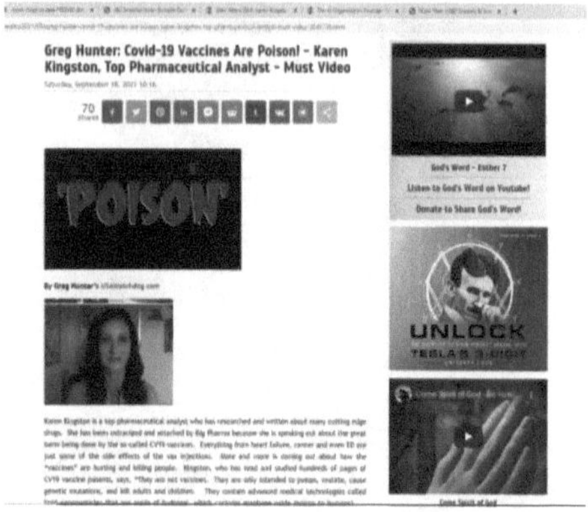
Greg Hunter: Covid-19 Vaccines Are Poison! - Karen Kingston, Top Pharmaceutical Analyst - Must Video
POISON
UNLOCK

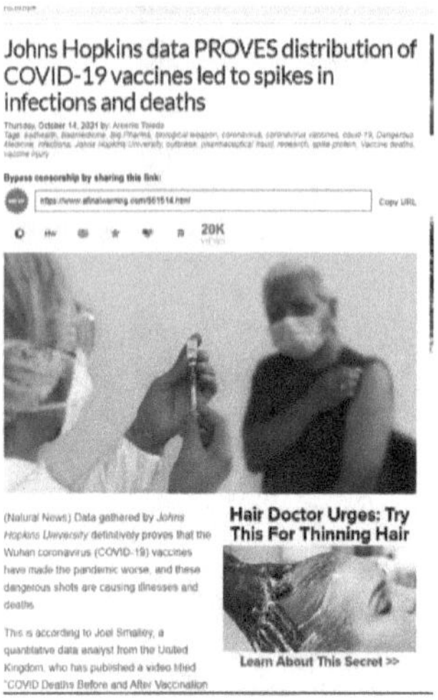

This is from their own camp. Johns Hopkins data proves distribution of Covid-19 vaccines led to spikes in infections and deaths. And now, even people who work for these companies are starting to speak out. And they are saying please don't do it. Even Johnson & Johnson, who always seems to get a pass, is saying it's not safe. J&J scientist Durrant says "Don't get J&J Covid vaccine." And it just continues. Pfizer, same thing.

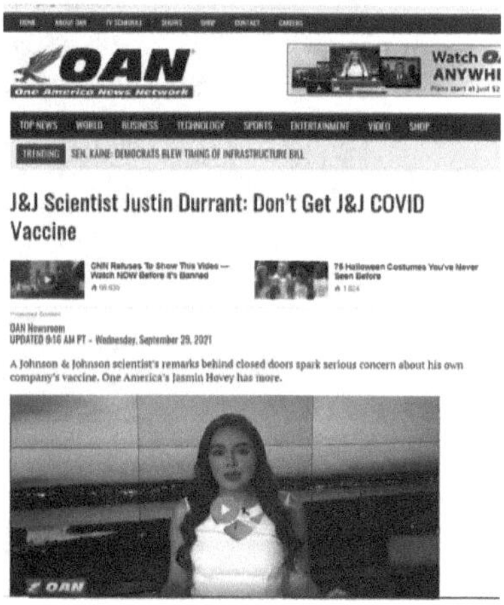
OAN
One America News Network
J&J Scientist Justin Durrant: Don't Get J&J COVID Vaccine
OAN Newsroom
UPDATED 9:16 AM PT - Wednesday, September 29, 2021
A Johnson & Johnson scientist's remarks behind closed doors spark serious concern about his own company's vaccine. One America's Jasmin Hovey has more.

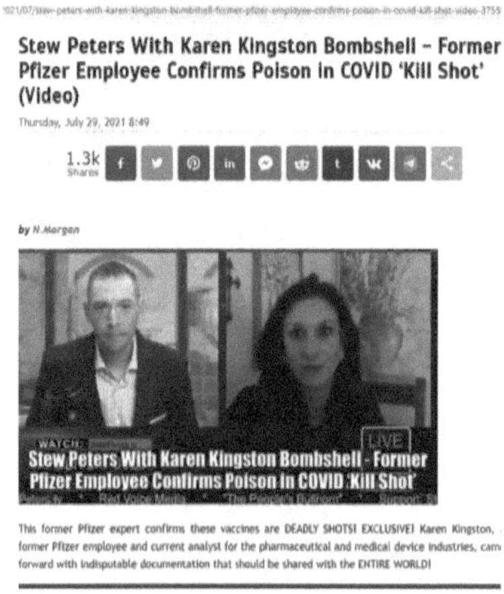

They are calling it a kill shot. Other organizations are saying that these vaccines are an "Extinction Agenda." What else would you call it?

And that's why more than 3,000 doctors and scientists, have signed a Declaration accusing Covid policymakers of "Crimes Against Humanity." You know, like what Hitler did? Except it's happening in our time.

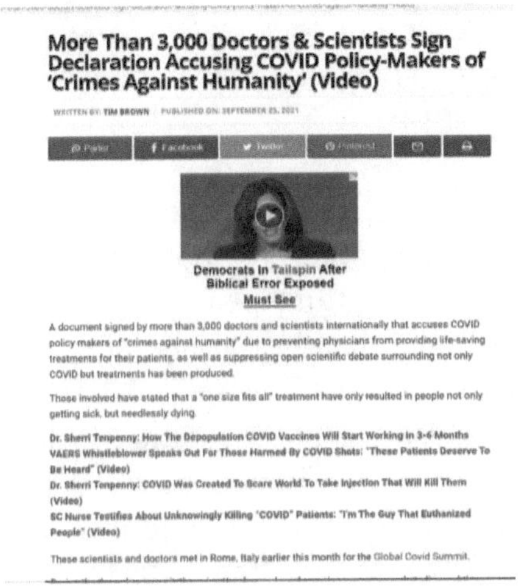

More Than 3,000 Doctors & Scientists Sign Declaration Accusing COVID Policy-Makers of 'Crimes Against Humanity' (Video)

WRITTEN BY: TIM BROWN PUBLISHED ON: SEPTEMBER 25, 2021

Democrats In Tailspin After Biblical Error Exposed
Must See

A document signed by more than 3,000 doctors and scientists internationally that accuses COVID policy makers of "crimes against humanity" due to preventing physicians from providing life-saving treatments for their patients, as well as suppressing open scientific debate surrounding not only COVID but treatments has been produced.

Those involved have stated that a "one size fits all" treatment have only resulted in people not only getting sick, but needlessly dying.

Dr. Sherri Tenpenny: How The Depopulation COVID Vaccines Will Start Working In 3-6 Months
VAERS Whistleblower Speaks Out For Those Harmed By COVID Shots: "These Patients Deserve To Be Heard" (Video)
Dr. Sherri Tenpenny: COVID Was Created To Scare World To Take Injection That Will Kill Them (Video)
SC Nurse Testifies About Unknowingly Killing "COVID" Patients: "I'm The Guy That Euthanized People" (Video)

These scientists and doctors met in Rome, Italy earlier this month for the Global Covid Summit.

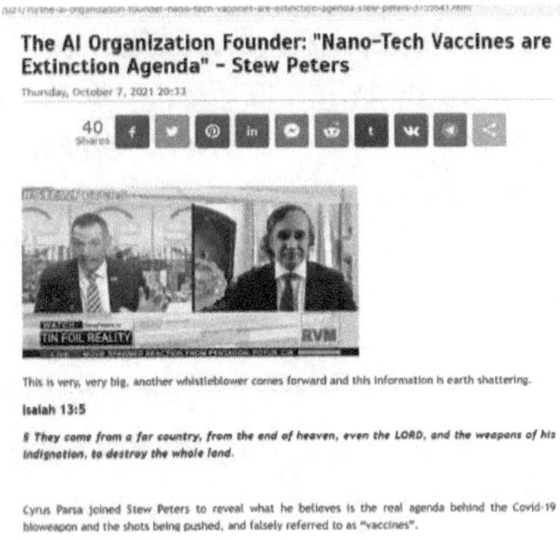

The AI Organization Founder: "Nano-Tech Vaccines are Extinction Agenda" - Stew Peters

Thursday, October 7, 2021 20:33

40 Shares

This is very, very big, another whistleblower comes forward and this information is earth shattering.

Isaiah 13:5

5 They come from a far country, from the end of heaven, even the LORD, and the weapons of his indignation, to destroy the whole land.

Cyrus Parsa joined Stew Peters to reveal what he believes is the real agenda behind the Covid-19 bioweapon and the shots being pushed, and falsely referred to as "vaccines".

Now how many of you would say, we've been lied to just a wee bit? Would you put your life, your health, your family's health, your future into somebody's hands that lied this much, this often, repeatedly? I don't! And it's not a conspiracy theory. This is exactly what is going on, in fact if you don't think these people aren't coming after the church, you better think again. They are splitting the church right down the middle. Dividing us as Christians. They are coming into the church, and they're saying those of you that did get the shot, you better pressure those other ones in the church that didn't. And you need to become our apostles. Because the vaccines are from God. Now that sounds ridiculous and blasphemous. Right? This is a clip of a video of the New York governor, in a church. Look at what she said on tape.

New York Governor goes on vaccine rant, says the vaccine came from God, and she asks the vaccinated audience to become her "apostles."

Governor: *"I prayed a lot to God during this time and you know what? God did answer our prayers. He made the smartest men and women, the scientists, doctors, researchers, He made them come up with a vaccine. That is from God to us! And we must say thank you God. Thank you. And I* *wear my vaccinated necklace all the time to say, 'I'm vaccinated.' All of you, I know you are vaccinated. You are the smart ones. But you know there are people out there who aren't listening to God and what God wants. You know who they are. I need you to be my apostles. I need you to go out and talk about it, and say we owe it to each other, we love each other. Jesus taught us to love one another. And how do you show that love? To care enough about each other to say please get vaccinated because I love you. I want you to live. I want our kids to be safe when they are in school. I want you to be safe when you go to the doctor's office or to the hospital."*

Well, that's going to happen by not getting the shot, based on the data. In the church they are trying to get us at each other's throat. And that is sick! You talk about satan coming into the church, this is nuts. So, why are they doing this? I think we have demonstrated that they are lying, but why? There has to be an agenda, right? Again, to make Trump look bad, they had to get him out of office because he wasn't going to go along with it. Yes, they had to have an excuse to bring in the mail-in ballots, so they can pad the election to make sure he doesn't stay in office. Yes, to bring in the Great Reset. To usher in this global order, which the Bible calls the antichrist kingdom, that will culminate during the 7-year Tribulation. Yes, so they can bailout big pharma, but there are two more things that I want to give you.

They have done this because they have found out another way, to use their lies, to get a massive amount of not just money to bail them from going bankrupt, but to have a never-ending supply of cash. Because now the secular doctors are admitting, the more of these shots that you get, the more it destroys your immune system, until you have no immune system, and you are literally walking around, in essence, with AIDS. You have no immune system. The only way for you to survive, is to get endless booster shots. So, you are a customer for life. Take a look at this clip. This health practitioner is not ready to share her identity at this time but her presented information is invaluable.

"So, I am a natural doctor and I have 1,600 patients. Many are vaccinated. Just to give you a little bit of back story about my credibility. What I have seen so far and what I have learned, is all information from physicians, medical physicians, natural physicians, and also immunization virology doctors, and also nurses. What I am about to share with you is the first vaccine, the second vaccine, and then the boosters, and what it does to your body.

The first vaccine, as it goes into your body, it has a small amount of saline and a bunch of ingredients that are very catastrophic to your cellular system. What that does to your immune system, which is your bone marrow, your thymus gland, your spleen, and all other systems associated with your immune system, it decreases the ability to produce white blood cells by 50 percent from your first vaccine. Then 8 weeks later, which is the white blood cells reproductive system. So, your ability to make another generation of white blood cells is 8 weeks. That is why they set it up for 8 weeks later, to hit it again. You hit the white blood cell ability while its down.

So, now they decrease the saline in the second one and increase the harmful ingredients. So, now you have a shift in ingredients. And then what they do is they decrease the ability to produce white blood cells by an additional 25 percent. So now you have the ability to make white blood cells functioning at 25 percent. So, you just wiped-out 75 percent of your military, and the ability to make that military.

Then what they do is set in the booster. The booster has 81 strands of foreign bacteria that your cells have never come across and you don't have the antibodies to fight it, because you only have 25 percent of your white blood cell production to fight it, so it's a losing battle. So, now what starts to happen is that you get chronic inflammation that goes to the area that you had predisposition. So, if you were someone that had gut health issues, that is the area that it is going to focus on. You are going to have inflammation in that area. If it's respiratory, or a tumor, or cancer, or endometriosis, or a skin condition, whatever that is, it's going to inflame that area, because now the body has hit the sympathetic nervous system, which is fight or flight, and the body is in a chronic inflammatory state, with a low immunity and a low immune response.

Then you get your second booster. The second booster has 8 strands of HIV, and what that does is it completely shuts off your ability to make white blood cells, and you can Google what that disease is, it is HIV. Now we have people who are walking around with no immune system, no ability to make an immune system, 81 strands of foreign bacteria, and also 8 strands of foreign HIV, along with all the other harmful ingredients and then they remove all the saline from the first and second booster.

Now, to make matters worse, during this process, 20 to 30 percent of the population is going to die, every single series of this process. There are four series. There are three more boosters that are coming out, and the reason why is because, once they make you so that your immune system can't make white blood cells anymore, you become dependent on the boosters just to survive like someone becomes dependent on insulin.

Big pharma is looking for people that either die off, to protect our population control or those that don't die off, they will have reccurring customers for life, with the boosters so they will maintain income and collect the money back for all the funding that they put in to make these vaccines in the first place. So, I hope that was helpful. I hope you listened to this properly and I hope you take the time to do your own critical thinking just give it two-three years."

That is satanic. You're going to see a lot of people die, and they know it. What was the word that she used? Population control. That is what they want to do. They want to annihilate 90 percent of the population. It sounds nuts. We talk about this as a church. I feel unfortunate about other churches that don't, and I don't mean to boast, but God has us equipped. We know better. We know what's coming. But there are other churches out there still talking about that fluffy cat and how to be a better you. They have no clue as to what is coming. And that's sad! And dare I say that those shepherds are going to stand accountable to God, even if they are a real Christian or not. But this is really what they want to do, and it's an endless supply of customers and those that even survive, and most are going to die, a lot of them are going to die, but you are going to have to keep going back for boosters.

So, why else are they doing this? You just saw, for an endless supply of customers. Not just bailing you out, now you have figured out a routine for those that survived this onslaught, is you are going to have a never-ending supply of cash. That is sick. The love of money is the root of all kinds of evil. But the other one is that satan is not only a liar, but he is a murderer. This is literally mass genocide that we haven't seen since the days of Hitler. And to prove that I'm going to show you a video clip from Dr. Zelenko. He's one of the top doctors on the planet. He's got clout coming out of his ears. He's the guy that treated President Trump, Rudy Giuliani, he's not a fly by night guy. He's a Jewish doctor, and he warned his own Jewish community, that this is nothing but a poison death shot. If you give it to kids, you are into child sacrifice, and this is mass genocide that we haven't seen since Hitler, and we better wake up.

"So, I'll just give you quickly my experience, my team has directly treated successfully six thousand patients. I have trained hundreds of physicians, who are now training their students, and as our little group we have treated millions of patients successfully. President Trump was my patient, lawyer Rudy Giuliani was my patient, Yaakov Litzman, the health minister of Israel, last year, was my patient. I'm just telling you which people have contacted me here, including President Bolsonaro of Brazil.

Now my experience has given me a very unique perspective in approaching Covid-19, which is basically keeping people out of the hospital. Regarding children, the only reason you would want to treat a child, is if you believe in child sacrifice. There would have to be a very good reason to treat a child otherwise there would be no necessity. Let me explain. Any time you have any therapeutic, you have to look at it from three perspectives. Is it safe, does it work, and do you need it? Just because you have the capability it doesn't mean you have to use it. There has to be a medical necessity. There has to be a need for it. If you look at the CDC, the statistics for children under the age of 18 that are healthy, the survival rate is 99.9998 percent. The survival rate with no treatment. The influenza virus is more dangerous to children than Covid-19. It was estimated that out of a million, 100 children would die from the vaccination. I feel the number would be significantly higher. And I will explain the rationale for it.

If you have a demographic, that has no risk of dying from an illness, why would you inject them with a poison death shot? Now let's see if this thing works. Two countries in the world that have the most vaccinated citizens are Israel, with an 85 percent rate of vaccination and an island nation in the Indian Ocean called Seychelles, also for 80 percent. Both countries are experiencing a Delta Variant outbreak. So, let me ask you a question. If you vaccinated the majority of your population, why are you still having an outbreak? That is number one. Number two, why would you even give a third shot of the same stuff if it didn't work the first two times? That's whether or not it works.

Now, let's talk about safety. It's the real issue. There are three levels of safety or depth that we need to look at. One is acute, one is subacute, and one is long term. The acute, I'll define from the moment of injection to 3 months. The number one risk of the shot is blood clots, according to the Salk Institute. By the way, everything I'm saying I will defend with documentation and please don't take my word for it, do your due diligence. And I can provide proof of everything that I am saying. According to the Salk Institute, when a person gets an injection of these vaccines, the body becomes a spike producing factory making trillions of spikes which migrate to the epithelium, the lining of your blood vessels, and is basically little thorns on the inside of your vasculature. When the blood cells flow through it, they get damaged and cause blood clots. If that happens in the heart it causes a heart attack, if it happens in the brain, it causes a stroke. So, we are seeing the number one cause of death, in the short term, is blood clots and most of it is happening within the first 3 or 4 days, 40 percent of it is happening within the first 3- or 4-days of injection of this poison death shot.

Now the other problem is that it is causing myocarditis, inflammation in the hearts of young adults. And the third problem is the most disturbing is according to the Newman Journal of Medicine article, their preliminary data, is the miscarriage rate in the first trimester, if the woman gets vaccinated in the first trimester, miscarriage goes from 10 percent to 80 percent. I want you to understand what I just said. The miscarriage rate in the first trimester of pregnant women when they get vaccinated, goes up by a factor of 8. That is preliminary data, it may change with time, but I am just telling you what it is as of today.

That's the smallest of the problems. The second problem is the subacute issue. Which is the following. The animal studies that were done with these vaccines showed that all the animals responded well in generating antibodies. When they challenged with the virus that they were immunized against, a large percentage of them died. When that was investigated it was found that their immune system had killed them. It's called antibody dependent enhancement or pathogenic priming or paradoxical immune enhancement. But the point is that a lot of those animals died. So, you can make an argument that maybe human beings are different. My answer to you, however, is that those studies were not done, you are the studies right now. The Pfizer CEO said Israel is the largest laboratory in the world. So, those long-term studies to rule out, Luc Montagnier, who won the Nobel prize in medicine for the discovery of HIV, said that this is the biggest risk to humanity and the biggest risk of genocide in the history of humanity. So, the risk of a reaction in human beings which happens later has not been ruled out. So, my question is, why would I vaccinate somebody with a potentially destructive lethal substance without ruling that out first?

And the third component here is the long-term consequences. There is definite evidence that it affects fertility, damages ovarian function, and reduces sperm count. It definitely increases the amount of autoimmune diseases. Who knows over time, how that is going to reduce life spans? And just last week a paper came out showing that it increases the risk of cancer. Any way you want to look at it, whether it is in an acute setting where it is causing blood clots, inflammation of the heart and miscarriages, or in the mid-term setting where it could result in a pathological disastrous immune reaction or in the long-term whether it causes autoimmune diseases like cancer and infertility. Now that's a big concern. Actually, I will say it this way. In my opinion, the current Israeli government is a gilgul of Josef Mengele. They have permitted human experimentation on their own people.

I have received daily death threats, I risk my life, my career, my financial life, my reputation, almost my family, everything, just to sit here and tell you what I am telling you. So, I will just summarize it. There is no need for this vaccine, the protection is of no need to anyone. And I will explain. Children, I have already told you; they have a 99.9998 percent of getting better. Young adults from 18 to 45 have a 99.95 percent of getting better. This is according to the CDC. Same concept. Somebody that has already had Covid and has antibodies, naturally induced immunity, is a billion times more effective than artificially induced immunity through vaccines. So, why would I vaccinate someone with a poison death shot that makes inferior or dangerous antibodies, when I already have healthy antibodies?

And then if you look at the high risks. The population has a 7.5 percent death rate, so my data was the first one in the world that I published in the Pier Review Journal that has become the basis of over 200 other studies and I have corroborated my observations that if you treat people in the right timeframe, you reduce the death rate by 85 percent. So, out of 600,000 Americans we could have prevented 510,000 from going to the hospital and dying. And by the way, I presented this information to Bibi Netanyahu, directly into his hands in April of 2020 and I informed every single member of your ministry of health as well. So, my question to you is, if I can reduce the death rate of 7.5 percent to less than half of a percent why would I use a poison death shot that doesn't work and has tremendous horrific side effects? If everyone on the planet were to get Covid and not get treated, the death rate globally will be less than half a percent. I'm not advocating for that. There are a lot, 35 million people would die, however, if you follow the advice of some of the 'global leaders' like Bill Gates said last year, 7 billion people need to be vaccinated, the death rate will be over 2 billion people. So, wake up! This is WWIII, this is a level of malfeasance and malevolence that we have not seen, probably in the history of humanity. There is zero justification for using this poison death shot unless you want to sacrifice human beings."

Top doctor in the world warning his own Jewish people. Now that is exactly what they want to do, population control. What I found very interesting, knowing the scripture, not saying thus sayeth the Lord, but he said if these guys get their way, they vaccinate 7 billion people all over the planet, how many people are going to die? 2 billion. Now you fast forward to the first half of the 7-year Tribulation…

Revelation 6:7-8 "When the Lamb opened the fourth seal, I heard the voice of the fourth living creature say, "Come!" I looked, and there before me was a pale horse! Its rider was named Death, and Hades was following close behind him. They were given power over a fourth of the earth to kill by sword, famine and plague, and by the wild beasts of the earth."

So, if that were to happen today, based on the statistics it would be nearly 2 billion people. How come these guys can't survive? How did 2 billion people die so quickly after this global war, the second seal? Sword, famine, wild beasts, did they mention pestilence? Not saying thus sayeth the Lord, but is that why they couldn't survive that time frame because they have no immune system? That is the event that happens in the first half of the 7-year Tribulation. We leave prior. The other thing that takes place there is, he is warning his own Jewish people. The other people that get decimated during the 7-year Tribulation is the Jewish people, unfortunately, it's the second holocaust that is coming.

Zechariah 13:8 "In the whole land," declares the Lord, "two thirds will be struck down and perish; yet one-third will be left in it."

Well, how is that going to happen? How are two thirds of the Jewish people going to die? Maybe it is the antichrist going after them, hunting them down. Maybe it's that and this. Who's the number one vaccinated country in the world? What did he say? This is mass genocide; we better wake up! And our own government is in on it. That's the event that will happen in the 7-year Tribulation, but we leave prior. We don't know the day or the hour but it's getting close. Are there really people out there, a population control guy, elite, that is behind this Great Reset issue, pushing the Covid narrative to usher all this in? Did he really want to annihilate 90 percent of the population on the planet? And by the way, what's the other country that is being pushed? Not only the United States of America, every citizen, the military, the kids, why are they pushing so hard in America? What's going to be left of our own country and is this the reason why you don't find America mentioned in Bible Prophecy?

Chapter Four

The Murders of Covid

I don't know if you have been watching the news lately, (unfortunately, if you want to be brainwashed) but have you heard on the news, "Omicron" is coming to get you? Of course, it's the next scariant, I mean variant that they are launching on us. And it's already started the doom and gloom with Omicron. The Dow Jones report, it's taken a big giant tumble and we're all going to die. Then of course, you have Joe Biden. He's already restricted travel to South Africa. That's right, hypocrite. Because that's the same thing he

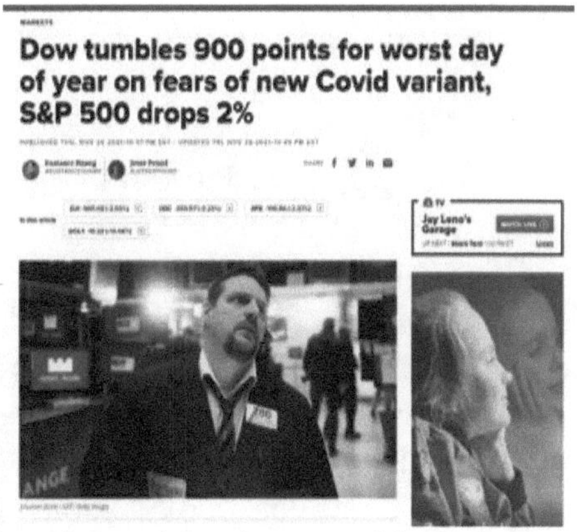
Dow tumbles 900 points for worst day of year on fears of new Covid variant, S&P 500 drops 2%
Jay Leno's Garage

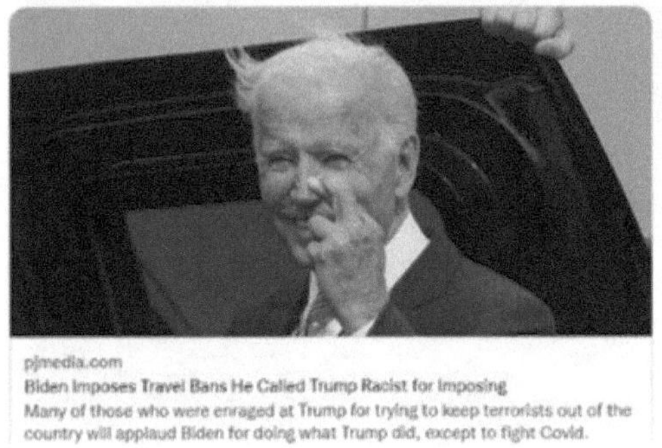

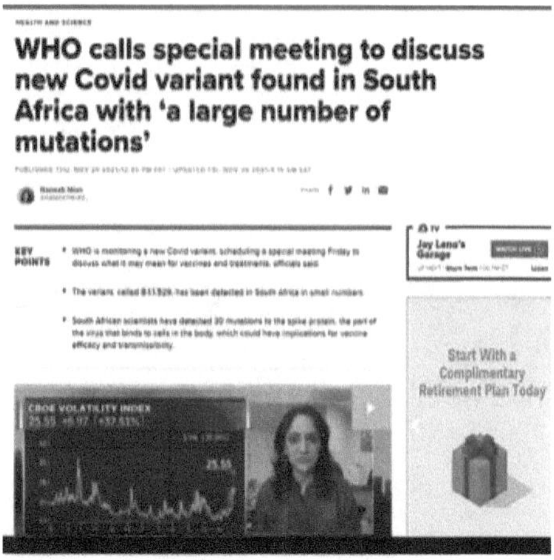

WHO calls special meeting to discuss new Covid variant found in South Africa with 'a large number of mutations'

Start With a Complimentary Retirement Plan Today

called Trump a racist for doing. But I guess that's okay for him. It's the scariant, you are supposed to be scared to death.

And apparently, it's supposed to be so scary and dangerous that he left the southern border wide open, but let's not talk about that. WHO says there's large mutations and we are all going to die, and you better be afraid! It's going to come and get you. Your only hope is the shot. Because that's exactly what this is all

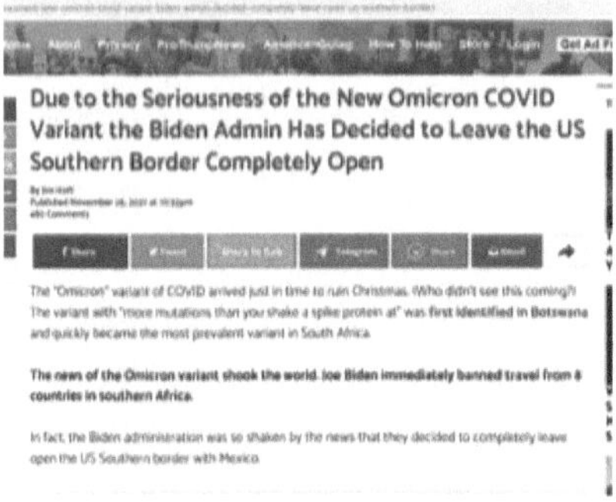

Due to the Seriousness of the New Omicron COVID Variant the Biden Admin Has Decided to Leave the US Southern Border Completely Open

about. It's the endless cycle of this fear-based pressure, manufactured by the media, to get us to take the jab. Fear is what they used to start this pandemic and here's the phrase, if you haven't caught on yet, it's a "Never ending fear" that they will continue to drum up, until we bend and fall in line with their ultimate goal. We're going to see what that ultimate goal is, and frankly it's sick and it's satanic. But this is what's going on with the latest Omicron scare. Now why are they doing it? What's the big deal? Well, there are a lot of people out there saying there's several different things. I don't think it's just about one of these things that I am going to tell you about, I think it's probably a compilation of several. But a lot of people are asking why are you doing this Omicron and specifically right now with this latest scariant? Well, **reason number one**…

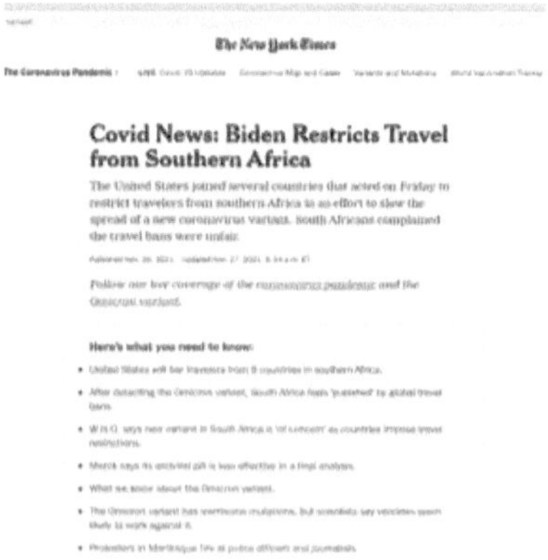

The New York Times

Covid News: Biden Restricts Travel from Southern Africa

What? Yeah, because if you read the news, right before it came out South

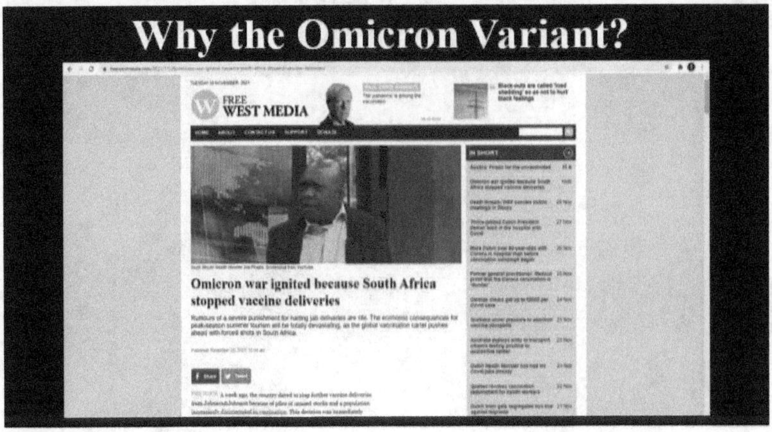

Africa was saying, "We are done with this!"
Omicron war ignited because South Africa stopped deliveries.

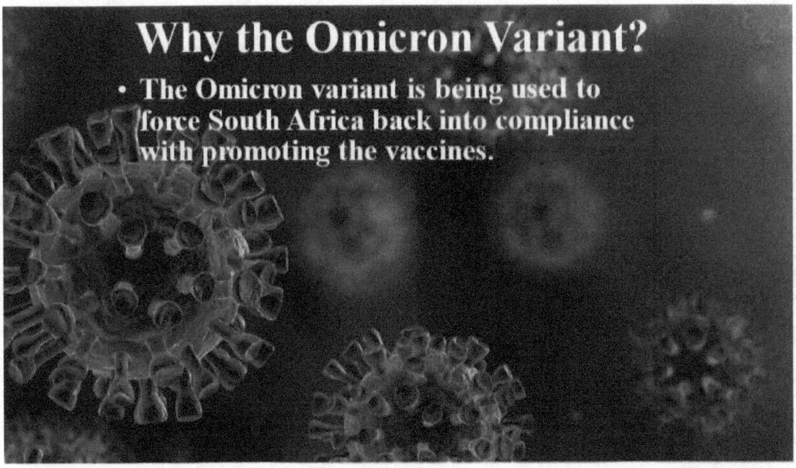

Why the Omicron Variant?
• The Omicron variant is being used to force South Africa back into compliance with promoting the vaccines.

We don't want to do this anymore. And then all of a sudden, the new scariant comes out. Do you think that is by chance? It is to force them back into compliance. Another reason why is **reason number two.**

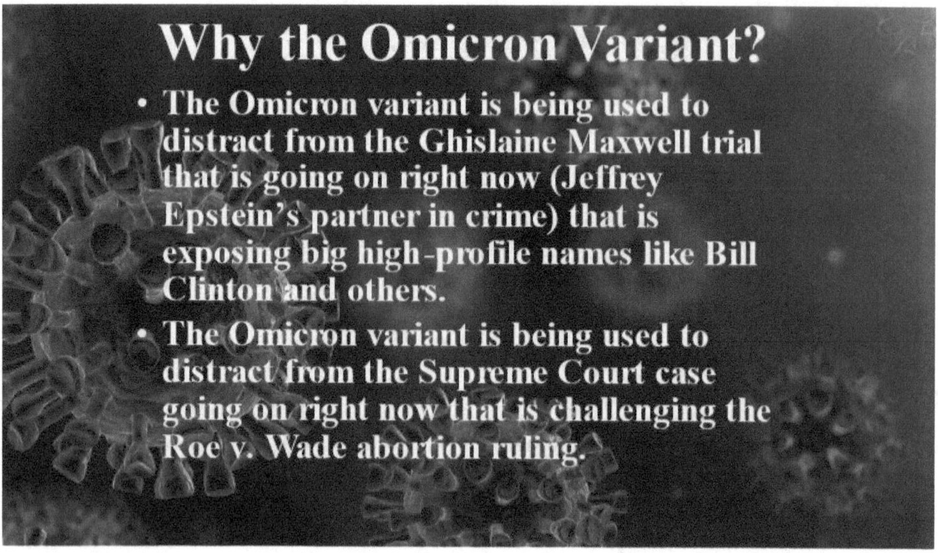

Why the Omicron Variant?
• The Omicron variant is being used to distract from the Ghislaine Maxwell trial that is going on right now (Jeffrey Epstein's partner in crime) that is exposing big high-profile names like Bill Clinton and others.
• The Omicron variant is being used to distract from the Supreme Court case going on right now that is challenging the Roe v. Wade abortion ruling.

Now, don't think of these. Don't encourage the people to vote. You know Omicron is coming to get you. **Reason number three**.

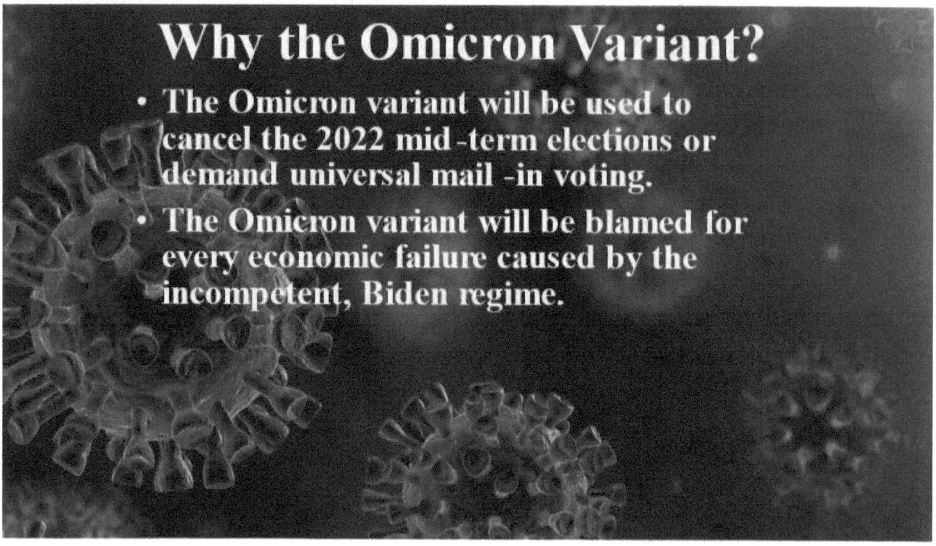

Why the Omicron Variant?
• The Omicron variant will be used to cancel the 2022 mid-term elections or demand universal mail-in voting.
• The Omicron variant will be blamed for every economic failure caused by the incompetent, Biden regime.

They are getting such horrible numbers; they are going in the tank. That is "Build Back Worse" which is their campaign. It's so bad they are going to have to figure out how to rig it and cheat even more than they did last time. And they need to blame Covid for the economic failure because it sure wasn't Biden's bad decisions to destroy our country on purpose. Because they are a part of the Great Reset globalist agenda. Oh, by the way, if it's so bad, then the South African Association debunks the global hysteria. Keep reading, it's a scam, that's what's going on.

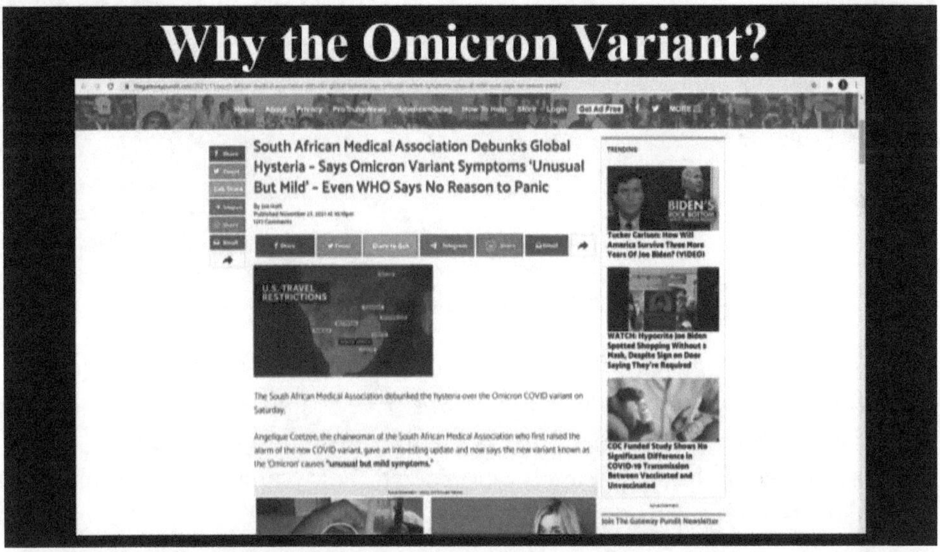
Why the Omicron Variant?
South African Medical Association Debunks Global Hysteria - Says Omicron Variant Symptoms 'Unusual But Mild' - Even WHO Says No Reason to Panic
U.S. TRAVEL RESTRICTIONS
The South African Medical Association debunked the hysteria over the Omicron COVID variant on Saturday.
Angelique Coetzee, the chairwoman of the South African Medical Association who first raised the alarm of the new COVID variant, gave an interesting update and now says the new variant known as the 'Omicron' causes "unusual but mild symptoms."
Tucker Carlson: How Will America Survive Three More Years Of Joe Biden? (VIDEO)
WATCH: Hypocrite Joe Biden Spotted Shopping Without a Mask, Despite Sign on Door Saying They're Required
CDC Funded Study Shows No Significant Difference in COVID-19 Transmission Between Vaccinated and Unvaccinated
Join The Gateway Pundit Newsletter

Reason number four.

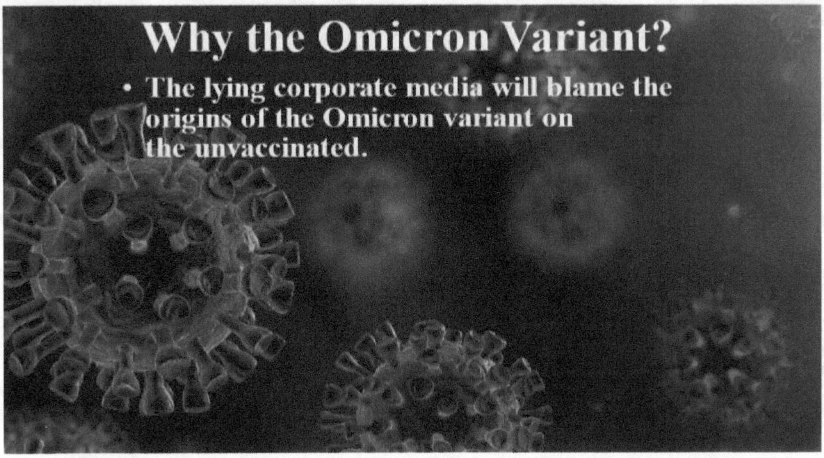
Why the Omicron Variant?
• The lying corporate media will blame the origins of the Omicron variant on the unvaccinated.

Because you and I didn't get in line, we're the ones that brought this on.

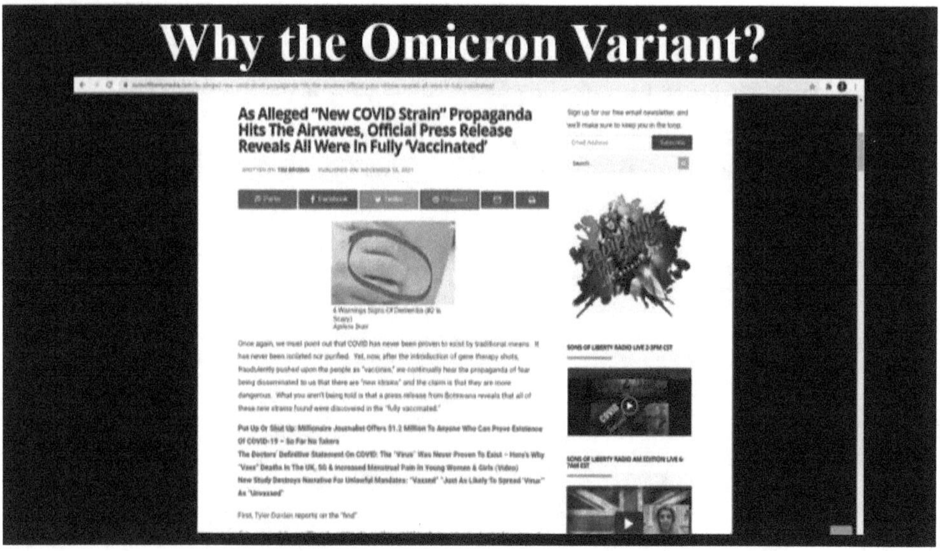

Look at it, check it out yourself, 100 percent of the Omicron cases were fully vaccinated people. 100 percent! Every single one of them was fully vaccinated. That's where this is coming from, but if you just keep lying to people and say it is the unvaccinated then you can make them look bad. **Reason number five**.

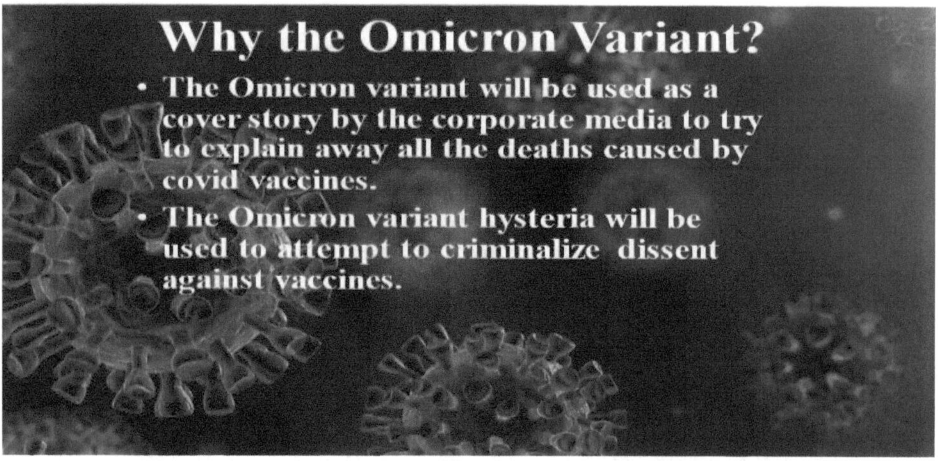

Why the Omicron Variant?
• The Omicron variant will be used as a cover story by the corporate media to try to explain away all the deaths caused by covid vaccines.
• The Omicron variant hysteria will be used to attempt to criminalize dissent against vaccines.

It's just this new variant. That's why people are dropping like flies from the jab, and we will see some other lame excuses shortly. Surely, it's not the vaccine. But they are going to use it to criminalize us and then they will have to take legal action. **Reason number six**.

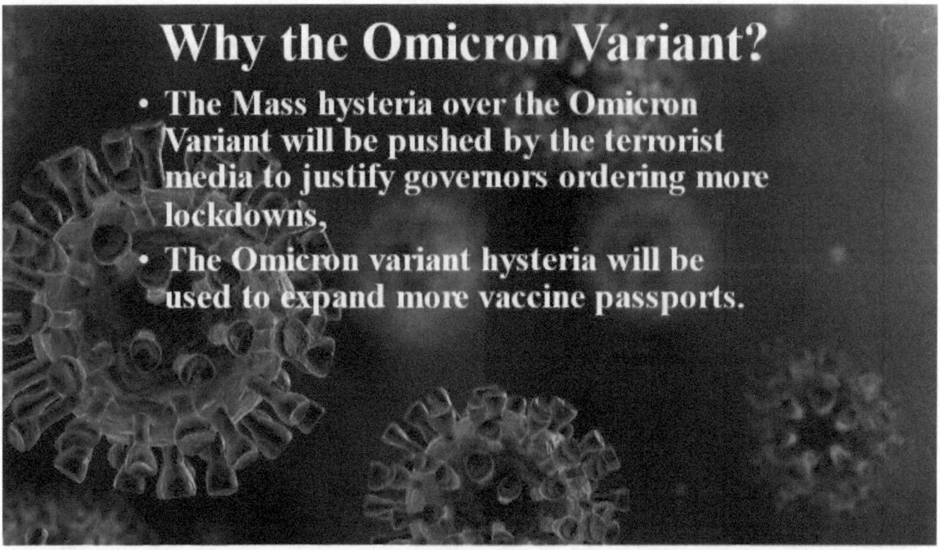

Why the Omicron Variant?
• The Mass hysteria over the Omicron Variant will be pushed by the terrorist media to justify governors ordering more lockdowns,
• The Omicron variant hysteria will be used to expand more vaccine passports.

Now, did you see it's coming to California? **Reason number seven**.

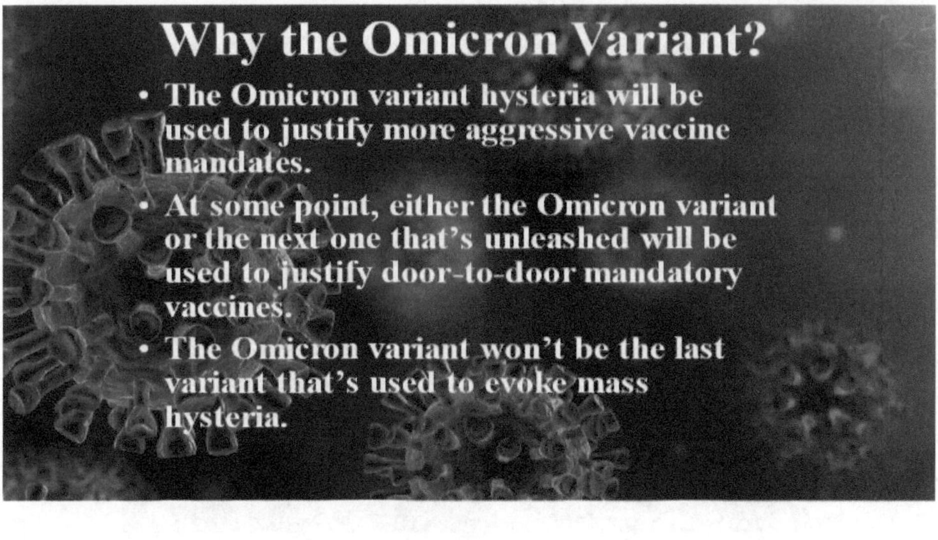

Why the Omicron Variant?
• The Omicron variant hysteria will be used to justify more aggressive vaccine mandates.
• At some point, either the Omicron variant or the next one that's unleashed will be used to justify door-to-door mandatory vaccines.
• The Omicron variant won't be the last variant that's used to evoke mass hysteria.

Again, it's comply, comply, comply and get the jab whether you want it or not. Have you seen the reports about what is going on in Australia? They are rounding people up, including kids, and forcing them to get it. So, it's already happening in other places as well. I like what this guy says.

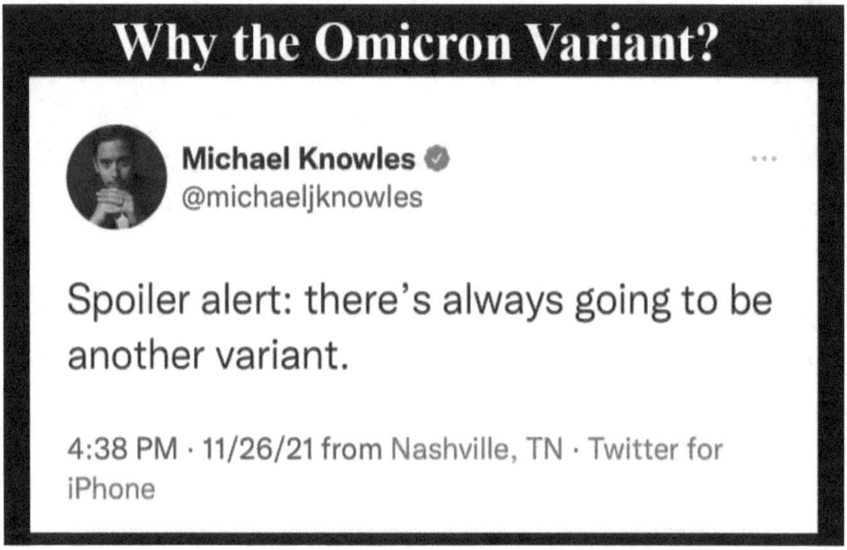

Anybody see a pattern here? It keeps happening again and again and again. I also like what this guy says.

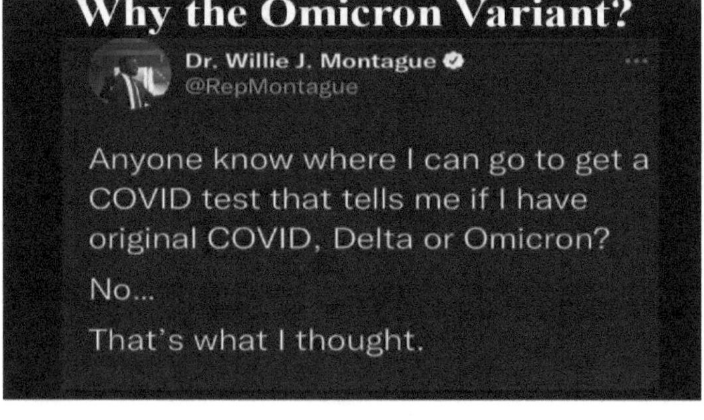

Why the Omicron Variant?
Michael Knowles
@michaeljknowles
Spoiler alert: there's always going to be another variant.
4:38 PM · 11/26/21 from Nashville, TN · Twitter for iPhone
Dr. Willie J. Montague
@RepMontague
Anyone know where I can go to get a COVID test that tells me if I have original COVID, Delta or Omicron?
No...
That's what I thought.

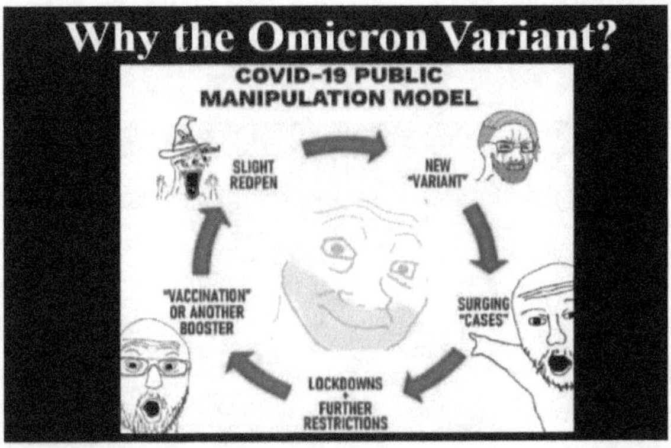

There is no test. How do you know you even have Omicron? You don't. We are being lied to. Now this is the model. Have we not caught on yet? How many scariants do we have to go through before we catch on? Here's the pattern.

First you start off with the new variant, the original then the Delta, then Omicron, what's coming next? And then it starts in one area, and it spreads around the world. It starts in South Africa and then to the UK, then oh no, now it's in California, it's in the US. Then that's the excuse. We have to have more lockdowns, more mandates, more restrictions, are you sick and tired yet? The only hope is if you get the jab. Get the jab, get the booster, get more boosters and then you finally start to relax, and you have to go around the horn again. It's a new scariant. They're running out of letters. Maybe they will go to the Egyptian language. Have you caught on yet? It's the same cycle of fear to manipulate. And look at what this guy admitted.

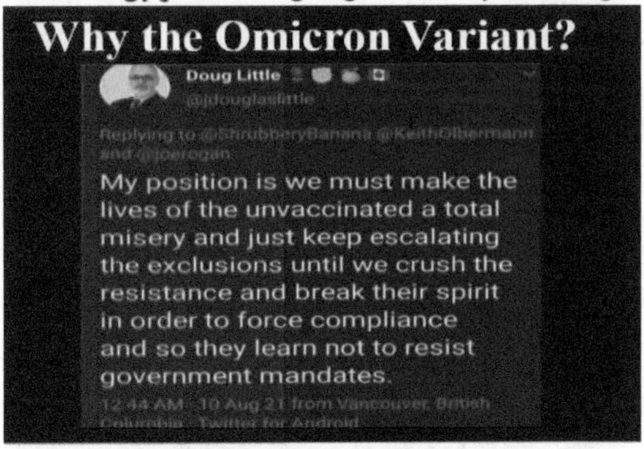

Why the Omicron Variant?
Doug Little
My position is we must make the lives of the unvaccinated a total misery and just keep escalating the exclusions until we crush the resistance and break their spirit in order to force compliance and so they learn not to resist government mandates.

That's sick but at least he was honest. But that is really what is going on.

Of course, I like what this one says.

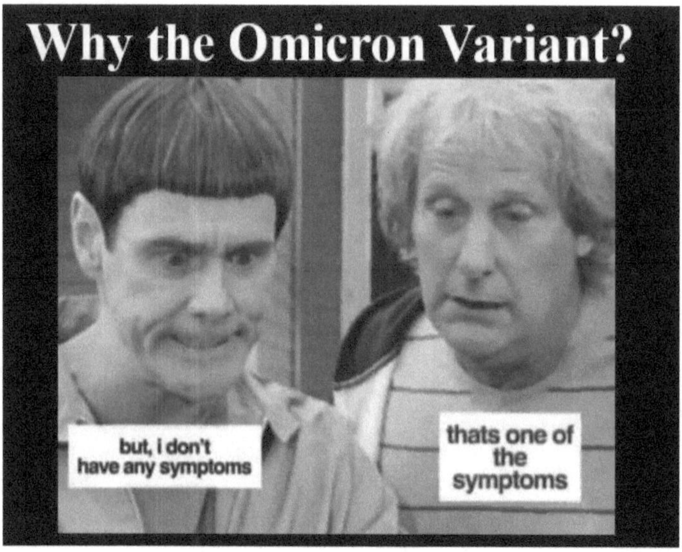
Why the Omicron Variant?
but, i don't have any symptoms
thats one of the symptoms

When speaking of dumb and dumber. I don't know if you ever noticed this, but have you heard of an anagram? It's a word you can scramble into another word. Well, it just so happens with Omicron. It spells moronic. Showing a lack of good sense; stupid or idiotic:

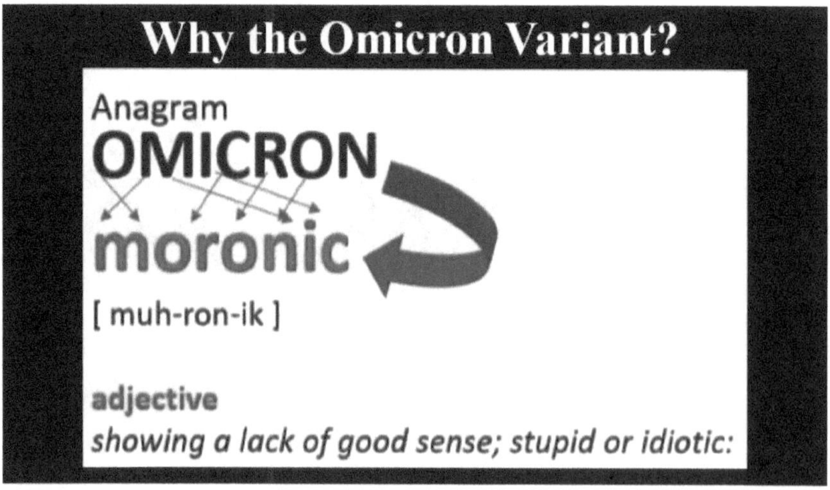

But speaking of idiotic, this stuff is why we did our documentary, "*Subliminal Seduction, How the Mass Media Mesmerizes the Minds of the Masses*" That is why we put it out just a couple months ago. We exposed it all. These guys are controlling the mass media. They own it all around the world, and they are using it to scare people to comply. It's a joke! I'm not saying that this Covid thing is not real, it's real. But the reasoning for it and what they are doing to justify what they are trying to get people to do, is the joke. It's not just a joke, it's a sick joke. But this media, media, media, what you stay plugged in to, people just stay freaked out. In fact, when you run into people that are so freaked out over this, here is how they are acting. Look at this and see if it looks familiar.

There are three girls in the video. One with a T-shirt with a big rainbow and she is wearing a black cap. Different emblems are on her shirt and her cap. (She is vaccinated) The second girl has on a blue shirt, and she is drinking a cup of coffee. (She is unvaccinated) The third girl is the therapist. She has on a white sweatshirt, glasses, and is holding a paper and pen.

Rainbow girl: *"I just don't feel safe around her. I mean look at her."*

Therapist: *"Okay, tell me why you don't feel so safe around her."*

Rainbow girl: *"She's dangerous. She's clearly mentally unstable."*

Coffee girl: *"Me?"*

Rainbow girl: *"She is trying to kill me."*

Coffee girl: *"No I'm not!"*

Therapist: *"You've taken steps to protect yourself, right?"*

Rainbow girl: *"Of course, but she's putting me in danger by not protecting herself."*

Therapist: *"That's just not very logical."*

Coffee girl: *"That's what I keep saying."*

Rainbow girl: *"She is a danger to society. She shouldn't be allowed to have a job or have access to health care or be around in the same spaces as me."*

Therapist: *"So because she is different from you, you think she should be an outcast from society?"*

Rainbow girl: *"Yes, she is unclean."*

Coffee girl: *"I am a perfectly healthy, sane person. Why are you treating me like a second-class citizen?"*

Therapist: *"Actually, that's a great question, and to be totally honest you are kind of sounding like a bigot."*

Rainbow girl: *"What? I am not that! Look at me, look at what I support. I am inclusive and tolerant."*

Therapist: *"Except for her and those like her."*

Rainbow girl: *"She's dirty."*

Therapist: *"This behavior of yours is what we call unvaxedaphobic."*

Rainbow girl: *"You just made that up."*

Therapist: *"Your words are making you sound very vaxist and you are exhibiting signs of vaxism."*

Rainbow girl: *"Vaxism?"*

Therapist: *"Yes. You believe certain people are better than others and should have more rights than others based on their vaccinated status."*

The coffee girl clears her throat.

Rainbow girl: *"Did you hear that?"* She grabs her mask and puts it on.

Therapist: *"What?"*

Rainbow girl: *"She just cleared her throat. I told you she was dirty. Her very purpose is infecting all of us."*

Therapist: *"It's completely normal for one to clear one's throat."*

Rainbow girl starts to light a religious candle.

Rainbow girl: *"Please help me St. Fauci, these people are crazy."*

The coffee girl and the therapist are staring at the rainbow girl while she is in such a panic and even has put on a face shield.

Rainbow girl: *"I just need a booster hit; it will make me feel better."*

Coffee girl: *"I'm going to go. I don't think I am the actual problem here."*

Therapist: *"Yes, you can go."*

Rainbow girl is pounding on her phone looking for some soothing news. Coffee girl is gone, and the therapist is looking at her, trying to figure out how to help this girl.

Do you know anybody like that? That is what happens when you certainly don't open up your Bible. When you don't plug into anything but the media. The news is just hysteria. It's crazy, we laugh about it because it's so true. If racism is wrong, vaxism is wrong too. Hey, have they brainwashed you? Who's the one brainwashed? Where it's all coming from is just drummed up fear.

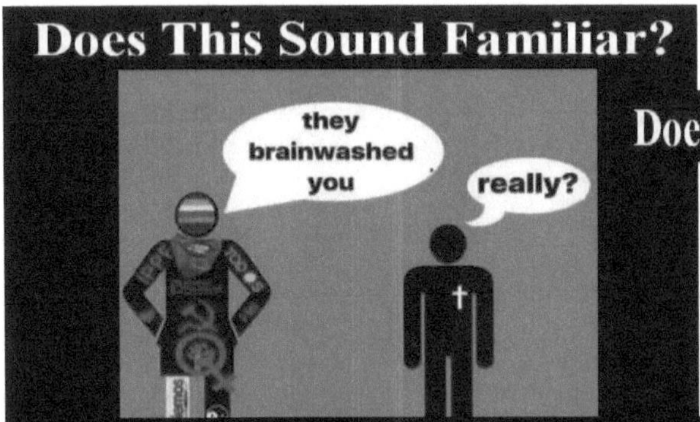

Does This Sound Familiar?
they brainwashed you
really?

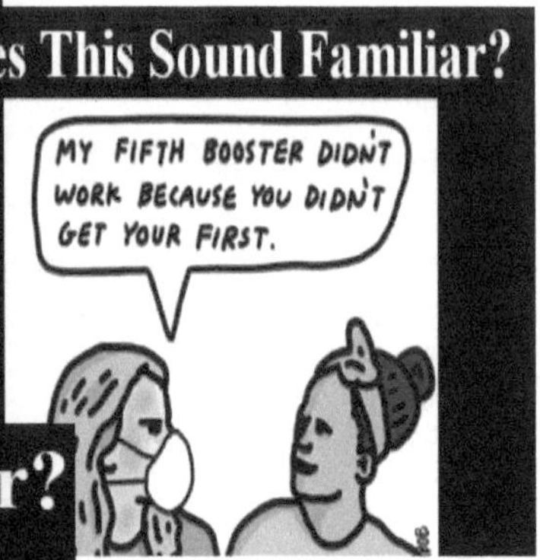

Does This Sound Familiar?
MY FIFTH BOOSTER DIDN'T WORK BECAUSE YOU DIDN'T GET YOUR FIRST.

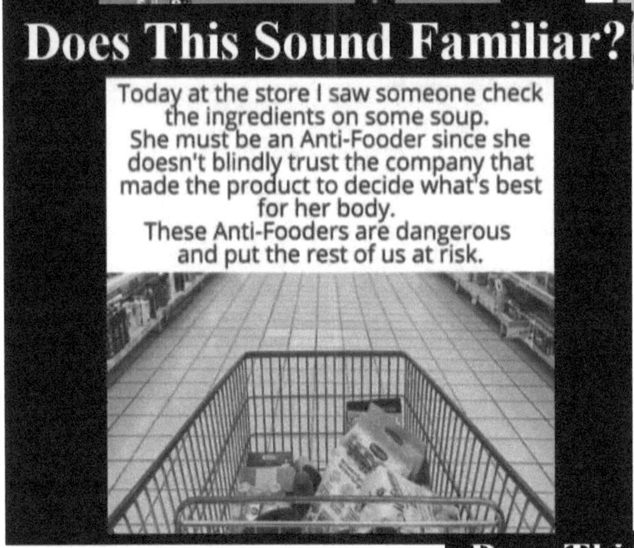

Does This Sound Familiar?
Today at the store I saw someone check the ingredients on some soup.
She must be an Anti-Fooder since she doesn't blindly trust the company that made the product to decide what's best for her body.
These Anti-Fooders are dangerous and put the rest of us at risk.

This is the mindset. This is what is being created with this media hysteria and this scariant. Now I like this one.

It's funny but isn't that true. I'm just questioning what is inside that shot that is going inside my body. But everybody has been conditioned. We have been told for decades to read the ingredients on labels, what's good for your body, but I can't with something else going on. It's very interesting. It's the media. I'm not here to do a

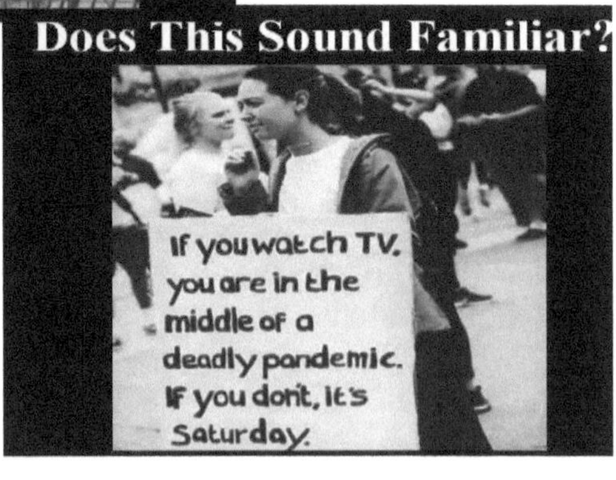

Does This Sound Familiar?
If you watch TV, you are in the middle of a deadly pandemic. If you don't, it's Saturday.

commercial, but again, "*Subliminal Seduction, How the Mass Media Mesmerizes the Minds of the Masses.*" That's what it produces. Which not only answers the last election cycle but what we are dealing with right now. We exposed the whole thing on a global basis.

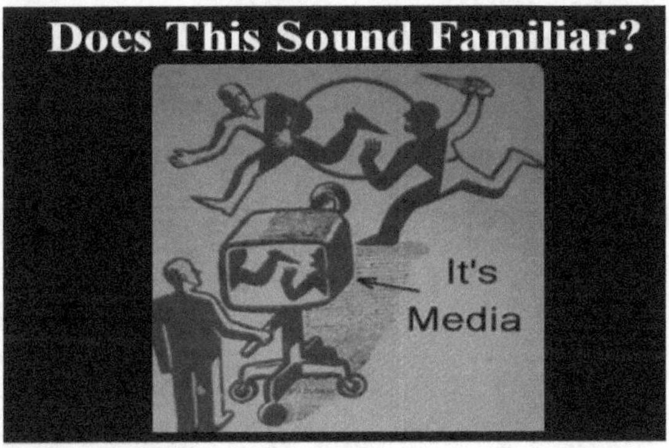
Does This Sound Familiar?
It's
Media

But what you can see there, that is what was really going on, but notice how they cropped the picture. It actually makes the guy being chased look like he's the one trying to kill the other guy. Or this classic shot.

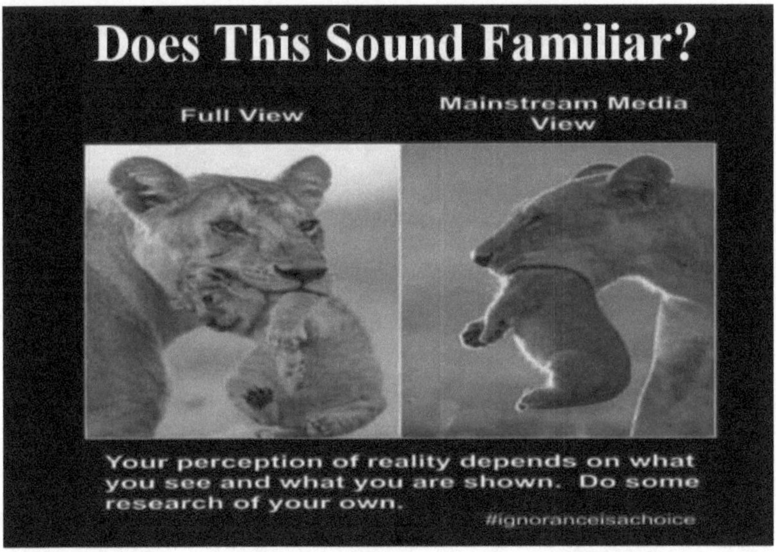
Does This Sound Familiar?
Full View
Mainstream Media View
Your perception of reality depends on what you see and what you are shown. Do some research of your own.
#ignoranceisachoice

That's the real view on the left but the one on the right is the one shown to the public. And you get a completely different perspective. This happens all the time. And that's why we have Misinformation here.

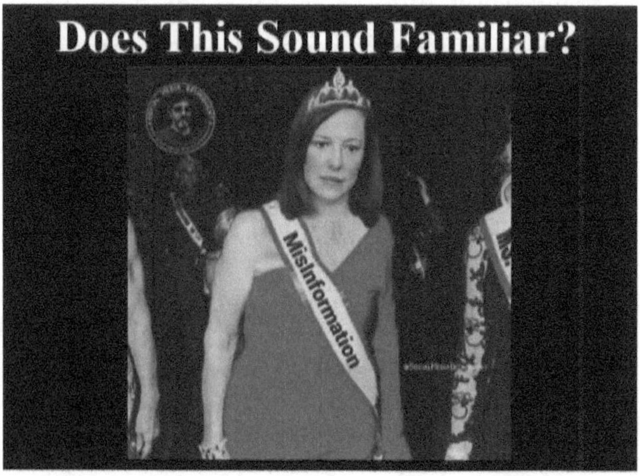
Does This Sound Familiar?
Misinformation

She won that award, right? That's pretty clear. But that's not funny because we have fact checkers.

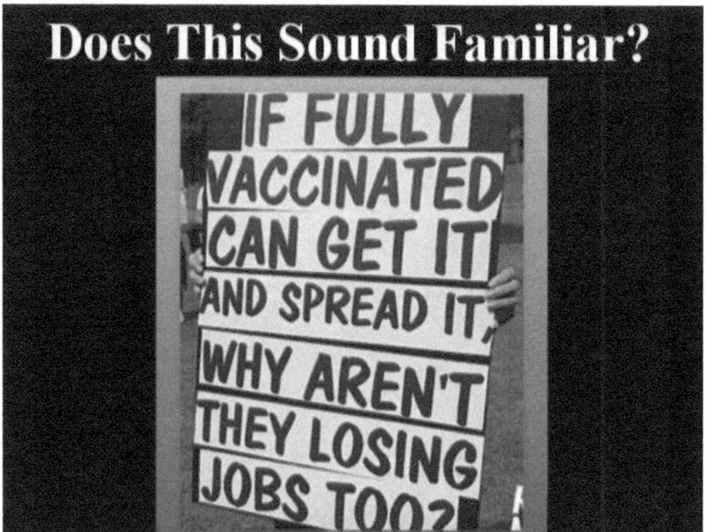
Does This Sound Familiar?
IF FULLY
VACCINATED
CAN GET IT
AND SPREAD IT,
WHY AREN'T
THEY LOSING
JOBS TOO?

None of this makes sense. It's because it's misinformation, it's ramped up fear. Well, here are your fact checkers.

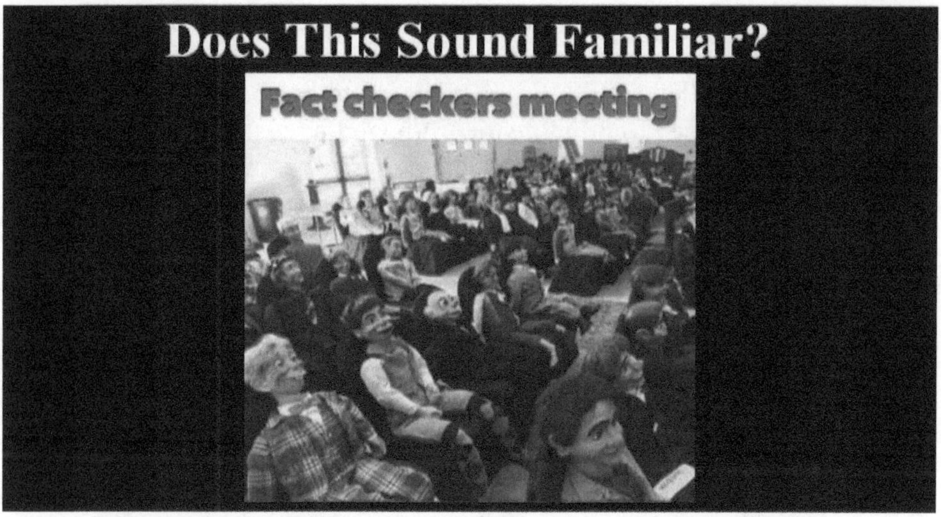

That's what's really going on there. I love this one. The Garden of Eden.

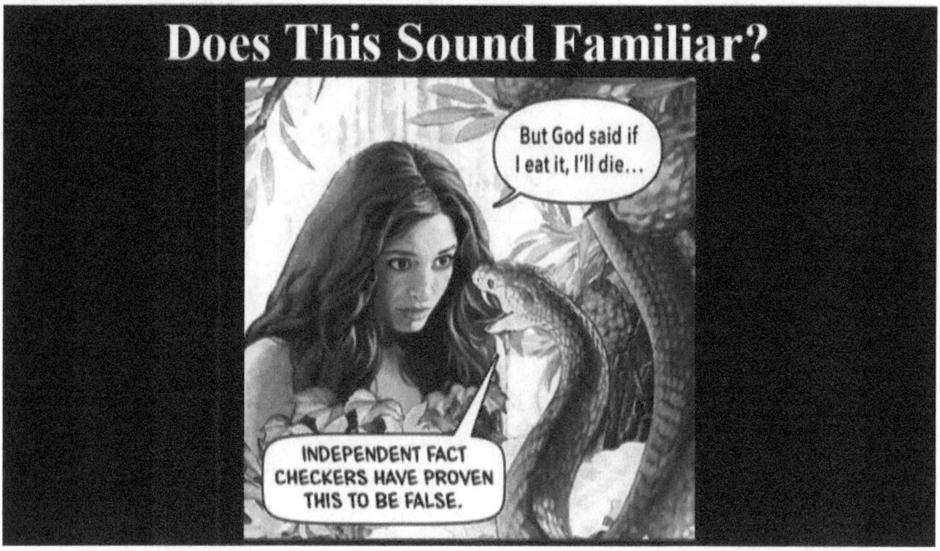

Does This Sound Familiar?
But God said if I eat it, I'll die...
INDEPENDENT FACT CHECKERS HAVE PROVEN THIS TO BE FALSE.

Now I like this one because that's not only what is going on right now, but that is exactly what's going on satanically, with this agenda with these murders. People are being lied to, and it's leading them down the path, as we are going to see. Now if you don't think the church is being brainwashed and being duped by this agenda, remember in the last chapter we dealt with lie, after lie, after lie, until we lost count. As Christians what are we supposed to be about? We're supposed to be about the truth. God's truth, we are supposed to promote the truth, and have nothing to do with anything that would harm somebody, let alone kill somebody. We would never promote that. Are we supposed to be on the side of abortion that kills and murders children? Then why would we be on the side of something that is not only full of lies, but also hurt people?

Watch what is going on with the church and you tell me if the churches are not unfortunately caving in. You would think that we would be the ones rising up in mass and speaking out, since we are the truth tellers. Watch what's going on with this.

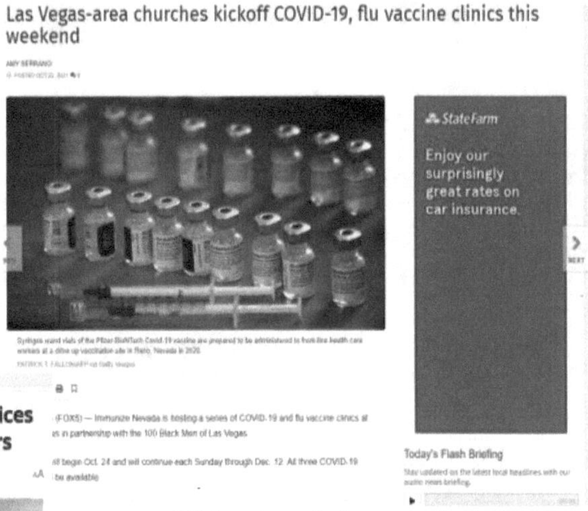
Las Vegas-area churches kickoff COVID-19, flu vaccine clinics this weekend
State Farm
Enjoy our surprisingly great rates on car insurance.
Today's Flash Briefing

So now you can go to these churches that want you to get the shot. Really? Have you done your homework? What are you promoting? And it gets even worse.

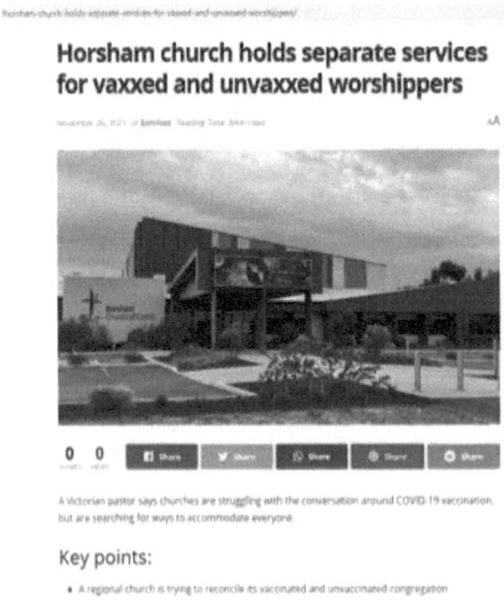

This church is even holding separate services for vaccinated and unvaccinated worshipers. Is that Biblical? Are you supposed to divide the body of Christ like that? But they are doing it and you know why? Because they are scared. They listen to the media. Last time I checked God is the one in control. Last time I checked; I don't care what is going on. "Oh, we need to social distance," Jesus touched lepers. Get back to the Bible. This is the Church not the world. Oh, it gets even worse than that.

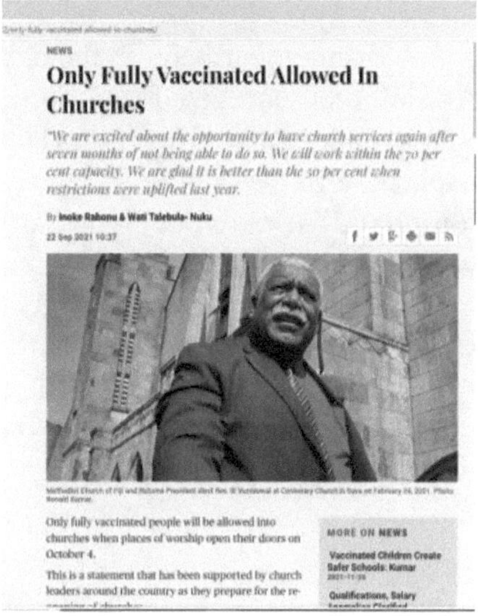
NEWS

Only Fully Vaccinated Allowed In Churches

"We are excited about the opportunity to have church services again after seven months of not being able to do so. We will work within the 70 per cent capacity. We are glad it is better than the 50 per cent when restrictions were uplifted last year.

By Inoke Rabonu & Wati Talebula- Nuku

22 Sep 2021 10:37

Only fully vaccinated people will be allowed into churches when places of worship open their doors on October 4.

This is a statement that has been supported by church leaders around the country as they prepare for the re-

MORE ON NEWS

Vaccinated Children Create Safer Schools: Kumar

Qualifications, Salary

Now in some churches, only the fully vaccinated people are allowed. Now they are starting to preach a different gospel. I like that photo. You might as well rip off the cross and put a syringe up there. A different gospel.

Now look at this. This is what is going on in America. Not just the world. This is what is going on with our fellow brothers and sisters in Christ, who are being brainwashed by the media, not reading their Bible apparently, and they are going along with the narrative. And I quote from

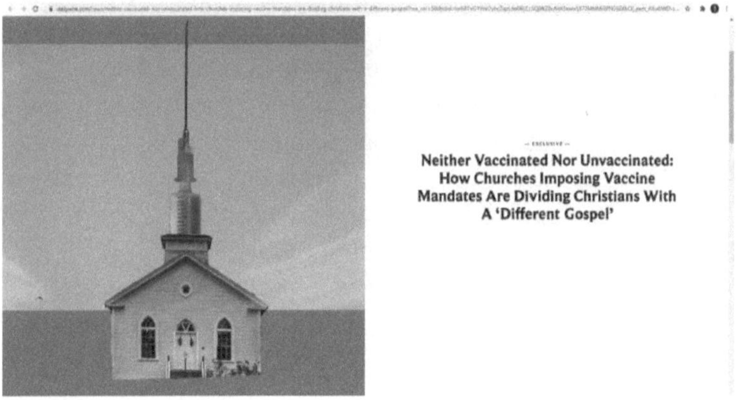

the article above, *"New York City's Redeemers Presbyterian, Tim Keller, so-called theologically conservative church, supposedly firmly embedded in the mainstream of American Evangelicalism, quietly posted a statement on their site about their service attendance. 'Individuals that are fully vaccinated are welcomed to sit on the main floor of the sanctuary without social distancing and masks will be optional. Individuals that are not fully vaccinated are welcome to sit in the balcony. This church's congregation is effectively segregated based on vaccine status.'"*

Remember back in the day when our country was really racist? And we had segregated seats, and restaurants and water fountains? That was wrong, that was horrible. This isn't happening in the world; this is happening in the church. If racism was wrong back then, vaxism is wrong for today. They are not alone. Anyone over the age of 12 years old that wants to attend the Episcopal Church in Rockland, Maine or St Luke in the Fields, in New York or Grace Cathedral in San Francisco, will have to show vaccine passports. And anyone looking for fellowship with the Atlanta Greater Piney Grove Baptist Church, not prepared to provide proof of vaccination, will be asked to provide a doctor's note, explaining why they can't get the shot. They also need to reserve a place in the sanctuary online and sign a waiver."

And the crazy thing that we saw last time, where did this whole thing come from? If you don't have your head in the sand, shut the TV off, "Hey, it's Saturday" open the Bible. This thing is full of what? Lies, so what in the world are Christians doing promoting something that is a whole pack of lies? And certainly, what we are going to see is the outcome? Now, again, how much more proof do we need to know that this is not just a lie, not just a pandemic, but a plandemic? And we have exposed several different obvious things that show that this really did happen. It was pre-planned. By the World Economic Forum, Bill Gates and the Rockefeller Foundation, and things of that nature, prior to it being released. But let me give you more proof. Here is another piece that has come out that this thing has been pre-planned. We are being lied to. Take a look at this clip.

OAN News reports: *"Newly uncovered video shows that Anthony Fauci and other HHS Officials discussing how a new virus from China could be used to enforce universal vaccinations back in October of 2019. Here's One America's Pearson Sharp."*

Pearson Sharp: *"As many of us have long suspected this pandemic and all the resulting chaos was never about finding a new virus and protecting public safety, this entire exercise has been a government sanctioned effort to strip Americans from their rights and force us to follow their orders without question or else. You are not allowed to question or raise any objections, or the full weight of the Federal Government will come down on you, no exceptions."*

We are supposedly, to be in the midst of the worst pandemic in the history of the world. Hospitals are overflowing with sick and dying patients, yet at the same time, we can afford to fire hundreds of thousands of health care workers who refuse to take the experimental vaccine. Imagine that. And all to fight the most dangerous virus humanity has ever faced. But you only have a 99.99997 percent chance of surviving. It's so deadly that when you are diagnosed, doctors just tell you to go home and take Dayquil, until it goes away.

Clearly, something is not adding up, and many now believe it's because this entire situation, may have been contrived, from the very start. Footage has just been uncovered from a panel at the Milken Institute, where the high profits of pharma, the good doctor and dog murderer, Anthony Fauci, was discussing viruses with other officials at the Department of Health and Inhuman Services. In the video Fauci complained that releasing a vaccine in the proper way, takes way too long, at least ten years, and how unfortunate it is that people don't take the regular flu seriously.

The other officials agree and suggest blowing the system up and finding a new way to impose a universal flu vaccine. They noted that people would be reluctant to take that kind of vaccine, when it hasn't been tried or tested. That's what another doctor, Rick Bright, also a member of the Rockefeller Foundation, proposed that they should disrupt the bureaucratic process somehow, and cut through all the red tape using what he called an entity of excitement. And then, Bright tops it all by suggesting, 'You know it's not crazy to think that there may be an outbreak of a novel Indian flu virus from China, and they could then use that to make a global mRNA vaccine to be tested out on the public'. And the best part of all, this happened in October of 2019. Watch it here for yourself."

Rick Bright: *"Why don't we blow this system up? I know obviously we can't just turn off the spigot on the system we have and then say everyone in the world should get this new vaccine that we haven't given to anyone yet. But there must be some way that we grow vaccines mostly in eggs, like we did in 1947."*

Fauci: *"In order to make the transition, from getting out from the tried-and-true, egg growing which we know gives us results that can be beneficial, we've done well with that, to something that has to be much better. You have to prove that this works and then you have to go through all of the clinical trials. Phase one, phase two, phase three, and then show that this particular product is going to be good over a period of years. That alone if it works perfectly is going to take a decade."*

Rick Bright: *"There might be a need or even an urgent call or an entity of excitement out there that is completely disruptive and not beholding to bureaucratic extremes and processes."*

Fauci: *"So we really do have a problem of how the world perceives, influenza is going to be very difficult to change, that unless you do it from within, and say I don't care what your perception is, we are going to address the problem, in a disruptive way and an innovative way. You need both."*

Rick Bright: *"It is not too crazy to think that an outbreak anomaly virus could occur in China somewhere. We could get the RNA sequence from that, beam it to a number of regional centers, if not local, if not even in your home at some point, and print those vaccines on the patch to self-administer."*

Pearson Sharp: *"It's hard to misinterpret what's being said here. They are essentially describing the pandemic. Everything we have seen in the* *last year and a half has been described right here in this video before it happened. This isn't the first time that Fauci has gone on the record to apparently broadcast his intentions about the pandemic. Back when President Trump first took office, Fauci came out with a suspicious prediction. That a major viral pandemic will strike the United States during Trump's administration."*

Fauci: *"The topic today is the issue of pandemic preparedness and if there is one message I want to leave with you today, based on my experience, and you will see that in a moment, is that there is no question that there will be a challenge with the coming administration in the arena of infectious diseases, both chronic infectious diseases and the sense of already ongoing diseases of which we have a large burden of that. But also, there will be a surprise outbreak."*

Pearson Sharp: *"And now, here we are today, living through the scenario that Fauci said was coming all the way back in 2017. The government has used this pandemic to enact sweeping, totalitarian changes to our everyday lives, seeking control faster than anyone thought possible. Never in the history of the world has the government taken power and then given it back voluntarily.*

So, while China gains strength, Taliban terrorists take over countries, our border collapses amid millions of third world illegal opportunists, inflation skyrockets, the supply chain dries up, we are being threatened with even more restrictions of our rights if we don't comply with the tyrannical vaccine mandates. Unless we the people, demand that our rights be preserved, and our civil liberties be protected, and our government be held responsible for its treachery, then this rogue administration will never stop encroaching on our freedoms."

So, in other words, we need to wake up, we need to get equipped, and as this is going on, it's real, get your head out of the sand. In an interview I had with a gentleman last week I said in my opinion, we are in WWIII. Our country has been invaded by outside sources. A lot of people are saying this is a bioweapon being done for a multitude of purposes.

Nobody wants to hear the news, but guess what? We've got to deal with it. We have to speak up and Lord willing that is what we are going to be doing in our next chapter. What do we do about this, as Christians? But we are doing our part, we are getting ourselves equipped, and we are also providing this information to try and share with as many as we can. But it's obvious, when you look at the facts, did this just happen by chance or just one of those unfortunate experiences? No. It's a plandemic. And that's not just a cutesy thing to say. When you deal with the facts that's exactly what is going on, it's a plandemic.

So, my question is, what is your ultimate goal? I think we've established it's a joke, it was preplanned, certainly a bail-out for big pharma, it's all full of lies. But what is your ultimate goal with all this media hype, all these lies, with all the fear mongering, all the misinformation, the intimidation? Well, believe it or not, their goal is global. We have heard Bill Gates say this on tape. This is a global plan. And the global plan is that he wants to vaccinate 7 billion people on the planet with this particular vaccine. 7 billion. That's the bulk of the planet, the goal of the vaccines. Crazy, but that is what they are really shooting for. But why would they want to vaccinate 7 billion people? Well, again they are using fear, this Covid generated fear. And again, I'm not saying it's not real, it is real. I'm not saying people haven't died, they have died, but I think it was preplanned.

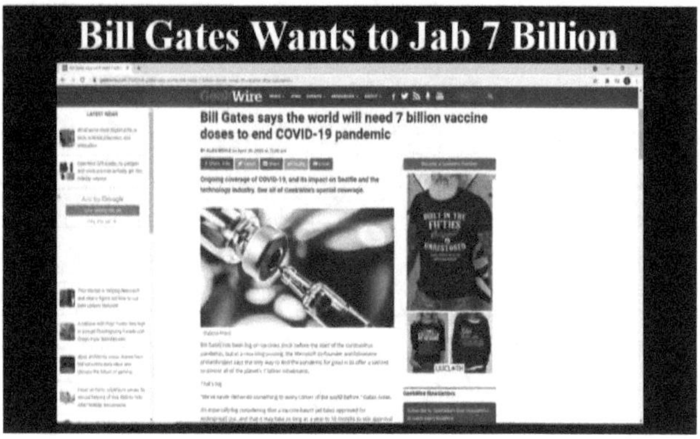

I think there is another agenda. Covid was just the first step to get people to take the jab, which was leading towards their ultimate goal. As we have seen before, it was released to make Trump look bad, it was an excuse to bring in mail-in ballots to steal the election, it was designed to begin to dismantle our country and the economies around the world, which they are still doing to usher in the Great Reset, The World Economic Forum, Klaus Schwab and the gang, which the Bible alone tells us what that is. The rise of the antichrist kingdom, the New World Order, you don't want to have anything to do with that. Yes, it was used as a bailout for big pharma that was going bankrupt by the billions. Then as we saw in the last chapter, it's reducing people. The more you give these shots, if you survive, it completely destroys your immune system which you have to go back endlessly for booster shots, which means you are a constant customer, which means you never stop the money supply. But what we are going to see is that they want to murder the bulk of the planet. And we are going to prove that with all kinds of things. But are you serious? Are these shots really that deadly? We are going to review what Dr. Zelenko, who treated Trump and others, worldwide famed noted Doctor, not some quack. He told us what is coming with these shots.

Dr. Zelenko: "*So, I will just summarize it. There is no need for this vaccine, the protection is of no need to anyone. And I will explain. Children I have already told you; they have a 99.9998 percent of getting better. Young adults from 18 to 45 have a 99.95 percent of getting better. This is according to the CDC. Same concept. Somebody that has already had Covid and has antibodies, naturally induced immunity, is a billion times more effective than artificially induced immunity through vaccines. So, why would I vaccinate someone with a poison death shot that makes inferior or dangerous antibodies, when I already have healthy antibodies?*

And then if you look at the high-risk population that has a 7.5 percent death rate, so my data was the first one in the world that I published in a Peer Reviewed Journal that has become the basis of over 200 other studies and I have corroborated my observations that if you treat people in the right timeframe, you reduce the death rate by 85 percent. So, out of 600,000 Americans we could have prevented 510,000 from going to the hospital and dying. And by the way, I presented this information to Bibi Netanyahu, directly into his hands in April of 2020 and I informed every single member of your ministry of health as well. So, my question to you is, if I can reduce the death rate of 7.5 percent to less than half of a percent, why would I use a poison death shot that doesn't work and has tremendous horrific side effects?

If everyone on the planet were to get Covid and not get treated, the death rate globally will be less than half a percent. I'm not advocating for that. There are a lot, 35 million people would die, however, if you follow the advice of some of the 'global leaders' like Bill Gates said last year, 7 billion people need to be vaccinated, the death rate will be over 2 billion people. So, wake up! This is WWIII, this is a level of malfeasance and malevolence that we have not seen, probably in the history of humanity. There is zero justification for using this poison death shot unless you want to sacrifice human beings."

Certainly, since the time of Hitler. But he wasn't the only one. Mao Tse-tung, Stalin, way more, it's happening. And he's not the only

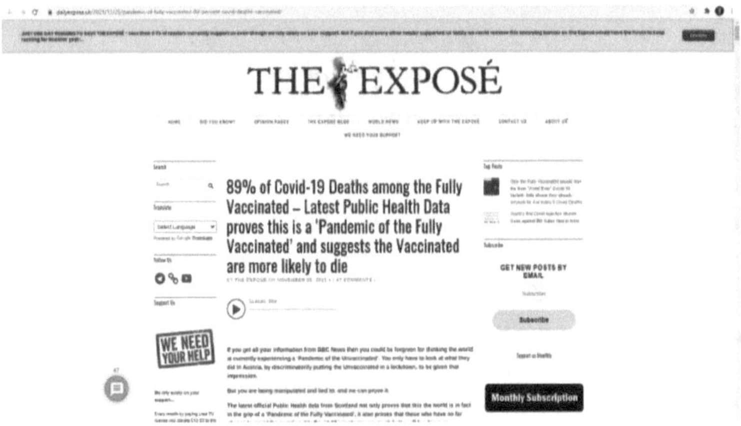
THE EXPOSÉ
89% of Covid-19 Deaths among the Fully Vaccinated – Latest Public Health Data proves this is a 'Pandemic of the Fully Vaccinated' and suggests the Vaccinated are more likely to die
WE NEED YOUR HELP
GET NEW POSTS BY EMAIL
Subscribe
Monthly Subscription

doctor saying what's coming with these jabs. All kinds of secular doctors are coming out and saying this is mass genocide.

89 percent of Cov-19 deaths are among the who? The fully vaccinated. Those are the ones who are really dying here. It's a pandemic of the fully vaccinated. A cancer expert in the UK is seeing a spike in non-covid deaths. Nobody is willing to call out the vaccine elephant in the room.

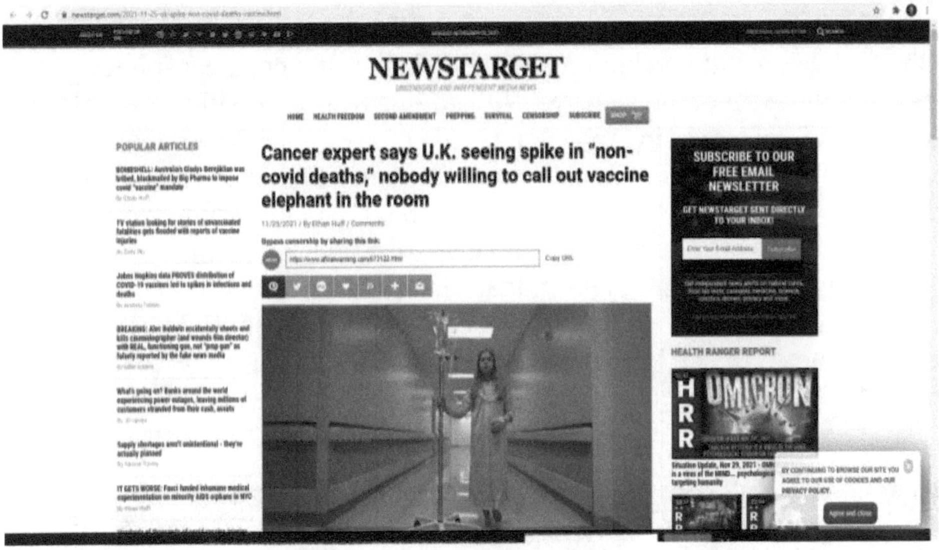

Remember what we saw, that even if you survive, it destroys your immune system, especially the more you get, now you are susceptible to anything. And if you already had a predisposition to cancer, you're going to get it like a firestorm. If you had a predisposition to something else, that is what people are dying of. This is a doctor saying this. And they are secular people. You can't say it's some Christian Conspiracy Theory, blame it on the devil. The stillbirth rate is going through the roof.

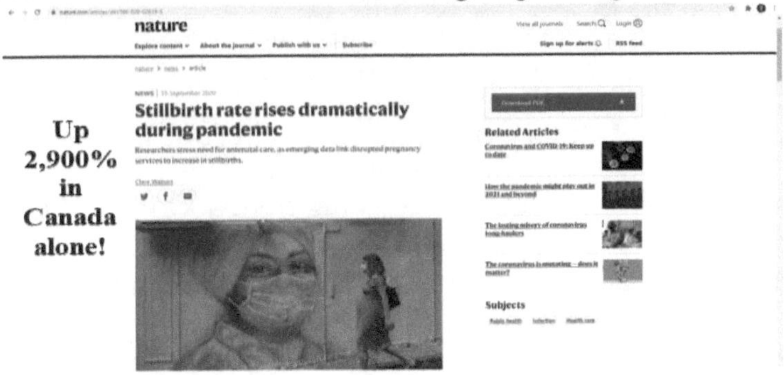

As for you and I, are we supposed to support abortion, as Christians? Did you know that, just in Canada, alone, the stillbirth rate has gone up 2,900 percent? That's just in Canada. I just got that yesterday.

2,900 percent and yet you have churches that say come here and get the jab. And this is killing children. That's verified. It's not a conspiracy. And this is still the tip of the iceberg. With all due respect, I will be just a little bit blunt, if you are going to a church that refuses to deal with the truth, and you are a Christian, you better run for your life. I'm not a doctor, I don't play one on TV and this is not a hospital. I'm just saying you better do your homework. As a born-again Christian you should never be a part something that is promoting lies, that can easily be demonstrated and certainly harming and killing people, especially children. But here's another one. A doctor says study posted in AHA Journal is proof the mRNA jabs are murder.

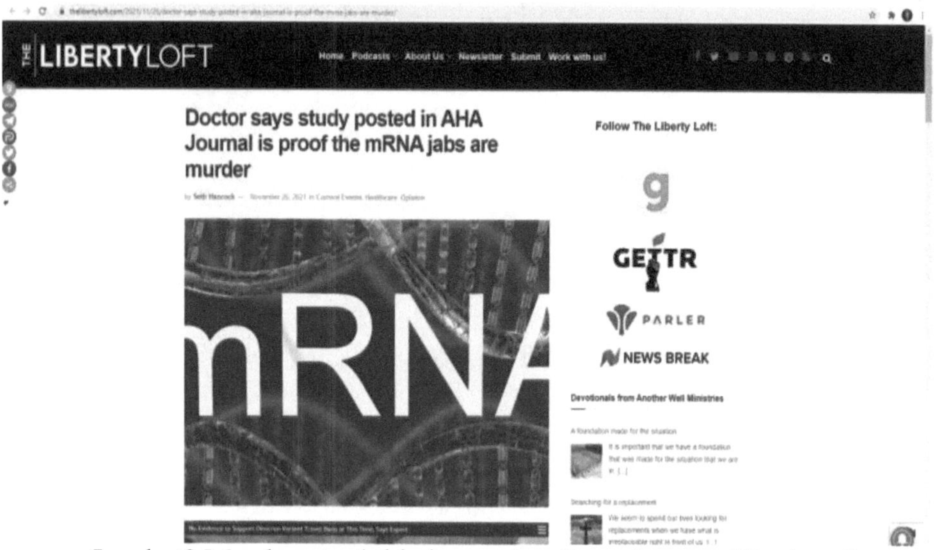

Is what? Murder. And this is coming from doctors. Not just Joe Shmoe dot com. MIT Scientist and Professor on Exposing Covid-19 vaccine injuries "You have to be careful because you could be eliminated."

They want to eliminate you. That's the agenda.

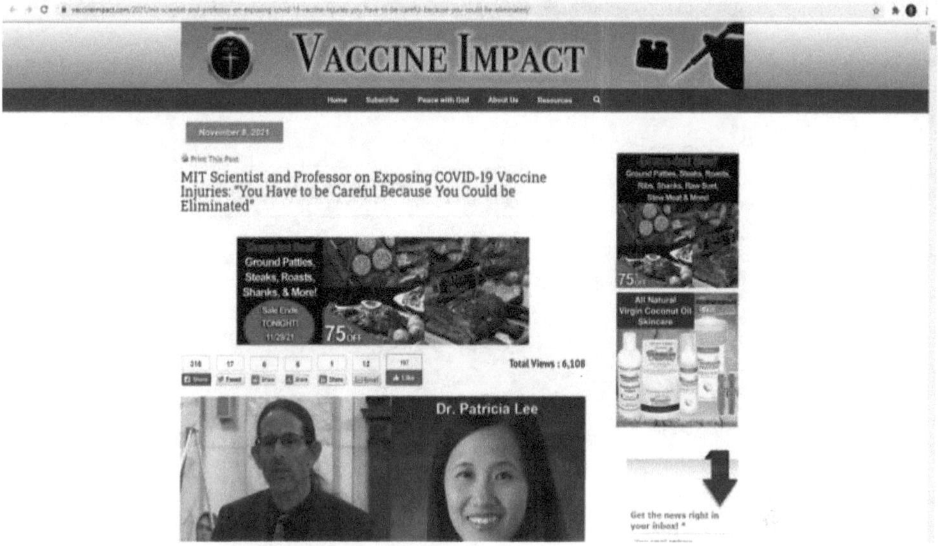

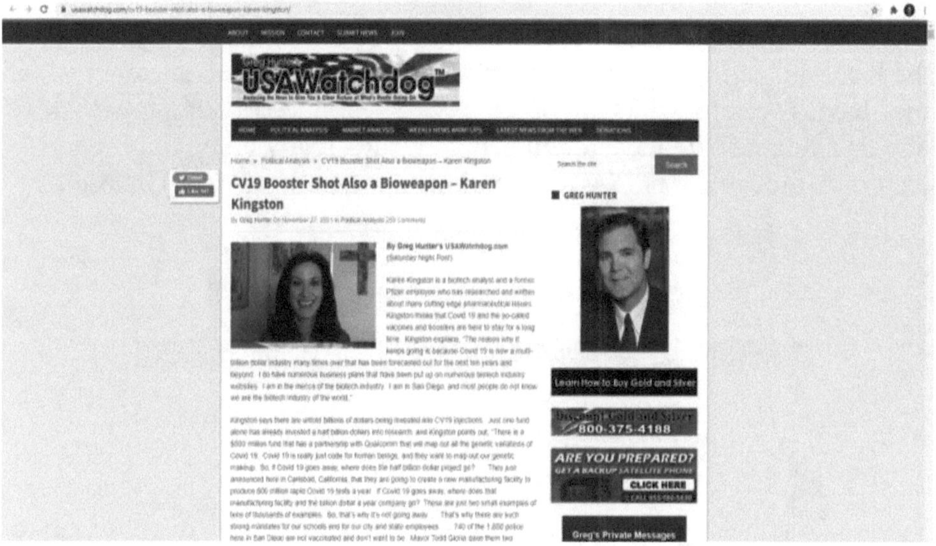

The CV19 booster shot is a bioweapon. It's designed to kill people. Another doctor says the CV19 injections will cause massive deaths.

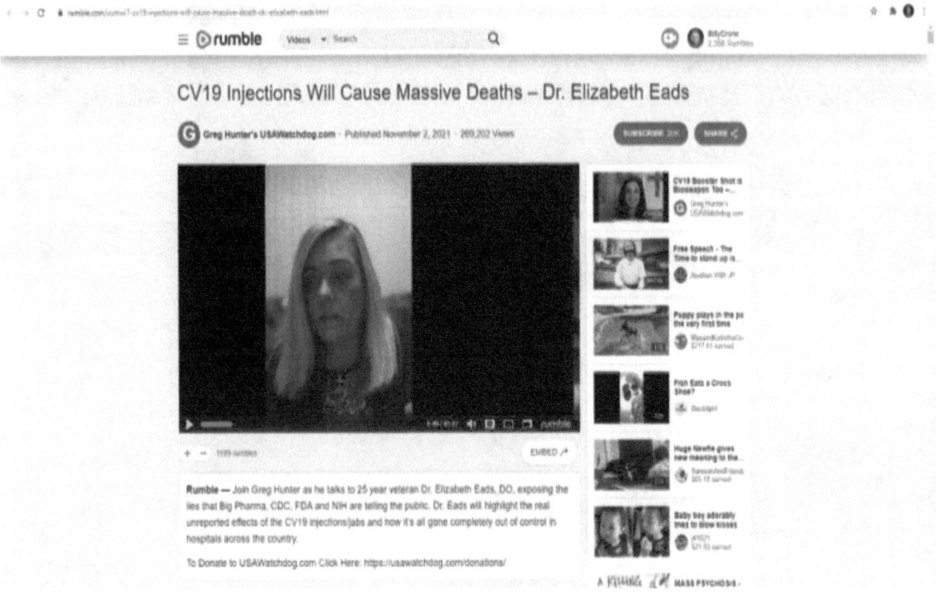

Is anybody seeing a pattern? These are doctors, that haven't drunk the Kool-aid and are coming out, and by their own Hippocratic oath which they have sworn to, which all doctors have sworn to, are saying we can't do this anymore. We have to tell people what's really going on, even in their own industry. And it is so apparent now that this is mass murder.

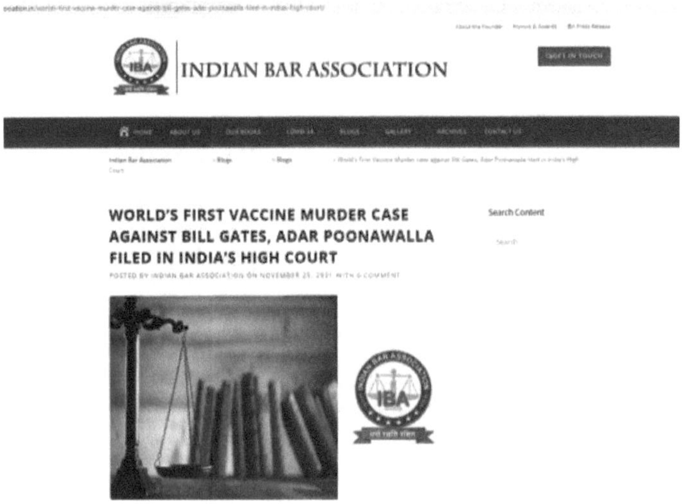
INDIAN BAR ASSOCIATION
WORLD'S FIRST VACCINE MURDER CASE AGAINST BILL GATES, ADAR POONAWALLA FILED IN INDIA'S HIGH COURT
Search Content
IBA

The world's first vaccine murder case against Bill Gates filed in India's high court. I believe that is November 25th. It just happened. They are suing him because it is so apparent that this is mass murder. In India, as we saw in the last chapter, was the country that said, excuse me we are going to pass out Ivermectin. And what happened to it? It went away. And they are cramming vaccines down the worlds throat and these guys say, "Oh yeah, you're killing people, we're taking you to court, we're suing you, Bill Gates." This is what's going on.

Now Omicron is coming to get you! Look over there. All this is going on to keep us scared. My point is, this is sick, this is gross, this is what is really going on. These people have an agenda. They want to depopulate, call it whatever you want, they want to murder the bulk of the planet. So, my question is, where in the world did they get that idea from? Well, let's go back to the Bible. God tells us, shocker, exactly in a text we saw last time. Let's remind ourselves where all of this is coming from. It's a spiritual battle. Where are these guys getting this idea? "Let's go murder some people." I wonder who came up with that thought.

John 8:42-45 Jesus said to them, "If God were your Father, you would love me, for I came from God and now am here. I have not come on my own, but He sent me. Why is my language not clear to you? Because you are unable to hear what I say, you belong to your father, the devil, and you want to carry out your father's desire. He was a murderer from the beginning, not holding to the truth, for there is no truth in him. When he lies, he speaks his native language, for he is a liar and the father of lies. Yet because I tell the truth, you do not believe me!"

What is the desire, ultimately of satan? He hates mankind. We are created in the image of God; he wants to kill us. I didn't say that Jesus did. And of course, in the context, if you keep reading, the Jewish people, when Jesus declared himself to be God, what did they want to do? He knew it was coming. They wanted to kill him. He called them on the carpet. Now why did Jesus say that satan is not only a liar and the father of all lies? Again, where are all the lies coming from with the pandemic? Who's inspiring it? I might not have been there, you might not have been there, but it's some sort of demonic input, that is where all this stuff is coming from. There is an agenda. What was the second one? Murder. Where does this idea of murdering people come from? It's satanic. It's some sort of demonic, satanic influence.

But what does Jesus say in the beginning? He's a murderer and has been one from the beginning. **Genesis Chapter 3** is our next text. This is what he was referring to. The very first murder in the beginning was in the Garden of Eden which was led by satan. Let's see why Jesus said he has been one from the very beginning.

Genesis 3:1-5 "Now the serpent was craftier than any of the wild animals the Lord God had made. He said to the woman, "Did God really say, 'You must not eat from any tree in the garden?' The woman said to the serpent, 'We may eat fruit from the trees in the garden, but God did say, 'You must not eat fruit from the tree that is in the middle of the garden, and you must not touch it, or you will die.' 'You will not surely die,' the serpent said to the woman. For God know that when you eat of it your eyes will be opened and you will be like God, knowing good and evil.'"

What did he do first? Caused doubt. Here are the facts, but did he say that really? God said you can have everything that you want but with the one tree, keep your hands off it. And He told them in advance, if you do it you will die. So, what did satan do next? He called God a liar. But why did he cause doubt and then lie? Because he had a goal in mind, to kill them. Unfortunately, Eve listened to satan, disobeyed God, gave some to her husband, and what happened? They died right there on the spot. No, they didn't die on the spot, but did they die?

Yes, death entered the world through one man, Adam, when he listened to satan. That's why Jesus said he had been a murderer from the beginning. He's a liar, he's the father of all lies. He didn't just want to mess up Adam and Eve's relationship with God, he doesn't just want to mess up our relationship with God, ultimately, he wants to kill you. He hates us. He hates mankind. And he knew it wasn't going to happen right then, but he knew it would happen, because God is not a liar. God said, you do it and you are going to die. So, satan is a murderer.

But notice, here's my point, in the Genesis account, when it all started, that explains why he is a murderer from the beginning. But notice what kind of a death it was. It was a satanic delayed death. It didn't come right away, but it came sure enough, after a while. Now, believe it or not, this is exactly what Dr. Zelenko and other secular doctors are saying. It's coming. And basically, what they are saying is, we ain't seen nothing yet! The true death fall-out, is going to be a delayed death. And that's part of the illusion. You think you are okay; you think you're fine, but oh no, the big goal is coming. The decimation of the planet.

And again, he gave us the phases of what happens when people get these shots. He said the first phase was the acute phase, and people can die within just a matter of hours or a couple days. Well, there is a second phase, he said, that happens is the subacute phase, and there are people that will die a couple months later, after getting the shot. The third phase, if you recall, he said, was the long-term phase, and that is a couple years down the road, is when you die. The first two phases are well under way. Including kids, that they are now just starting to vaccinate, and they are dropping like flies.

This is mass murder, and as one guy says, even if the kids can survive with the side effects, this is child abuse. Do we support child abuse? Do we support murder? What in the world are we doing lining them up to get the shot? Do your homework, get your head out of the sand and you better run for your lives from those places. Look at this clip, people are dropping like flies.

News from various TV stations:

"A high school senior is in the hospital after collapsing on the tennis courts."

"We're bringing you the details of the death of a high school soccer player."

"Finland Denmark's star man, Christian Erickson collapsed towards the end of the first half."

"The Kennedy Heights Community is mourning tonight after one of their high school football players died."

"A South Carolina high school football player died during football practice."

"Star college basketball player collapsing on the court. I have to warn you the video may be difficult to watch."

"Florida Gators star Keyontae Johnson collapsing during the game."

"A West Catholic high school student has died after a collapsing during a scrimmage."

"On mile eight she suddenly felt fuzzy and blacked out."

"Seventeen-year-old Ryan Jacobs heart stopped."

"Unexpectedly he suddenly collapsed on the field."

"Megan went into cardiac arrest."

"Collapsing after Friday night's football game."

"Florida high school football player dies after collapsing during practice. The football player, a student at Citrus High School in Inverness, about 75 miles north of Tampa, Florida, the principal said."

BBC News: *"Josh Downie: Cricketer, 24 dies after heart attack at practice. A mother has paid tribute to her 'beautiful' 24-year-old son who died after suffering a heart attack while playing cricket."*

Hvg.hu News: *"An 18-year-old Hungarian football player collapsed on the field and died. Viktor Marcell of Violin became ill during the training of Andrashida."*

Newsy Today: *"He collapsed in the middle of the game. The young Flemish player collapsed at the end of the first half, he owes his salvation to the efficiency of the various actors present on the lawn and to the rapid intervention of the emergency services."*

"Footballer collapsed in match. In Eltendorf on Sunday a player collapsed during the football game Eltendorf against Gerersdorf-Sulz. The 18-year-old was flown to the hospital by emergency helicopter."

Pennlive: *"Pa. boy, 12, collapses, dies at middle school basketball practice. The Latest: Cause of death in on Pa. boy 12, who died at basketball practice. 'We never expected anything like this.'"*

Newswep: *"Jens (27) collapses on the football field and dies."*

Golf Digest: *"Latinoamerica tour suffers another tragic loss after caddie collapses and dies."*

Fanreport.com: *"Player collapses in lower house game. Dramatic scenes played out on the weekend in 2nd class Triestingtal in Lower Austria during the match between SC Berndorf and ASV Baden. In the eighth minute of the game, an ASV Baden player suddenly collapsed on the field and had to be reanimated and stabilized. An emergency doctor's helicopter was requested because there was a suspicion of heart failure, the SC Berndorf described on Facebook page."*

Mittelhessen News: *"C-league: Player collapses, game in Flammersbach ends. Football C-League Dillenburg: Weidelbach celebrated his first* *victory in Group 1, and a player from Hirzenhain lost consciousness in Group 2."*

Augsburger Allgemeine: *"Aborted game after collapse. The game between Emersacker and Pfersee is canceled after the collapse of the assistant referee. TSV Dinkelscherben takes over the top of the table."*

Sportbuzzer: *"After a collapse on the pitch: 17-year-old soccer player on the mend. After the drama about a 17-year-old soccer player who lived in Hann. Munden had collapsed on the square and had to be reanimated, there is a cautious all-clear. The player should be doing well according to the circumstances. His first question didn't just surprise the coach."*

Spox News: *"Danish second division player Wessam Abou Ali collapses on the pitch – the game is abandoned."*

Developing Now: *"The reason he collapsed is unknown."*

RTL Boulevard: *"Kjeld Nuis very sick after vaccination: 'The body is not cooperating.'"*

Team Tucker Carlson: *"24-year-old Hockey player dies after collapsing on ice in cardiac arrest – 80% of league is vaccinated. Last Friday, Boris Sadecky collapsed in the middle of the ice during the match in Dombim. Even after days of intensive treatment, Sadecky passed away."*

The Covid World: *"Pedro Obiang: 29-year-old Professional Footballer Suffers Myocarditis After Covid-19 Vaccines, Possible End of Career."*

"You might be wondering how someone in such great shape could suffer cardiac arrest."

"It's a rare thing that happens."

Kendte News: *"Got two heart attacks in a few hours. Died only 37 years old. Only 37 years old, the former French professional footballer Franck Berrier has died."*

"A player suffered a double cardiac arrest! Atletico Goianiense confirmed through its official channels that the youthful Felipe de Jesus Moreira suffered a double cardiac arrest. His condition is serious, and he may lose his life."

Independent News: *"Emil Palsson: Footballer collapses from cardiac arrest during game in Norway. Emil Palsson's on-field cardiac arrest is the second such incident this year."*

Free Press: *"Madhya Pradesh: Teen player's death due to cardiac arrest triggers concern. Doctors warn of change in lifestyle, stress. The sudden death of 17-year-old Shruti Soni, an athlete from Betul due to a cardiac arrest on Thursday has raised concern."*

People Magazine: *"Grand Slam Champion Murphy Jensen Recovering after Suffering Sudden Cardiac Arrest While Playing Tennis."*

Indy Star: *"The story of LaPorte football's Jake West who died of sudden cardiac arrest. Jack West sings in a video with friends. He died shortly after at the age of 17 after suffering sudden cardiac arrest at a LaPorte football practice."*

"Barcelona star Sergio Aguero admitted to hospital for 'cardiac exam' after chest pain during match."

"3 high school athletes died of sudden cardiac arrest. Their moms are fighting back."

Mirror News: *"FA Youth Cup match abandoned as player 'suffers cardiac arrest' on pitch. Three ambulance crews were called after a player collapsed during the game between West Bridgford and Boston United as paramedics rushed to administer life-saving treatment."*

The Hindu: *"Young Saurashtra cricketer Avi Barot dies after suffering cardiac arrest."*

Euro Weekly: *"Runner in Bilbao half-marathon suffered three cardiac arrests. A 53-year-old man who was participating in the Bilbao half-marathon race on Saturday, October 23, died after suffering three cardiac arrests. This was confirmed last Sunday, 24th."*

La Gazette: *"Soccer player goes into cardiac arrest before Saint-James vs Avranches match. Just before the start of the Saint-James game against Avranches, a player suffered cardiac arrest on Sunday October 10. He was rescued by a firefighter who plays for the opposing team."*

LaProvincia: *"Cardiac arrest on the track. The Colverde athlete is still serious, saved by the defibrillator."*

Handball World: *"Sad news from Belgium: 19-year-old player dies surprisingly of cardiac arrest."*

Donauworther Zeitung: *"Referee suffers cardiac arrest: shock for amateur football. The game between Laub and Buchdorf / Daiting must be abandoned after the referee has suffered cardiac arrest. The rescue service reanimated the Altisheimer."*

Father who lost his son to the Covid vaccine: *"I'm from Edinburg, Texas. I'm the father of a 16-year-old son. A single parent. I raised my boy since he was a baby. He meant the world to me. I got the vaccine to protect my son. In March or April, they were saying it was safe for teenagers. Me and my son have never been apart. We are always together. He was my best friend. He always told me it was you and me against the world. At the age of 7 he wanted to play baseball.*

So, I ended up coaching little league baseball for 7 years. He was a heck of a baseball player. Then he was telling me he wanted to join the Air Force. So, I said good, that's good, I would back him in anything that he wanted to do. He joined the ROTC in high school. He was always full of smiles. Anybody who knew my son would see he was happy. I wasn't rich but I gave him everything he wanted. We didn't lack for anything. We used to go fishing, camping, we did everything. He got the covid vaccine because I thought it would protect him. I thought it was the right thing to do. It was like playing Russian roulette. My government lied to me. They said it was safe. Now I go home to an empty house.

When I used to wake him up, I'd give him a hug and a kiss, time to go to school, don't miss school. I'd get home from work he would come running out, he knew when I'd get home. He'd run out and give me a hug. I'd give him a kiss and a hug. What do you want to eat today? He was my baby boy. Everybody knew we were always together. Like I said, next week is his birthday. You know where I am going to celebrate his birthday at. (He holds up a picture of himself standing over his dead son in a casket.)

While everybody, once we leave here, are going to forget about what we are doing, or what we said here, they will be enjoying time with their family and kids. Thanksgiving, I'll be spending time in the cemetery, Christmas in that cemetery. They need to quit pushing this on our children. I lost mine, you need to protect yours. They are trying to target the 5- to 12-year-olds. We are going to have more deaths on our hands, than they planned, and they say it's worth the risk. It wasn't worth the risk to me.

My son meant the world to me. They can never give him back to me. That's all I want is my son back. So, don't make the mistake that I did. I did it because I thought it was the correct thing to do, it wasn't. It was not. I always said I loved the hell out of my country, but I don't trust my government anymore. Everyone of us that are going through this deal, what they did to my son, they knew what was happening. I consider that murder.

Because on December 17th, 2020, they did a study, and they knew it caused heart conditions in a teenager. So, why wasn't this information released until October 1st of this year? If we had of known this, my son would be here with me. So, I figure, like I said, they murdered my son, and the other people that are suffering, these kids with all these side effects, that's child abuse right there. Why isn't something being done? This should be pushed, that we don't let anybody hurt our children. We put our lives in front of our children. Why are they doing this to our kids?

Because these people want to kill off a huge portion of the populace. It's sick, it's satanic, it's twisted, it's evil, and they don't care who it is. Kids or adults. That's what's going on. And you have churches today that are not only saying, come here and get the shot, but if you don't get the shot, you're not welcome here. They will stand accountable to God. But hey, don't worry about these deaths, you might be catching on and all of a sudden, these people are dropping like flies. But hey, it's not the vaccine. If you watch the media, they have the real answers for you. I'm going to catalog some of them. But they are out there saying this stuff. Let's get back on the theme of Dumb and Dumber.

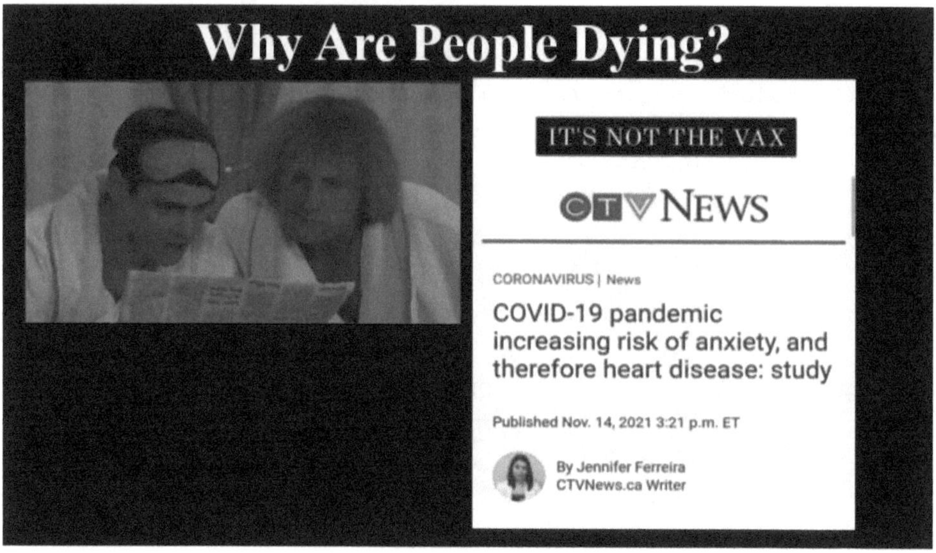
Why Are People Dying?
IT'S NOT THE VAX
CTV NEWS
CORONAVIRUS | News
COVID-19 pandemic increasing risk of anxiety, and therefore heart disease: study
Published Nov. 14, 2021 3:21 p.m. ET
By Jennifer Ferreira
CTVNews.ca Writer

Why are people dying? Covid-19 pandemic increasing risk of anxiety and therefore heart disease. They are just anxious about the pandemic, they just had a heart attack. That's all it is. Not the vaccine, don't look over there. It's the anxiety, it gets worse as you go. No, the mysterious rise in heart attacks from blocked arteries is from not trusting the science hard enough. Somehow apparently you don't trust that science is going to kill you.

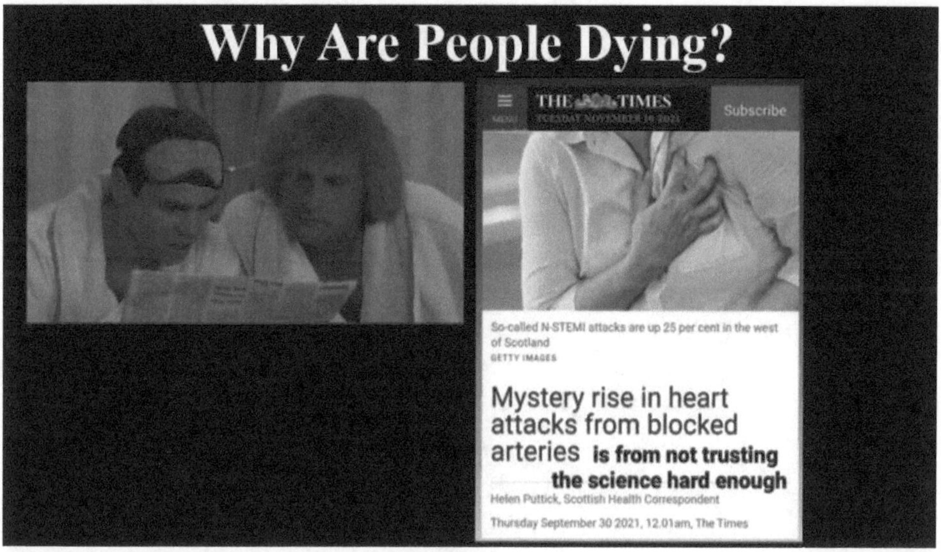

Why Are People Dying?
Subscribe
So-called N-STEMI attacks are up 25 per cent in the west of Scotland
GETTY IMAGES
Mystery rise in heart attacks from blocked arteries is from not trusting the science hard enough
Helen Puttick, Scottish Health Correspondent
Thursday September 30 2021, 12.01am, The Times

Here's one and I kid you not, it's marijuana, cannabis may be linked to the growing number of heart attacks. Those kids are smoking

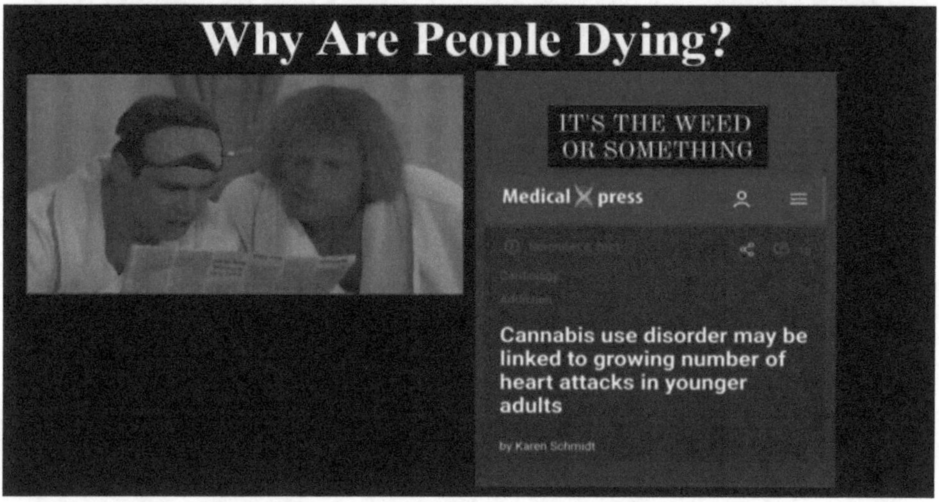

weed man. It's not the vaccine. Shhhh! That is a joke. Oh, by the way, if you don't have something murderous and evil up your sleeve, it has now come out that the FDA needs 55 years to release Pfizer vaccine safety and efficacy data.

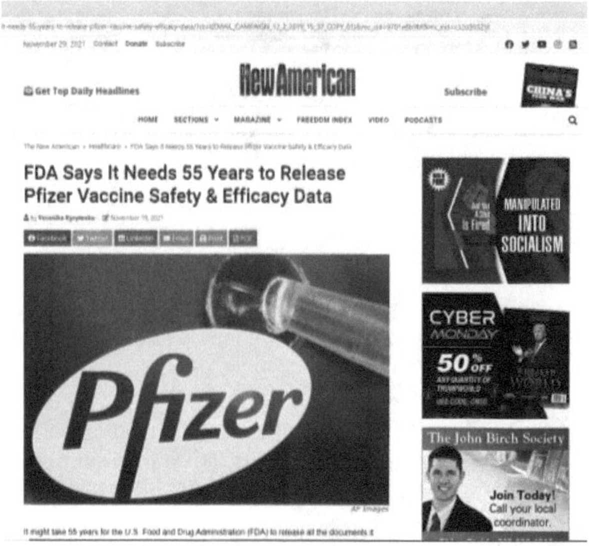
Get Top Daily Headlines
NewAmerican
Subscribe
HOME
SECTIONS
MAGAZINE
FREEDOM INDEX
VIDEO
PODCASTS
FDA Says It Needs 55 Years to Release Pfizer Vaccine Safety & Efficacy Data
Pfizer
MANIPULATED INTO SOCIALISM
CYBER MONDAY
50% OFF
The John Birch Society
Join Today! Call your local coordinator.

55 years before you tell us really what's going on. Do you smell a rat? I like how this lady put it. Common sense analogy here.

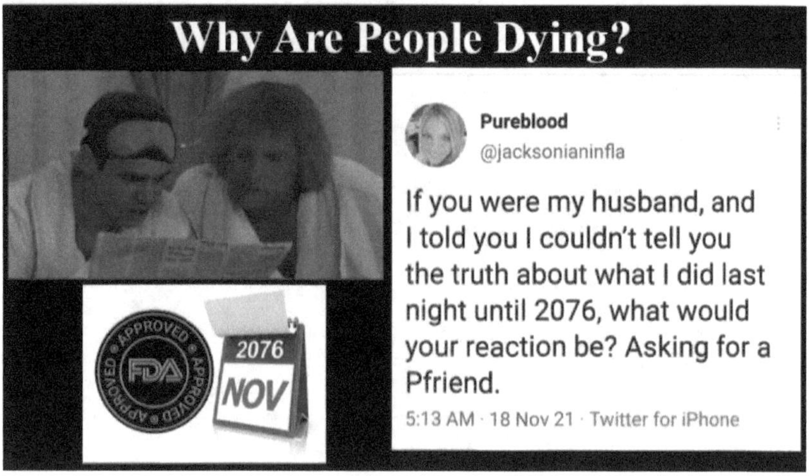
Why Are People Dying?
Pureblood
@jacksonianinfla
If you were my husband, and I told you I couldn't tell you the truth about what I did last night until 2076, what would your reaction be? Asking for a Pfriend.
5:13 AM · 18 Nov 21 · Twitter for iPhone
APPROVED
FDA
2076
NOV

This is exactly what is going on. And not so surprisingly, shocker, the ones who have already demonstrated this, the current administration, they bought into this, "Build Back Better" that's a Great Reset slogan. Biden's all in on this, that's why the media is all in on this. They are all in on this and are out there continually lying to us all to make sure kids, adults, children, they even want to inject the babies now. Get this shot!! But watch these lies from the current administration.

Biden: *"If you're vaccinated, you are not going to be hospitalized, you're not going to be in an ICU unit, and you're not going to die."*

"If you have been fully vaccinated you no longer need to wear a mask. Let me repeat, if you are fully vaccinated you no longer need to wear a mask."

"If you are vaccinated you shouldn't wear a mask but if you aren't vaccinated you should be wearing a mask."

"You're okay, you're not going to get Covid if you have these vaccinations."

"The vaccines are effective against the variants currently circulating the United States."

"Earlier today our medical experts announced a plan for booster shots for every fully vaccinated American. The plan is for every adult to get a booster shot eight months after you got your second shot."

Dr. Rochelle Walensky: *"We can almost see the end. We are vaccinating so very fast. Our data from the CDC today suggests that vaccinated people do not carry the virus and don't get sick."*

"Vaccines work, right now they are working, and they require two doses to be vaccinated to work well. So, I would encourage all Americans to get their first shot and then when you are due get your second shot and then you will be protected against the Delta Variant."

Yahoo! Finance: *"Do you anticipate it getting worse in the winter weather?"*

Bill Gates: *"Yes, the amount you spend indoors and the fact that it is colder, your upper respiratory tract doesn't do a good job compressing the virus."*

Anthony Fauci: *"Really quite impressive, a 94.5 percent efficacy."*

"Certainly, with breakthrough infections, breakthrough infections is when you have been vaccinated but you still get infected."

"When people are vaccinated, they can feel safe that they are not going to get infected whether they are outdoors or indoors."

"That's the bottom line of it. To get people to appreciate you can get vaccinated and you are really quite safe from getting infected."

"Even if you do get a breakthrough infection when you are vaccinated the chances of you transmitting it to someone else is exceedingly low."

"The ability of individuals who are infected through breakthrough infections, namely vaccinated people who ultimately get infected, they are generally without symptoms."

"Minimally symptomatic, however it is clear that they are capable of transmitting the infection to uninfected individuals."

"We are starting to see waning immunity against infection and waning immunity in the beginning aspect against hospitalization and if you look at Israel which has always been a month to a month and a half ahead of us in the dynamics of the outbreak in their vaccine response and in every other element of the outbreak, they are seeing a waning immunity, not only against infection but against hospitalizations and to some extent, death, which is starting to now involve all age groups. It isn't just the elderly."

Bill Gates: *"These vaccines, will allow us to save millions of lives. They will also have another enormous benefit that will allow us to develop a plan for the world to globally eliminate Covid-19."*

Globally eliminate people. Notice, he mentioned this whole thing is a "global plan." These elites have a global plan, he admitted it on tape. Also, they admit it doesn't work, you still can get it, and you can still transmit it, but somehow, it's safe and effective and you better get one. It's our only hope. Anybody buying this? I'm not buying this. In fact, this guy in Australia said out of 8 employees that got the shot, all 8 are either dead or have serious side effects.

Bob Katter: *"I just want to say that we have eight cases in our office. Two, they got the immunization, they died. Two, they got the immunization, and they are crippled for life. Three, have serious problems that will remain with them for the rest of their lives, and one was rushed to ICU, Intensive care almost straight after he got the inoculation. So, don't tell me there's no problem. If one small member of parliament's office has eight in eight weeks there is one huge problem."*

Yeah, it's a huge problem. In fact, if it's so good and safe and effective, then why do you have to chase people down, and force them to get the jab? Or threaten them with their livelihood, their job? If it's so good people would be lining up. Why do you have to resort to that? Why are they doing this? I'm telling you, it's to kill off a massive amount of people. And that kill off is coming in this third phase, that the secular doctors are warning about, that we saw that satan did at the very beginning. A delayed death response. In fact, Bill Gates even said, you're not even going to find the real aspect of this until two years later. Isn't that crazy? If you want to see if a side effect shows up it takes

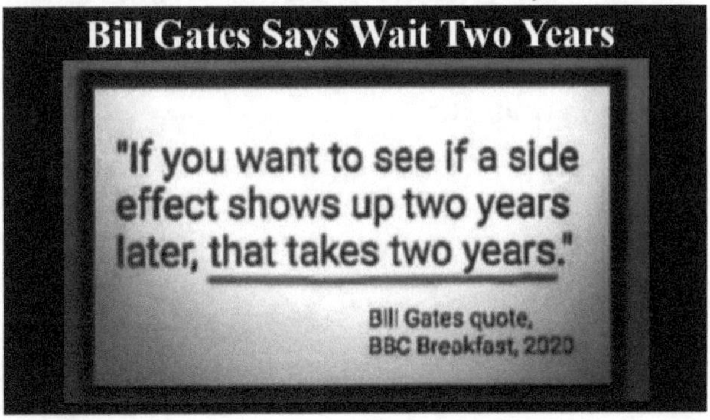
Bill Gates Says Wait Two Years
"If you want to see if a side effect shows up two years later, that takes two years."
Bill Gates quote,
BBC Breakfast, 2020

two years. We're not even going to see the real results until two years. In fact, here he is on tape.

Bill Gates: *"We are doing everything we can, we will write checks for those factories faster than governments can. It should be all the best constructs full speed ahead. Science limited."*

BBC Interviewer: *"So as I understand it, what you are saying, is that there may be need to be some compromise in some of the safety measures, that would normally be expected to create a vaccine because time is so crucial."*

Bill Gates: *"Well of course if you want to wait and see if a side effect shows up two years later, that takes two years, so ahh."*

Ahh! Is right, Bill. So, you admit, that you are cramming this down our throat. You are doing everything you can to just cram this thing through, skip all the regulations, all the normal safety medical procedures, hurry up and get it done, cut those checks as fast as you can. Why? When you admit you're not even going to see the real ultimate effects of this for two years. I'm telling you what it's going to do, this delayed death result. And this is what they are warning us about. Does that sound like a good plan to you? I don't think so either. It's a delayed death result.

And not so surprisingly, guess who's out there pushing people over the edge, like I guess I'd better get it. These guys are getting it. They know what they are doing. Right? Hollywood. Hollywood who is a part of the same camp, the same current administrations agenda, the Great Reset, they are all in on it. They're out there, encouraging people to get this poison death shot. I like what one person said, shouldn't they be held liable for murder? By encouraging people to do this. Look at this clip, this is crazy.

YOU MAY NEVER TRUST ANOTHER CELEBRITY AFTER WATCHING THIS VIDEO!

"Hundreds of thousands died after taking the advice of these celebrities. Should they be tried for murder? Aiding and abetting mass murder through vaccination, all for population control."

Morgan Freeman: *"I'm not a doctor but I trust science, and I'm told that for some reason people trust me. So here I am to say I trust science and I got the vaccine. If you trust me, you will get the vaccine."*

The next clip is of a person having seizures in the car right after getting the jab. The paramedics have been called to find out what is wrong, and she struggles to tell them "I got the vaccine. I can't breathe."

Jimmy Fallon: *"The good news is that these vaccines are being rolled out and you're on the list."*

Ricky Gervais: *"I can't wait to get it. I would fight an old lady. I will be like a deranged junkie; I will grab the needle out of her arm"*

Another clip is of a lady in bed moaning shaking uncontrollably. Someone is sobbing while trying to comfort her, knowing there is nothing he can do. He asks her, "Can you talk to me?" But all she can do is moan.

Another clip shows a man in the hospital on a ventilator. At first, he is laying there peacefully but then he starts shaking and someone comes to hold his arm down.

The Daily Show: *"To keep that variant from taking hold, America needs to vaccinate people as quickly as possible."*

Another clip shows a little boy laying in the arms of his mother as she is wiping his mouth and saying, "Come on baby, breathe, breathe, while his sister is sobbing watching him gasp for breath."

Actor: *"There are still nearly 20 million children around the world who are not getting the routine vaccines they need to be safe. So, please don't wait. Vaccinate yourself. Vaccinate your children."*

Girl on TikTok: *"I've been hiding a lot, not showing what this has done to me, but I'm done hiding, and I'm done being scared. There are several stories like mine. The same doctors who told us it was safe, are the same doctors brushing us off, as if we didn't matter. It is now time that we are heard, seen, and believed."*

During the time of her doing this clip, she showed videos of her in the hospital bed on a ventilator, at home unable to do anything because she was shaking so badly, and how she got out of the hospital bed, hardly able to walk.

Fauci: *"The younger kids are vulnerable. You don't want to put something into younger children until you know it's safe and effective. So, we know we are good to go for the 12 to 15, so now we are going to go 12 to 9, 9 to 6, 6 to 2 years, and 6 months to 2 years."*

Tucker Carlson: *"More people, according to VAERS have died after getting the shot in 4 months during a single vaccination campaign, than from all other vaccines combined for over a decade and a half."*

Elton John: *"More people of society that get vaccinated the more chance there is of eradicating the national Covid pandemic. It's really important to know that all the vaccines have been through and met the necessary safety and quality standards."*

Clip from a video of a lady in her car wearing a mask: *"This is for all of you clowns out there that say that you have to take the shot. Don't take it! I'll tell you why. As a grieving mother, I'm going to tell you why my daughter took that shot yesterday in Las Vegas and she is dead! She took the Pfizer vaccine and she's dead. They couldn't even revive her. I'm begging you people, don't take it! They are killing us!"*

If Hollywood should be held complicit with this, and I'm going to say it again. Of all people who should know better, what about the churches? Telling you to come line up to get this thing. And we are supposed to be the people of the truth. We are supposed to be on the right to life. Not promoters of death. But is that lady, right? Right here in Las Vegas? Are they trying to kill us? Yes, she is. Now, real quick I'm going to give you a history lesson, in case you feel this is just a conspiracy theory. These people don't really want to annihilate the planet. They are and the phrase that is out there is "population control." How many have heard of that? It's been out there for a long time. For decades. We have been brainwashed to think that the planet is overpopulated. It's not! Here is an easy acid test. This year I am breaking the record.

Believe it or not, if I am still alive next week, I will have made 50 flights in one year. It's crazy, I've been flying all over the place. I'm not saying it to boast but guess what? I had it drilled in my head, I always get a window seat. And you know what I do every time? I look out the window. I look out the window and there's nothing but open land everywhere. Are you kidding me? We are not overpopulated! So, why do they brainwash you with the media, showing you Beijing, China? Of course, it's populated! Go outside the city, another city. There's plenty of room. It's all a lie, to condition us to go along with this.

These people are putting into place, with this Covid-19 agenda, they really want to depopulate, 90 to 95 percent of the planet. Now if you want to do more homework, watch our study on Satanism, and The Rise of Devil Worship. In the history section, we traced the trail. The idea of a New Age of Aquarius came from early satanists. And they believe that we need to build our own peace on earth, our own millennial kingdom. We need to follow a One World Leader, they say, and we need to annihilate most of the planet and those they decide that get to live, get to serve them. Isn't that a wonderful utopia? Isn't that a great plan? This is where they are getting it.

We traced the trail. Satanism, it's coming in, mixed with New Age. It's the same root. It's all coming from satan. This is why no matter what we do, or what we say, or how we speak up against it, wars, feminism, birth control, homosexuality, abortion, forced sterilization, are allowed to continue on a global basis. Why? Because they all have one thing in common. They reduce the population. Put it all together. There is an agenda behind the agenda, behind the scenes. That is their goal. In fact, I just checked it out, abortion, murdering children, has killed more than 1.63 billion people since 1980. They want to literally annihilate the bulk of the planet, with this Satanic lie that they have bought into. Of course, it's not them and their families. It's everybody else's families. They are the elites, like Bill Gates, the rich and the powerful, it's their duty to do this, to save humanity. Haven't you heard of global warming? It's all part of depopulating the planet. If you don't believe me, it's a plan in place that has been here for quite some time. And I think they are now putting into play with Covid. Margaret Sanger is the founder of what? Planned Parenthood. Here is what she said, it's on record.

Margaret Sanger called for, "The elimination of 'human weeds,' for the 'cessation of charity,' because it prolonged the lives of the unfit. And she called for the segregation of 'morons, misfits, and the maladjusted,' and for the sterilization of genetically inferior races"

Now we dealt with this in our other documentary called "Hybrids, Super Soldiers and the Coming Genetic Apocalypse", and we traced the trail of the eugenics program, and these population control people, and believe it or not, when she was alive in our country at that time promoting this, our own Supreme Court, it was big into eugenics. The church was going along with it, and it was called the social gospel. Let's all feel good, let's improve humanity with all our technology. But our own Supreme Court had ruled at that time, for forced sterilization in many of our states in the United States of America. We exposed all of this amongst other stuff.

But what happened was, it hopped the pond from our own country and went to Germany. Hitler got his ideas of sterilization and eugenics, from population control from here in America. What he did was wrong. But this has been embedded in our country for quite some time.

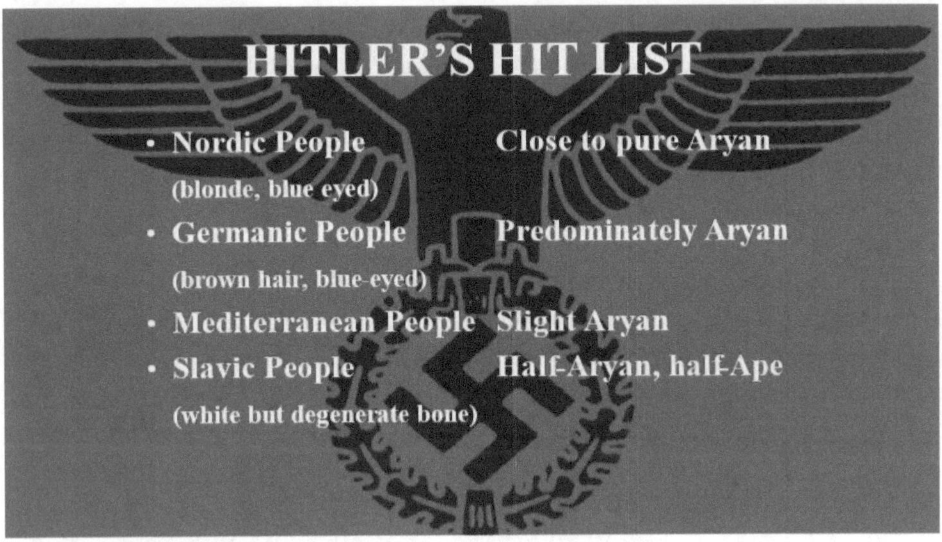

.

That is also why Hitler was annihilating the Jewish people. Because it was his duty to create a utopia, and he had to get rid of the lesser races. That is why he started with the Jewish people, because they were at the bottom of his hit list. If Hitler was to have his way and God didn't intervene, he wasn't going to stop with the Jewish people, he was going up his list. Annihilate the bulk of the planet, left with a pure race creating his own utopia.

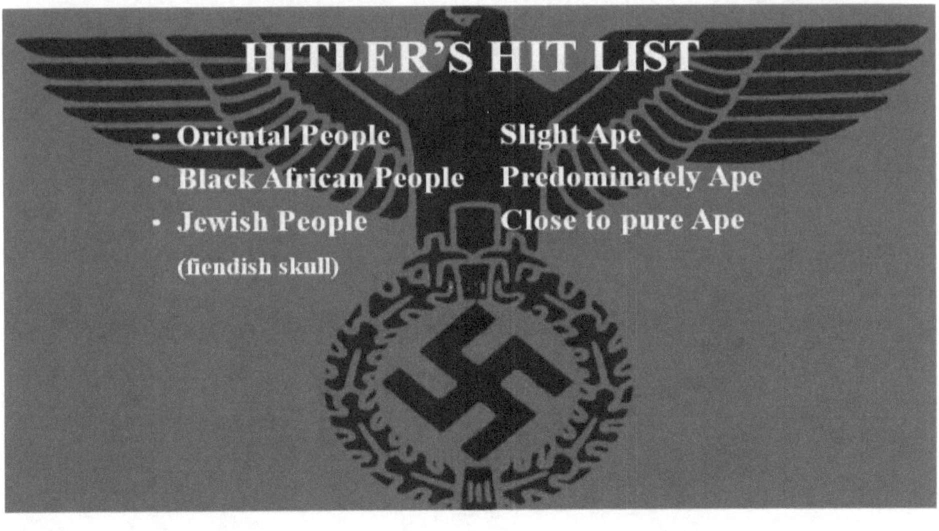

That's why today, Klaus Schwab, the World Economic Forum, the Great Reset, you know his background, tied directly to the Nazis and they are calling it the 4th Reich. Learn the history. It's the annihilation of the bulk of the planet. Now even modern people in secular society, you know the elites, those guys with degrees on top of their degrees, who know better than us say this.

David Graber, a research biologist with the National Park Service: *"We have become a plague upon ourselves and upon the earth. Human happiness is not as important as a wild and healthy planet. Until such time as homo sapiens should decide to rejoin nature, some of us can only hope for the right virus to come along."*

Jacques Cousteau: *"The damage people cause to the planet is a function of demographics – it is equal to the degree of development. One American burdens the earth much more than twenty Bangladeshis. This is a terrible thing to say. In order to stabilize world population, we must eliminate 350,000 people per day. It is a horrible thing to say, but it's just as bad not to say it."*

Bertrand Russell: *"At present the population of the world is increasing. War so far has had no great effect on this increase. I do not pretend that birth control is the only way in which population can be kept from increasing. There are others. If a Black Death could be spread throughout the world once in every generation, survivors could procreate freely without making the world too full. The state of affairs might be somewhat unpleasant, but what of it? Really high-minded people are indifferent to suffering, especially that of others."*

Because it's not them, it's the rest of us that need to go.

Prince Phillip, Duke of Edinburgh: *"If I were reincarnated, I would wish to be returned to Earth as a killer virus to lower human population levels."*

These are elites around the world and a lot of them are still alive pushing this murderous satanic agenda.

Ted Turner: *"People who abhor the China one-child policy are dumb-dumbs, because if China hadn't had that policy, there would be 300 million more people in China right now."* And then he later advocated that we would reduce the world's population from 6 billion to 2 billion.

Okay Ted let's start with you and your family. But it's the elites, not the rest of us, it's their duty to annihilate and cull the planet of these weeds.

John Holdren, Obama's Science Czar: *"Forced abortions and mass sterilizations are needed to save the planet. Women could be forced to abort their pregnancies, whether they wanted to or not;* (Isn't that what the shot is doing right now?) *the population at large could be sterilized by infertility drugs* (Isn't that another side effect of the shot?) *intentionally put into the nation's drinking water or in food. And people who contribute to social deterioration,* (i.e., undesirables) *can be required by law to exercise reproductive responsibility* (that is, be compelled to have abortions or be sterilized) *and a transnational Planetary Regime should assume control of the global economy and also dictate the most intimate details of American's lives using an armed international police force."*

Dr. Eric Pianka, a scientist: *"The need to exterminate 90 percent of the population through the airborne Ebola virus. We're no better than bacteria!"* Standing in front of a slide of human skulls, he gleefully advocated airborne Ebola as his preferred method of exterminating the necessary 90 percent of humans. Choosing it over AIDS because of its faster kill period. At the end of Pianka's speech the audience erupted not to a chorus of boos and hisses but to a wild reception of applause and cheers.

Send your kids to college and this is what they come out with. We need to save the planet, haven't you heard? Recycle or we are all going to blow up. This is what's all behind this. It's a smoke screen for the satanic agenda.

Dr Sam Keen, a New Age writer and philosopher: *"We must speak far more clearly about sexuality, contraception, about abortion, about values that control the population, because the ecological crisis, in short, is the population crisis. Cut the population by 90 percent and there aren't enough people left to do a great deal of ecological damage."*

Dr. Michael Berliner wrote of the Environmentalist's utter contempt for mankind, *"Such is the naked essence of Environmentalism. It mourns the death of one whale or tree but actually welcomes the death of billions of people. Is there a more malevolent man-hating philosophy than this?"*

And I wonder who is behind it all? Rhymes with satan. If you wondered. He is not only a liar but the father of all lies and he's a murderer and he has been one from the beginning. Now, believe it or not, these guys are so bold and brazen about this depopulation of the planet, that they have a monument. Did you know that? That monument is right outside of, of all places in the United States, the CDC., Atlanta, Ga. There's a little town out there called Elberton. It's like a Stonehenge thing. And they say as the very first thing on their list, is that they want to reduce the population down to 500 million. I was on location. This is not photoshopped. It's the real deal. It's called the Georgia Guidestones. Here is a clip.

The video begins with Billy getting out of the car and walking to a field of freshly cut grass and in the middle of the field are 4 white pillars, each facing north, south, east and west. He proceeds to walk around these pillars looking at what is written on each one. They are each written in a different language.

"This is wild, folks, no wonder these people don't repent in the 7-year Tribulation. They actually think they are fulfilling ***Revelation 6****. The pale horse rider, death. In fact, they are so brazen about it that they set up an actual monument right here in the United States. It's called the Georgia Guidestones. In fact, I'm standing in front of it right now as we speak. It's a New Age stone monolith similar to Stonehenge, where we just came from. If you go about 90 miles east, outside of the city of Atlanta, to the*

town of Elberton, you will find off to the right, the Georgia Guidestones. Again, it's kind of an American version of Stonehenge, and this was done by a guy who came in and paid cash. He had this company come in and set things up in 1980. He called himself R.C. Christian, but that's not his real name. It says on the stone it's a pseudo name or a false name. On the Georgia Guidestones it basically gives the ten commandments for the New World Order, in eight different languages. Here is what they are:

1. Maintain humanity under 500 million in perpetual balance with nature.
2. Guide reproduction wisely improving fitness and diversity.
3. Unite humanity with the living new language.
4. Rule passion, faith, and tradition and all things with tempered reason.
5. Protect people and nations with fair laws and just courts.
6. Let all nations rule internally resolving external disputes in a world court.
7. Avoid petty laws and useless officials.
8. Balance personal rights with social duties.
9. Prize truth, beauty, love, seeking harmony with the infinite.
10. Be not a cancer on the Earth, leave room for nature, leave room for nature.

Now let's go back to that first commandment. It was to maintain humanity under 500 million, just think about this, today's population is about 7.6 billion. They want to maintain humanity under one half billion, it looks to me like a lot of people have to die for their plan to work."

That's their plan, and I have wondered all this time how in the world were they really going to do it. We have known for years that this is what they really wanted to do. How are they going to do it? I'm convinced that we are seeing it right before our very eyes, with Covid, because of the delayed death action. People are already dropping like flies, but again, the doctors are saying you ain't seen nothing yet! Where are these guys getting it from? Just to remind ourselves.

John 8:44 "They're just like their father the devil, who's been a murderer from the beginning."

Now as I mentioned on that video, I came out of New Age and again, Satanism and New Age, you might as well merge the two together, it all comes from the same demonic source. But back in the New Age days, I was a part of this camp before I got saved. So, these people are real, and one of the things that they think, is that they are the ones who are going to decimate the planet in the 7-year Tribulation, except they think it's a badge of honor. It's a good thing. What they do is they look at the first part of this text the first half of the 7-year Tribulation, it talks about the annihilation of the planet.

Revelation 6:7-8 "When the Lamb opened the fourth seal, I heard the voice of the fourth living creature say, 'Come!' I looked, and there before me was a pale horse! Its rider was named Death and Hades was following close behind him. They were given power over a fourth of the earth to kill by the sword, famine and plague, and by the wild beasts of the earth."

What was the word there? Plague, and by the wild beast of the earth. Again, if that were to happen today, that would be the first half of the 7 year-Tribulation when that takes place. With the population today, that is nearly 2 billion people, are going to die just in that judgment right there. That is a horrific death toll. These people are believing in this satanic utopia, to build this utopia, they want to annihilate the planet. Why are they doing this? How can you sit there and have this Georgia Guidestone monument and literally celebrate with your monument? They want to bring the planet down to half a billion. They think it's their God given duty, because they are the Pale Horse Riders of Death. How twisted it is. But here they are admitting it.

Narrator: *"A New Age group called The Solar Quest, writes, 'And those who hinder will be removed – liquidated – (they) must be wiped clean off the face of the earth." The authors of a New Age Pamphlet called Cosmic Countdown, claimed to have received messages from a higher intelligence. The pamphlet says, 'The world should be forewarned to be on the lookout for (the decimation) of populations. These people will eventually be replaced by the new root race, about to make its appearance in a newly cleansed world.'*

But perhaps the most disturbing comment comes from New Age author, Barbara Marx Hubbard. Researchers John Ankerberg and John Weldon report that, 'due to her vast financial wealth and influence among leading world politicians, (and) industrialists – (she) is having a major impact behind the scenes. She has been influenced by spirits for almost two decades.' In her book titled 'Happy Birthday Planet Earth' Hubbard wrote, 'The choice is: do you wish to become a natural Christ, a universal human, or do you wish to die? People will either change or die. That is the choice.

Hubbard says, 'There have always been defective seeds. In the past, they were permitted to die a natural death. We, the elders, have been patiently waiting to take action, to cut out this corrupted and corrupting element in the body of humanity.' Hubbard's spirit guides gave her a vision of things to come. They told her, 'Out of the full spectrum of human personality, one fourth is electing to transcend, one fourth is destructive (and) they are defective seeds. Now as we approach the quantum shift from the creature – human to the co-creative human – the human who is the inheritor of god-like power, the destructive one fourth must be eliminated from the social body. Fortunately, you are not responsible for this act. We are. We are in charge of God's selection process for planet Earth. He selects, we destroy. We are the riders of the pale horse. Death.'"

That's not coming from the God of the Bible. It's the little god, satan. That's where they get this murderous twisted idea from. 2 billion, one-fourth of the planet, they think it's their duty, to be a part of that and pestilence is part of that. What was the number that Dr. Zelenko threw out there if Bill Gates gets his way and vaccinates 7 billion? The delayed death toll is 2 billion people. Is this a coincidence? I don't think so, but it's food for thought. Now if you don't think Bill Gates is part of the population control agenda, we saw this in our Satanism study, Bill Gates got his idea of population control from his dad, who worked for Planned Parenthood. And his wife Melinda, is into Satanism. Don't believe me look at this clip.

Bill Gates: *"The issue that really grabbed me as urgent is issues related to population, reproductive health."*

Bill Moyers: *"How did you come to reproductive issues as an intellectual?"*

Bill Gates: *"As I was growing up my parents were always involved in various volunteer things. My dad was head of Planned Parenthood, and it was very controversial to be involved in that."*

Today Exclusive: *"This pandemic has really exposed the weaknesses and strengths. You're focusing on one of the weaknesses that have been exposed here and that is how we take care of our caregivers. Why did you decide to take on this issue?"*

Melinda Gates: *"If we are going to look into reopening our economy, we have to take care of our most essential workers. 85 percent of nurses are women and yet who's the primary care giver at home?"*

She is wearing an upside-down cross which is one of the symbols of Satanism. So, Mr. Vaccine, Mr. Bill Gates' dad worked for Planned Parenthood, and his wife wears a satanic upside-down cross. I'm sure that's just a coincidence. It tells you where all of this is coming from, if you do the research. Remember the three phases, if you get the shot, it could be the first step, you could die within a couple hours or couple days, that's the acute. The subacute, maybe a couple months. Wow, made it past a couple months, means you are free and clear.

Maybe, maybe not, I'm telling you, other doctors besides Dr. Zelenko are coming out and saying, we ain't seen nothing yet! And what is so diabolical about this, is that it has permanently altered people's insides, their cell structure. But it's on a microscopic level. And you can hear them say this. Here is another video clip of them with their medical speak. They say you can't detect it on an X-ray or an MRI it is so microscopic, but it's there. They said what is coming in a couple years is the real fallout.

Dr. Sam Dube: *"You spoke to a potential mechanism of option of the injury, and you mentioned to me about the d-dimer test. We all know what it's for, but we have to explain it. Could you please speak to this a little bit and give us a relevant content and introduction? I think this is really groundbreaking and important."*

Dr. Charles Hoffe: *"Yes, thank you. So, one of the key things that really bothered me when I started to see serious vaccine injuries in my own patients, is that I had no idea what the mechanism of injury was and therefore as their doctor, I had no idea how to treat it. Because as their family doctor, they would come to me for help, and I needed to help them, so I was curious. This was an experiment, and I was aware that there was literally a medically induced disease being produced by this vaccine.*

So, I have asked this in my open letter to Dr. Bonnie Henry, our provincial health officer, what is the mechanism of injury and how do I treat this, as these people's doctor, and of course nobody knew. And as the vaccine manufacturers had told us, that the Covid spike protein does not go intravenous, it stays in the arm, the antibodies, to the spike protein are produced in the arm, and that is what we have found. Scientists now, as Dr. Brody has very clearly revealed, that only 25 percent of the vaccine actually stays in the arm. And the rest of it, these vaccines are a vast number of little messenger RNA strands.

The Moderna vaccine has 40 trillion messenger RNA molecules per vaccine dose. 40 trillion. So, these are wrapped in a little lipid capsule, the lipid capsule is to enable them to be absorbed into the cells. So, this is injected into the persons arm, in their deltoid muscle of the shoulder, and from there, as I mentioned, only 25 percent actually stays there, and the rest is taken up and collected through the lymphatic system and fed into the general circulation. So, it circulates around the entire body, and I think every doctor knows that absorption from the circulation occurs in capillary networks, because that's where the blood slows right down, that it's going through tiny, tiny vessels.

So, these little nano capsules containing these trillions of messenger RNA molecules are absorbed into the lining around the capillaries, what medically we call the vascular endothelium. So, these little packages are absorbed into the cells around the vessels, the packages open, the body recognizes these messenger RNA strands as a gene and gets to work making Covid spike proteins. So, in a virus, those Covid spike proteins form part of the viral capsule, but the problem, they're not in a virus, they're in the cells around blood vessels, so as a result they become part of the cell wall of that cell.

Normally, the cells that surround your blood vessels have to be very, very smooth to enable good and unimpeded flow of blood, but as soon as you've got all these little spike proteins that become part of the cell wall, it's going to be a rough surface. It's going to be like a very course sandpaper. It's now what the platelets are going to interpret as a damaged vessel. It's no longer smooth, it's rough. So clotting is inevitable, because the platelets that come down that vessel are going to hit a rough spot and assume this must be a damaged vessel. This vessel needs to be blocked to stop the bleeding, that's how our clotting works.

Because of this and the nature of this, clots are inevitable because of these spike proteins in the capillary network. So, I set out to then try and prove this. Could this theory be correct? So, the problem is, these little clots in the capillary networks are microscopic, and they are scattered so they're not going to show on any scan. They are just too small and too scattered. It's not like the big clots that cause strokes or heart attacks, they're too small and too scattered. So how on earth can we know if the person clotted?

The only way is with a test call a D-dimer. The D-dimer is a blood test that will show up a recent clot. It won't show up an old clot, it shows up a new clot, and it doesn't tell you where the clot is, it just tells you that the clotting mechanism has been activated. So, I have now been recruiting patients from my practice, people that have come into my office and others that have heard me speak about this and have asked people to do this D-dimer within one week of their Covid shot. So far, and this study is ongoing, these are preliminary results, so far, I've got 62 percent positive elevated D-dimer, which means, that the blood clots are not rare.

That's what the so-called experts keep telling us. The clots are rare, the big clots are rare, but the small ones are clearly happening in the majority of people, 62 percent. Now, I'll tell you what the real concern with this is, is that a clotted vessel is permanently damaged. That vessel never ever goes back to normal. So, if this theory is correct, which it really looks like by these D-dimer results, and I am being told it is being done in Australia, it's being done in the UK, and they also found elevated D-dimers. They discarded the information because they said there's no clinical evidence of clots.

Well, the clinical reason is because they're microscopic, and they're scattered, and so you're not going to see clinical evidence. In fact, all of the frequent side effects of the shot which are headache, nausea, dizziness, fatigue, could all be signs of cerebral thrombosis on a capillary level. I mean you could have thousands and thousands of tiny, tiny little clots in your brain, that won't show on a scan, but they will give those exact symptoms. So, the concern now is that I have six people in my medical practice who cannot exert themselves the way they used to, with what we call reduced effort tolerance. Six people, who now get out of breath doing things that they could previously do without any problem. I believe that these people, blocked up thousands and thousands of capillaries in their lungs. These six people.

So, I believe that these people now have permanently damaged their lungs, that is why they get out of breath. One fellow who used to walk two miles to my office every week for a shot for his arthritis, he says after a quarter of a mile, he is done. In other words, his effort tolerance is reduced to one eighth of what it used to be. I've sent some of these people for chest X-rays and CT scans, to see what it shows, and all it shows is distorted architecture, what the radiologist described as increased articulation, it's a very non-specific thing, and it's because it's microscopic.

The concern is that just because these vessels are now permanently damaged in a person's lungs, when the heart tries to pump blood through all those damaged vessels, there's increased resistance trying to pump the blood through those lungs. So those people are going to develop something called pulmonary artery hypertension, high blood pressure in their lungs and the concern with that, is those people will probably all develop right-sided heart failure within three years and die."

Delayed death! Just like in the very beginning. That's what satan knew he was up to. I just need you to take that first step, oh you won't die on the spot, but he knew you would die later. It's the same sick, twisted, lie. Do you see how it all comes around? He did it in the beginning and he's doing it here at the end. Just prior to the 7-year Tribulation. What are we going to do? Wait a second, if this is going to create a massive death rate around the world, and these population control guys really get their way, that includes America. Could this have anything to do with, and how strange it is, as much as we are a super world power now, why we don't find America mentioned in Bible Prophecy? What happened to America? How did America go out of existence before the 7-year Tribulation? Hey, great question but we are out of time. We'll have to deal with that in the next chapter.

Chapter Five

The Disappearance & Response to Covid

Strangely enough many would say America is not even mentioned in Bible Prophecy. Does this have anything to do with our disappearance and the big ending is the resistance. What are we supposed to do with all this going down? I don't know if you noticed or not, but our country has been radically changed over this covid issue. Have you noticed that? And if you have noticed, it has really drawn a line in the sand. We are really finding out people's true colors. Because overnight it would seem that many people that we know, even fellow Christians, have gone from a people of courage and conviction, who would gladly stand up as Americans for our God given rights and freedom, to a populace of sheeple and compliers which are exactly what these global elitists want. They don't want us to resist. Frankly we have to ask ourselves, what has happened to us, Jesus? Like this song declares:

CON Breaking News: This video clip starts off with people around the world and their reactions to what is going on today. When Trump was elected the scene of the two girls screaming and crying about what they thought was the most horrific thing that could ever happen. Guards are lined up in front of demonstrators holding up signs saying 'Our bodies.' A newborn baby is being handed to its mother with a face shield on it's little face. It's pink so it must be a little baby girl. The next scene is a group of masked people burning the American flag. Another is where a person is walking down the street and all the doors and windows are boarded up to keep out the looters.

Then we see two people embracing, but one is enclosed in a huge cellophane bag so not to spread germs. At the hospital, as the new mother is still laying in the bed after delivering the baby, they hand her the baby with a sheet of cellophane between. The mother cannot even touch her own baby. The next scene is the vials of the vaccine are spinning around on the holder and a woman with her mask on is covering her face with her hands like she can't take it anymore. And the song begins:

"Shut you mouth, get in line, just behave or pay the fine. They're pulling on your backbone and taking out your spine. They want you weak, don't speak, don't question, don't think. Keep staring at your smartphone, get dumber every week. Now give up your freedom and shush. Oh Jesus, what happened to us? Leave the church, kill your faith, judge the skin, learn to hate, make yourself the enemy, but call yourself a saint. Learn the rules, be a fool, remove your kid from school and apologize for everything, apologize for you. Now give the TV all of your trust. Oh Jesus, what happened to us?

*Mark, Jack, Bill, Joe, they'll tell you what you need to know. They'll give you your permissions and tell you where to go. Lights, camera, action, edit! We're so pathetic! You believe it 'cause you watched it, you believe it 'cause they said it. Now everybody stay home and rust. Oh, Jesus, what happened to us? We used to stand and fight; we had a voice alright. We had a life worth living, we had a da** worth giving. Now we're watching it fall, that's the truth of it all.*

So shut your mouth, get in line, just behave or pay the fine. They're pulling on your backbone and taking out your spine. They want you weak, don't speak, don't question, don't think. Keep staring at your smartphone and get dumber every week. Don't nobody put up a fuss. Oh, Jesus what happened to us? Oh, Jesus, Jesus what happened to us?"

During the song we see flags burning, people looting, people hugging through cellophane sheets, school children sitting in plastic compartments in their classrooms and past pictures of John F. Kennedy and Martin Luther King, Jr. when they stood up for what was right. The song ended with the girl from the beginning of the song taking off her mask and she has her face painted up like a clown.

Well, I'll tell you what, as you can see it turned us into a bunch of clowns in a very short amount of time. We have rolled over to a bunch of goof ball clowns. We have allowed these elites to take away our freedoms and our God given rights. I don't know about you, but our founding fathers must be rolling over in their graves. What has happened to us as Americans? But the good news is that not all of the great American spirit has gone away. I like this guy's song. He made it up as a good ol' American exposing the lie of Covid. Let's look at his version.

Singer: *"Hey folks I just thought I'd experiment with my creativity. I wrote a song for you. Would you like to hear it? Here it goes, and this is to Dr. Fauci.*

I had a couple friends who passed away today. They took the Pfizer, the Moderna and the J&J. They got to clutching on their chests with blood clots all in their veins and I stayed away, I stayed away. Now you see me, healthy and free. I wear a mask but now I have natural immunity. So, you keep talking to your sheep with every booster you can bring. I wish they knew with just one second Fauci funded this whole thing. Now you're back another year, another very thing is so scary that you are even here. Weren't you the one that said the vaccine was for me and if I took it, in no time it would get back to normalcy? So, you lied. I won't comply. As long as I avoid the shot, I know I'll stay alive. This experimental jab you came up with in a lab, don't even try. I won't comply.

Come on and dance with me Fauci!! Wooo!"

Dance with me, you lying murderer. Now if you still don't think that this covid plandemic was a preplanned murderous huge mass of lies after all the study we have been through and quoting them at their own words, I'm going to give you more. This just came out. This thing has been preplanned and staged. I don't know if you saw this, Glenn Beck was on the Tucker Carlson show. US doctors were reviewing Moderna vaccine in December 2019 before Covid even hit the US.

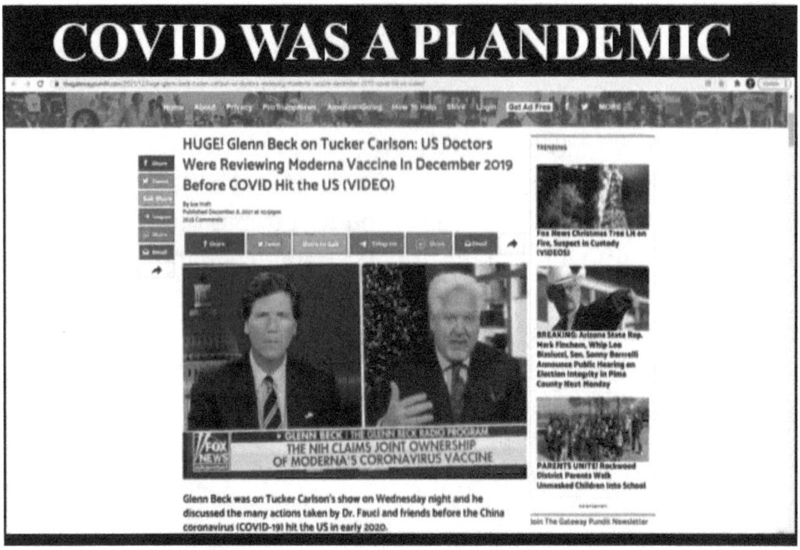
COVID WAS A PLANDEMIC
HUGE! Glenn Beck on Tucker Carlson: US Doctors Were Reviewing Moderna Vaccine In December 2019 Before COVID Hit the US (VIDEO)
THE NIH CLAIMS JOINT OWNERSHIP OF MODERNA'S CORONAVIRUS VACCINE
Glenn Beck was on Tucker Carlson's show on Wednesday night and he discussed the many actions taken by Dr. Fauci and friends before the China coronavirus (COVID-19) hit the US in early 2020.
Fox News Christmas Tree Lit on Fire, Suspect in Custody (VIDEOS)
PARENTS UNITE! Rockwood District Parents Walk Unmasked Children Into School
Join The Gateway Pundit Newsletter

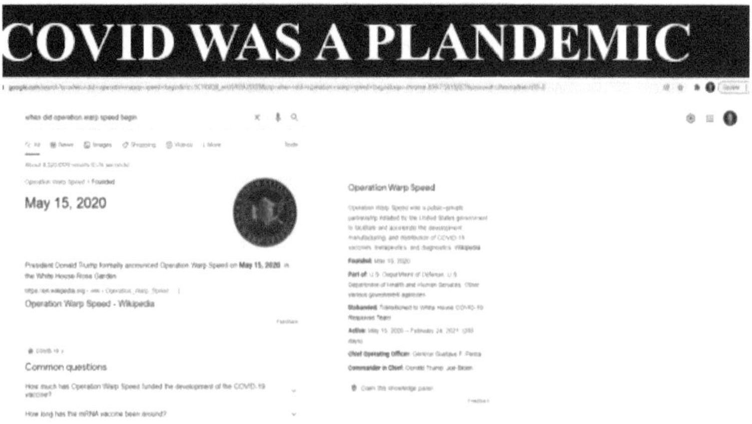
COVID WAS A PLANDEMIC
when did operation warp speed begin
May 15, 2020
Operation Warp Speed - Wikipedia
Common questions
How long has the mRNA vaccine been around?
Operation Warp Speed

Now, wait a second, how can you be reviewing a Moderna vaccine before it even hit? I thought the vaccines weren't even fast tracked until Operation Warp Speed came along. Check it out, it was May 15, 2020.

How are you reviewing a vaccine in December 2019 when you didn't even have a virus? Does anyone smell a rat here? How many times do we have to show that this thing was preplanned over and over again? And why? As we saw, yes, it was to make Trump look bad. Yes, it was an excuse to bring in the mail in ballots to get him out of office, to steal the election. Yes, it was to help, as we will see, to usher in the Great Reset which is basically the Biblical term for the antichrist kingdom; The One World Government, One World Religion, The One World Economy, the Mark of the Beast system that the Bible talks about. Yes, it was to bail out big pharma. Yes, it was to create an endless supply of booster shots for the endless supply of money. And as crazy as it sounds, these guys want to murder off the bulk of the planet. And this is getting the job done.

This is why many who are honest and are doing the research, including non-Christians, they are actually comparing Dr. Fauci to Joseph Mengele. Remember him? For those who aren't familiar with their history he was the guy who worked with the Nazis in the Jewish Holocaust, and he conducted human experimentation without their consent. But that's why Fauci is being compared to that guy. Look at this:

Fox News Reports: *"This is what you see on Dr. Fauci, this is what people say to me. He doesn't represent science to them. He represents Joseph Mengele. The Nazi doctor who did experiments on Jews during the second world war in the concentration camps. I am talking about people all across the world because of the response from Covid and what it has done to countries everywhere. What it has done to civil liberties, the suicide rates, the poverty, it has obliterated economies, the level of suffering that has been created because of this disease is now being seen in the cold light of day, i.e., the truth. And people see that there is no justification for what is being done."*

In other words, it's a big fat murderous lie. It's all starting to come out. And this is why I love this kid. Which by the way, as we saw before with what this is doing to kids, this jab.

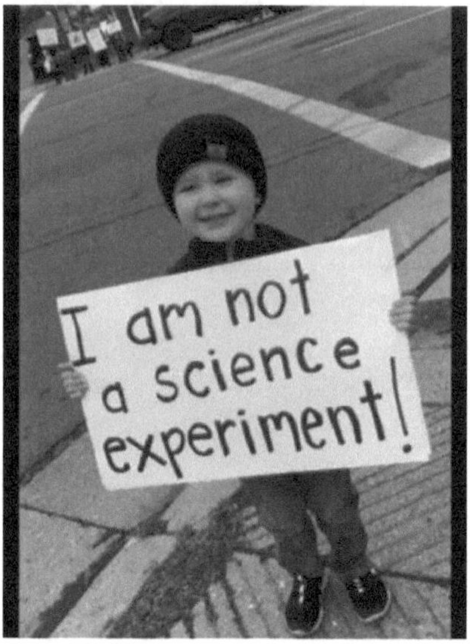
I am not
a science
experiment!

You need to ask yourself this question. What's the difference between these two pictures? Taking your children in for the jab or sacrificing your kid to Moloch of the Old Testament? They would sacrifice their kid to that idol. That idol was hollow inside and they would burn it with fire underneath so it would become red hot and then they would throw their child alive into Moloch's arms to give them favor and convenience to continue on with their livelihood. Answer, it's the same picture. And again, this is what the doctors are saying. If you do this to your kids, you are into child sacrifice. We saw that on tape. Even non-Christian's are saying that. That's what's really going on. And again, if you don't think over these

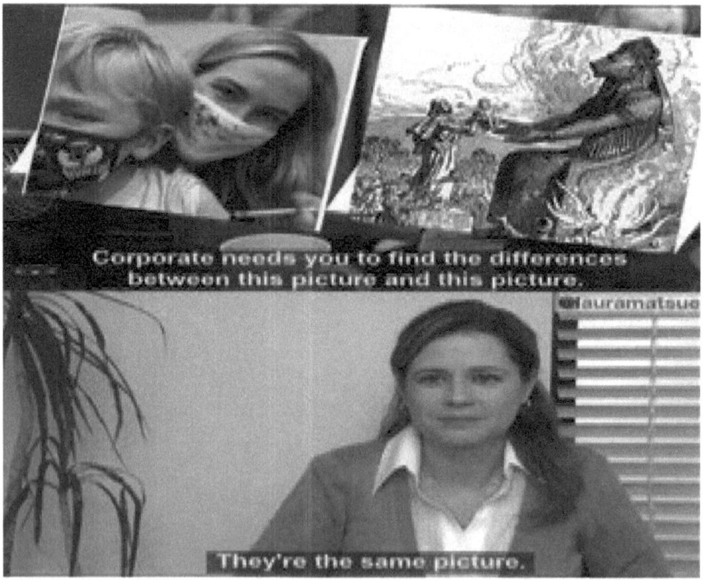
Corporate needs you to find the differences
between this picture and this picture.
@lauramatsue
They're the same picture.

covid issues, these jabs are not just one big giant murderous medical experiment thrust on people without their consent, like Joseph Mengele and the Nazis, this is why we have after what he did,

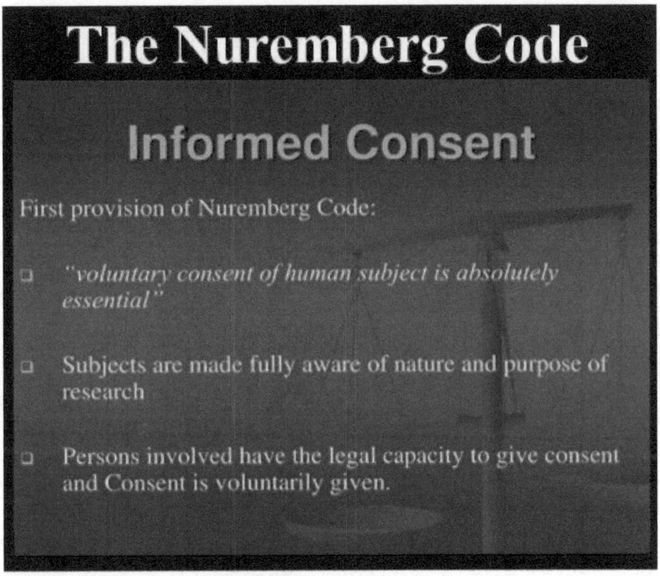

we have what we call the Nuremberg code and it's being violated on a massive scale.

After what he did, the medical experimentation on the Jewish people without their consent, the trial after WWII came up with this. It says that human consent is absolutely essential. So, what do you have to have? You have to have that person's permission. Subjects are to be made fully aware of the nature and purpose of the research. Are we being told what is really going on with this? No! So, strike two. Persons involved have the legal capacity to give consent and consent is voluntarily given. Is that happening? Absolutely not! So, this is a complete

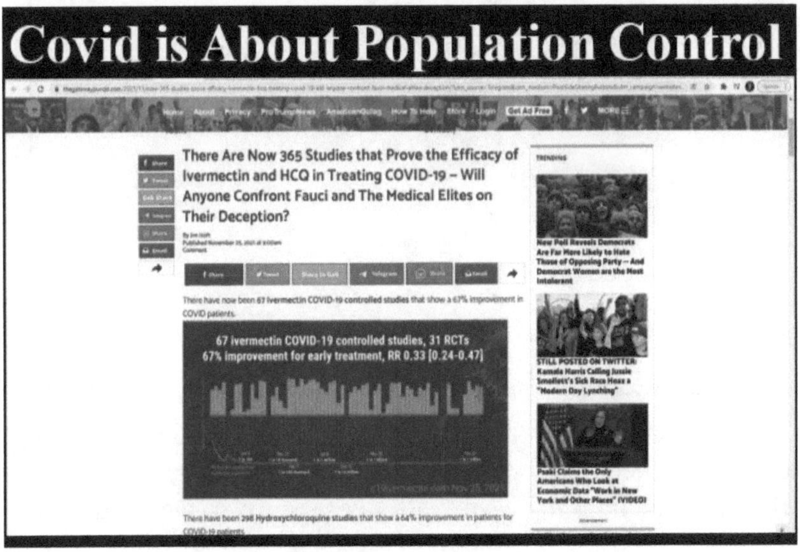

violation of the Nuremberg Code with this jab. And this has not been tested and as we see the effects are not just horrible side effects, it is causing mass deaths. So, once again, tell me if this is not something that is going on. We are being lied to! It's human experimentation on a global scale. We saw why they are doing it in the last chapters, it's murder and yes, it's for the money and they are lying through their teeth to get us to fall for it. This is a deliberate attack of human experimentation for a murderous agenda. It's now coming out that there are 365 studies that prove the efficacy of Ivermectin and HCQ in treating Covid-19. That's one for every day of the year. It works! So, even if you did come down with Covid, do you need to get the shot? No. You can do this, and it works. And by the way, never forget that the survivability rate is 99.98 percent.

As we saw statistically before, there are more deaths from the flu annually than due to Covid when you look at the true numbers. And then if you make it through without the shot, you're in great condition.

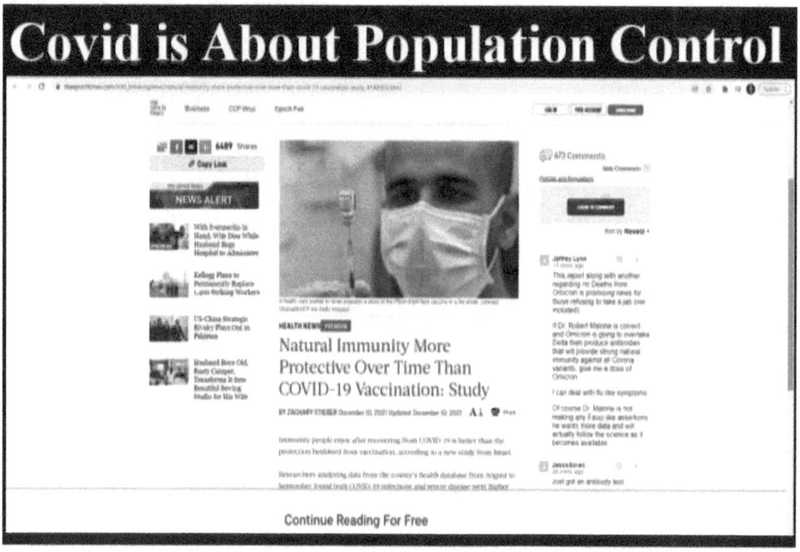

Natural immunity is more protective over time than the Covid vaccinations. So, here's my point. Why? Why would they even need to do a jab? If I survived it on my own, with my God given DNA structure, then

I'm sitting good. Right? Or if I do come down with it there are other medications, and they are very cheap by the way, but as we saw last time, they are keeping us from getting them. There is no reason for this. By the way, those who are dying, it's not the unvaccinated. It's the people who got the jab. I'm just going to share some headlines.

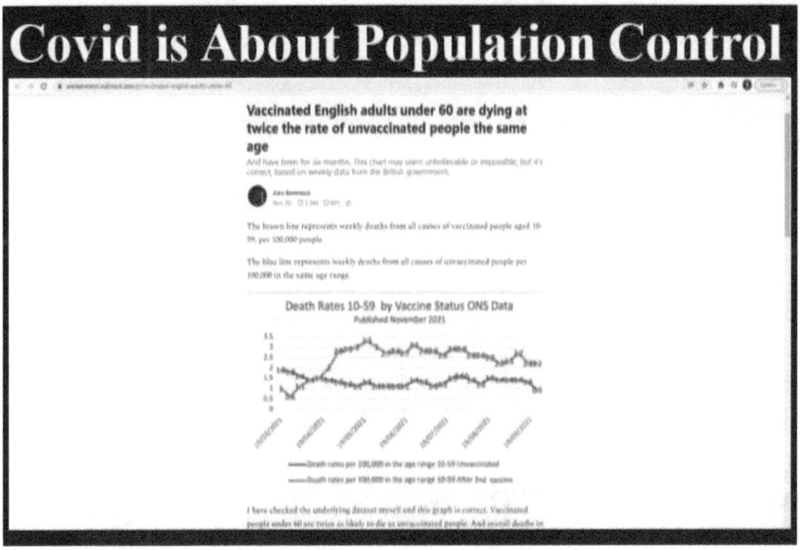

Vaccinated English adults under 60 are dying at twice the rate of unvaccinated at the same age. Official Data confirms "fully vaccinated" account for 9 out of 10 Covid-19 deaths since August! It's coming out and it's all around the world.

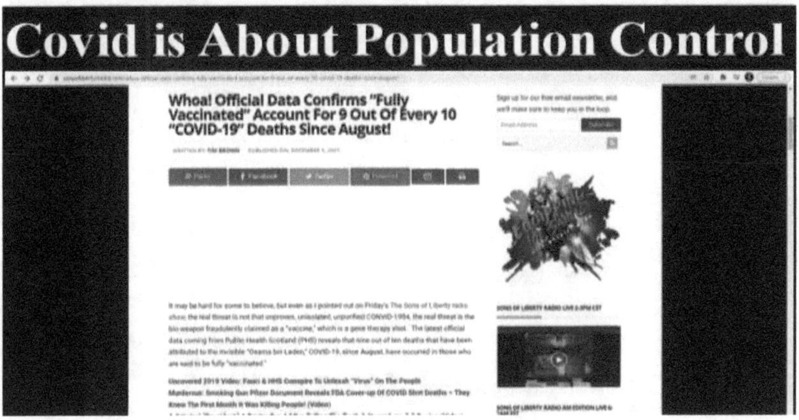

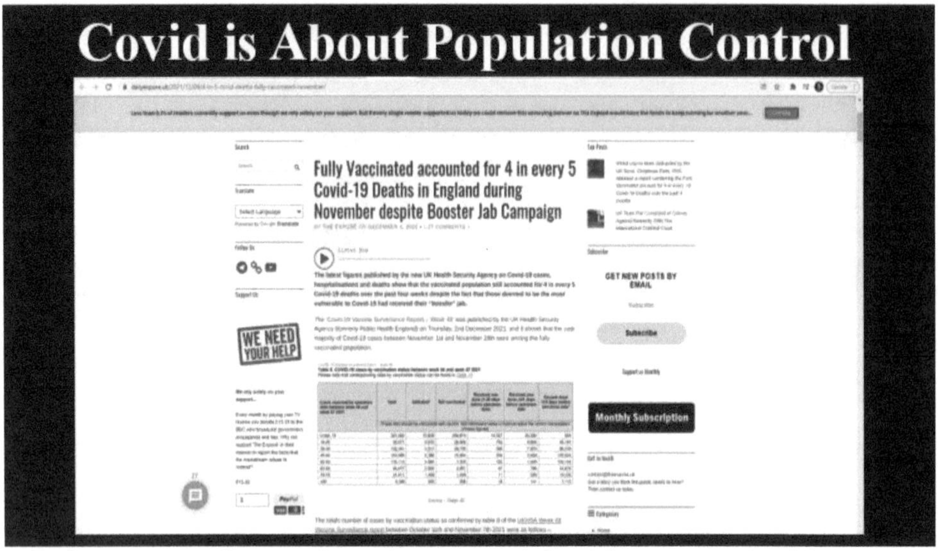

Fully vaccinated accounted for 4 in every 5 Covid-19 deaths in England during the November booster jab campaign. Get the booster and you'll be okay. No, you won't, it's why one person said this.

"The government has a difficult task simultaneously: Convince the uninjected that the injection works so they get the shot and convince the injected that the injection doesn't work so they get the booster shots."

As crazy as that is, that's what is going on. That's why it doesn't make sense. It's a joke and they know it, look at this.

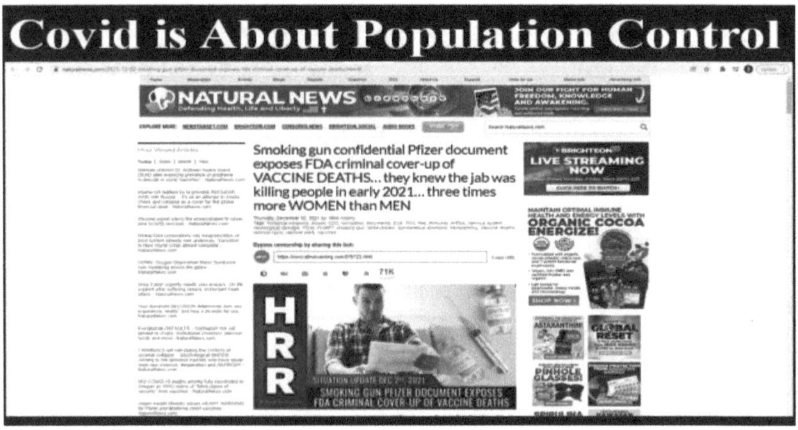
Covid is About Population Control
NATURAL NEWS
Smoking gun confidential Pfizer document exposes FDA criminal cover-up of VACCINE DEATHS... they knew the jab was killing people in early 2021... three times more WOMEN than MEN
LIVE STREAMING NOW
ORGANIC COCOA ENERGIZE!
71K
HRR
SITUATION UPDATE DEC 2nd 2021
SMOKING GUN PFIZER DOCUMENT EXPOSES FDA CRIMINAL COVER-UP OF VACCINE DEATHS

Pfizer document exposes FDA criminal cover-up of vaccine deaths, they knew the jab was killing people in early 2021. It's been almost a year now. And they knew it! This is murder! This is what's going on and by the way the guy that invented the mRNA vaccine, he is saying, stop this thing. This is the guy who invented it, saying that. It's in the press, it's all out there. And he is saying stop this thing. Oh, and did you know that something sneaky is going on.

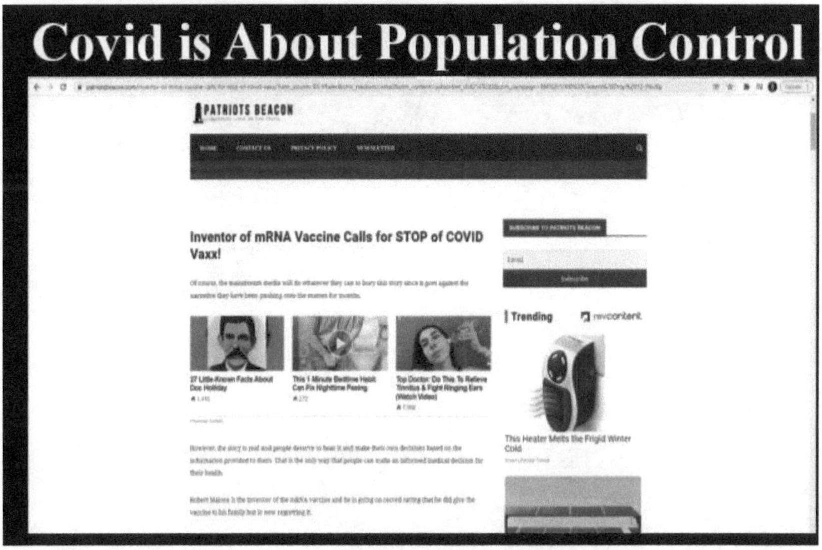

They said "Don't force us to release what is really going on with the deaths over these shots until 2076. Remember that? Oh no, now they are saying 2096.

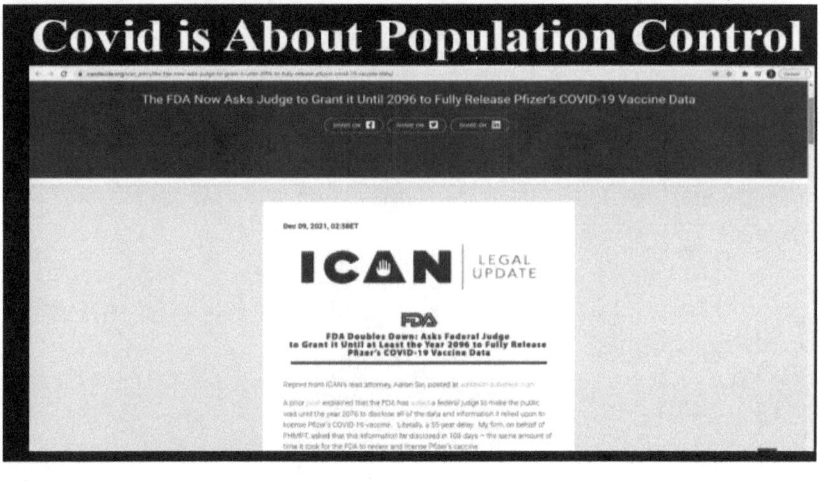

Now to make matters worse now they are saying if the jab doesn't kill you the hospitals will.

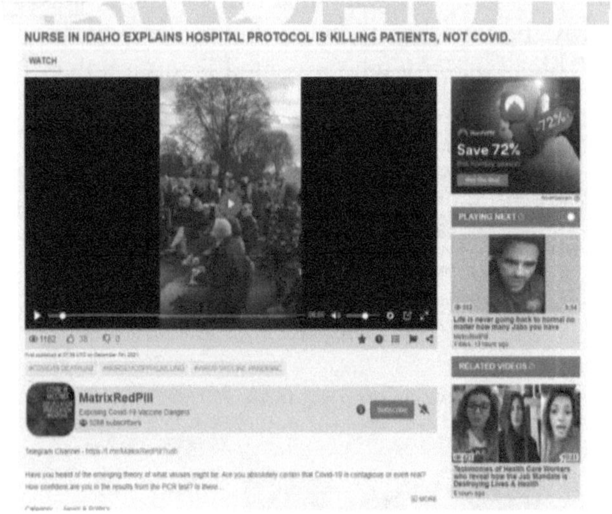

Apparently, the last place you want to go if you do get Covid is the hospital. I'm not joking, these are coming from nurses. A nurse in Idaho explains protocol is killing patients, not covid. Which is why one person said this:

"Yup, I live on Maui. We only have one hospital! I've taken care of 3 men now who have GBS after vax (Guillain-Barre' syndrome) 4 teenage boys with myocarditis (got vax to play sports) 1 lady had to cut off her leg because of clots. 13-year-old Bell's palsy after shot. 7-year-old with seizures after clots. Covid + patient with 3X booster. 2 ladies with spontaneous abortions after vax. 1 mid 30s woman with myocarditis and pericarditis ... the list goes on and on ... not to mention all the covid patients who've been killed by Remdesivir. And this is a small 240 bed hospital."

This is in one little, small hospital in Maui after they got the jab. One lady said this:

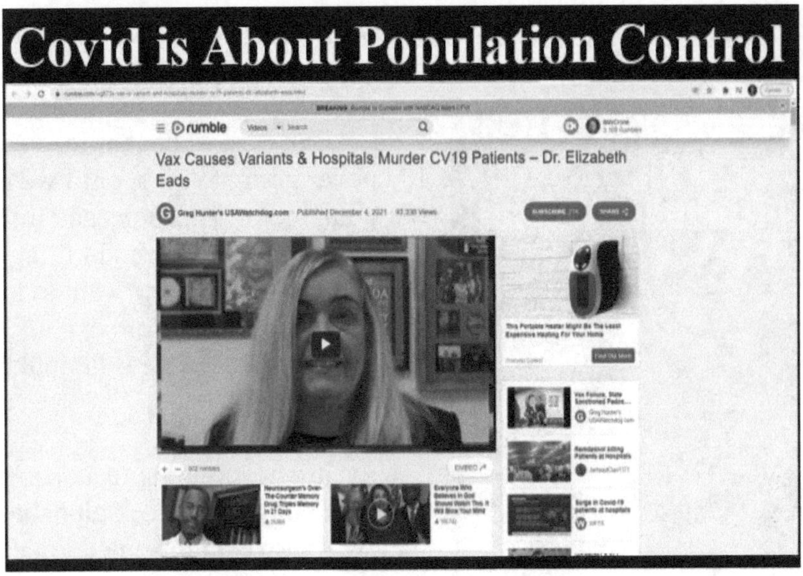
Covid is About Population Control
rumble
Vax Causes Variants & Hospitals Murder CV19 Patients – Dr. Elizabeth Eads
Greg Hunter's USAWatchdog.com

"Vax's are not only causing variants, like the Omicron, but hospitals are murdering CV19 patients." You don't want to go there. What has this turned into? There's this person who lives here and is literally fighting for his life. It's like a Twilight Zone episode. They are trying to get him out of there because they are killing him. This is going on in the United States of America and frankly it's going on all around the world. But hey you'll be happy to know that Bill Gates has informed us when the pandemic is going to end. And I quote, are you ready for some good news. This is crazy, this is what he said, *"In a couple years, it is my hope that the only time that you*

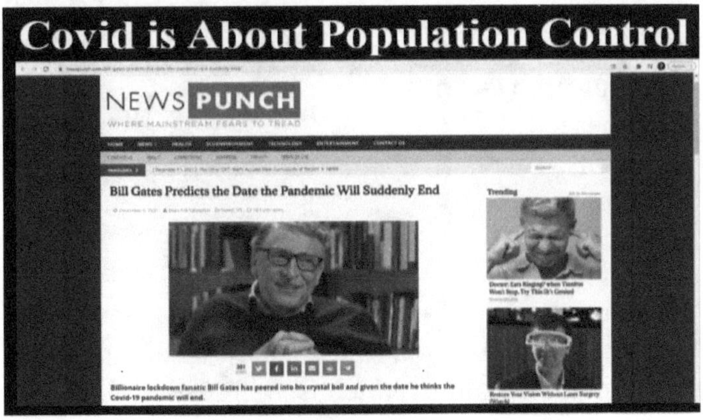
Covid is About Population Control
NEWS PUNCH
WHERE MAINSTREAM FEARS TO TREAD
Bill Gates Predicts the Date the Pandemic Will Suddenly End
Billionaire lockdown fanatic Bill Gates has peered into his crystal ball and given the date he thinks the Covid-19 pandemic will end.

think about the virus is when you get your joint covid and flu vaccine every fall."

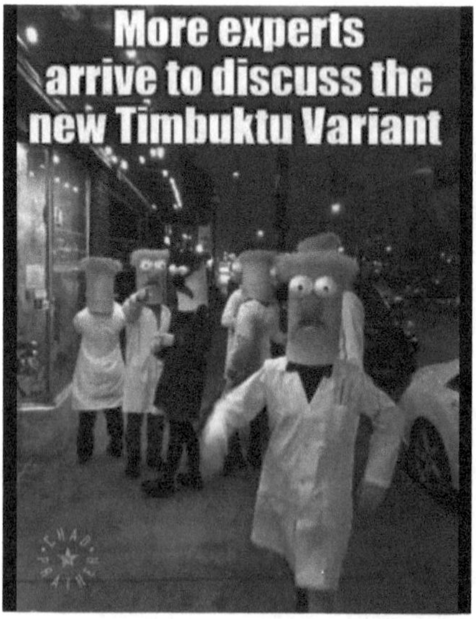

Can I translate that for you? It's never going to stop, until we reach our goal, making millions and millions and trillions of dollars and killing off the population that they want to kill. One guy said this: "More experts arrive to discuss the new Timbuktu Variant."

It's never going to stop. After they run out of the Greek alphabet, they will move on to something else. And it's getting worse. People are being forced to get the jab. Total violation of the Nuremberg Code.

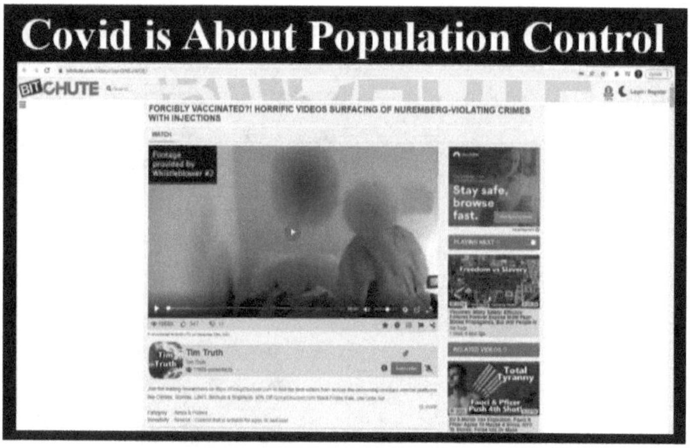

Forcibly vaccinated horrific video surfacing of Nuremberg violating crimes with these injections. There is no informed consent. I don't have time to show all the video clips, but you can go check them out, if you want to go cry and hopefully have some righteous indignation. Kids are being chased down screaming, adults are screaming no, but they are jabbing them anyway. This is sick. It's supposed to be a voluntary consent. But again, how much proof do we have to see that this is a lying murderous agenda, they really are trying to murder the bulk of the planet. How much proof do we have to see that this is a lying murderous agenda, they really are trying to murder the bulk of the planet.

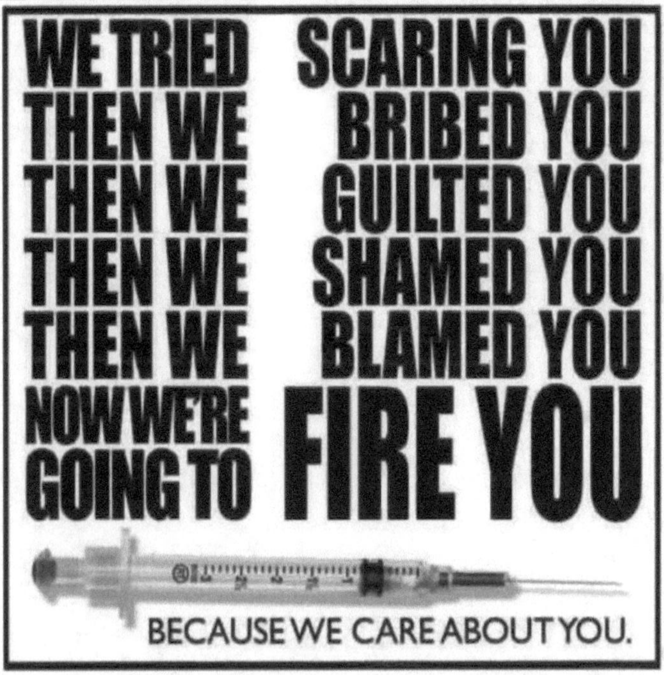
WE TRIED SCARING YOU
THEN WE BRIBED YOU
THEN WE GUILTED YOU
THEN WE SHAMED YOU
THEN WE BLAMED YOU
NOW WE'RE GOING TO FIRE YOU
BECAUSE WE CARE ABOUT YOU.

A massive holocaust, on a much grander scale than the last one, in violation of the Nuremberg Code, and again how is it being presented to us? So, we have an option? One guy puts it this way: First they try to scare you, you're going to die, you're going to die. Then they try to bribe you, hey you can win the lottery. Then they guilted you, how could you do this? Then they shamed you, it's your fault, it's your fault. Then they blamed you. And now they want to fire you, but it's because we care about you.

This is what is going on. It's a joke. And now people are being penalized with, you won't be able to buy and sell. What does that sound like? You can't go to concerts or movies, buy food or travel. We have someone right here at Sunrise that shared with me this week that they went to the hospital just for a check up and when they got there, did you get the jab? And because they come to Sunrise and we get you equipped with the facts, and so basically, they were told you better get it or you won't be able to go to the movies or concerts, whatever. And this is in America. Where is the informed consent on this? This is nuts but it's getting worse.

Remember, you start at the end of the spectrum, and you work your way in to your ultimate goal? This is what is going on in Canada. No more unvaccinated passengers on Canada's planes and trains.

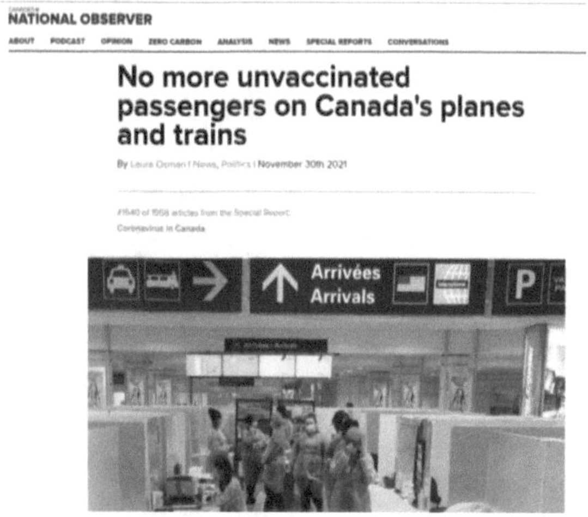
NATIONAL OBSERVER

No more unvaccinated passengers on Canada's planes and trains

November 30th 2021

First it was just the mask, right? But now you can't fly, this is happening in that country right now and look at this one:

No jab, no food mandates land quietly in Canada. Now let me read to you a portion from that article with that picture. *"Unvaccinated can now be banned from grocery stores in accordance with a new set of pandemic measures compiled by the Canadian Province of New Brunswick. Like the rest of Canada, they already forced vaccine mandates for places like restaurants and bars and gyms and entertainment centers. Now grocery stores will be permitted to ban those that cannot show proof of vaccination."*

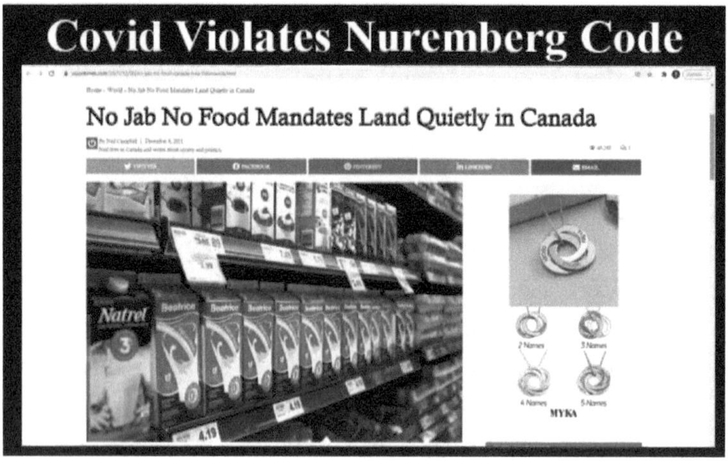

The guy writing this said, *"All Canadians should take note that when vaccine passports were originally rolled out in August, it wasn't long before the nations liberal media began to say that*

we need to do this across the country and then hop the pond over to Europe. Germany is initiating the practice of allowing grocery stores to bar the unvaccinated and then their Chancellor said they are now hopefully following in the footsteps of Austria, their neighbor with mandatory vaccinations. Israeli Minister of Health Nitzan Horowitz said that vaccine passports are not about public health but about coercing vaccine acceptance."

So they admit it! Is that informed consent? Absolutely not! Then in August for people that say, I just want to travel. *"In August, Israel was one of the first countries in the world to modify fully vaccinated passport status to automatically expire after 6 months after their last injection. A move that requires citizens by default to accept government booster injection mandates perpetually."*

So, those that complied because they just want to travel, I'll just get the jab one time and I'm good, no you won't. Do you see what they are doing? And in that article it says, *"The Nuremberg Code expressly prohibits this."*

They are right, this is an international law. Based on the last time this kind of satanic behavior happened with Hitler and the Nazis. Now it's happening on a massive scale even in our own country. This is what's going on. Now, if you don't think that this kind of forced behavior isn't coming here to America, you better think again. Schools. I've said this how many times? Get your kid out of public schools, not only for the filth being taught there but you better get them out now because the schools in the United States of America are vaccinating kids without parental consent. Here is just one example.

New reporter: *"Parents in the Los Angeles Unified School district are accusing schools of giving their kids the vaccine without their consent. One mother, Maribel Duarte, said her 13-year-old son, a student, at the Barack Obama Academy in South LA brought home this vaccine card after getting the shot at school. She said, he said yes after somebody offered him the vaccine in exchange for some pizza."*

Maribel Duarte: *"It started with him getting the shot without my permission, without me even knowing or signing any papers for him to get this shot."*

In the United States of America! Total violation of the Nuremberg Code, and the rationale that they have, well, it's implied because you send your child to public school. Total violation, which is why these vaccines are a giant human experimentation on we the people, we are their lab-rats. And the goal, as crazy as it is, they want us knocked off, 90-95 percent of the planet. This is what's going on. That is why Dr. Zelenko, the Jewish doctor who treated Trump and Giuliani and others, he now is saying, get your kids out of public school. And you better wake up, how many times do I have to say it? This is WWIII. Here he is saying it on another interview:

Dr. Zelenko: *"This is not a joke; this is really happening. This is WWIII. This is Hitler and Stalin on steroids with weapons of mass destruction. And the only reason why it's happening is because people don't realize it's happening. Wake up! Get your kids out of school. Take your kids and homeschool them. A few weeks ago, they showed us a paper, if your kids are in school that is an implied informed consent, and they can be vaccinated without you being told because you could have prevented them from going to public school. So, in other words, the fact that you send your kids to school it empowers the school and the government to inject them with this poison. So, not only are the souls of our children being assaulted in the public school system, with this debauchery and ungodly teaching but now they are lying to people as well.*

What a joke! We know the vaccine destroys the hearts of young people. You see all these athletes dropping dead. And now what they are trying to do is deflect the vaccine side effects and blame it on the new variant that the actual vaccine has caused. And what is interesting by the way, is I have a zero fear of new variants. You just have to use common sense, use early intervention, use prophylactics, stay away from the poison death shot and you will be okay."

It sounds like common sense to me. But that's not what is happening, right? We aren't given the choice. We are being forced to comply. You better get this poison death shot, or else. It's in total violation of the Nuremberg Code. But again, you put all this together and could this be why apparently, we see America disappear, from being mentioned in Bible prophecy? It's strange because we are the leading power on the world scene. I think we can agree we don't know the exact day or the hour, but man, we are getting close to the 7-year Tribulation, we leave prior in the Rapture. Something pretty quick has to happen to us. Could Covid and what's going on with it have anything to do with it? Well, again, let's take a look at that.

Again, doctors are saying you haven't seen anything yet with the death rate with this shot. There are three phases, just like we saw last time. The first phase is where the people die within a couple days. It's called acute death syndrome. The second phase is called the subacute death syndrome where they die a couple months later. And all of these are happening as we speak. But the doctors are warning that we ain't seen nothing yet. The real fall-out is coming in a couple of years. The long-term death rate.

Dr. Charles Hoffe: *"The concern is that just because these vessels are now permanently damaged in a person's lungs, when the heart tries to pump blood through all those damaged vessels, there's increased resistance trying to pump the blood through those lungs. So those people are going to develop something called pulmonary artery hypertension, high blood pressure in their lungs and the concern with that is those people will probably all develop right-sided heart failure within three years and die."*

So, we really haven't even seen it yet, according to these doctors, secular doctors as far as I know, but this is what they admit, a delayed death in a couple years is when it is going to happen. Could this be why we don't find America in Bible prophecy? Because what is happening in our country? Our country is now being pushed, even down to babies to get the death shot. And if there is going to be delayed death aspect in a couple years, what's going to remain of our country? Now I wanted to dispel this before we get into it, that there are some in the Christian community that say, oh no, America is in Bible prophecy. I don't think so. I want to bring up some popular ones, that they say we find America in Bible prophecy. Unfortunately, they are twisting things out of context.

Isaiah 18:7 "At that time gifts will be brought to the Lord Almighty from a people tall and smooth-skinned, from a people feared far and wide and aggressive nation of strange speech, whose land is divided by rivers – the gifts will be brought to Mount Zion, the place of the Name of the Lord Almighty."

So, there it is, Isaiah 18 says a tall and smooth skinned people and it's a nation who's feared far and wide and they are divided by a river, it's got to be America. I mean we are separated by the mighty Mississippi, right? And we are a powerful people and full of tall people, except for Pastor Billy. No, they have to be speaking of America. No, that's what you want it to say, but that's not even close to what's really going on here.

First of all, the context is talking about the land of Kush and if you do your homework, that is modern day Ethiopia which means the river they are talking about is the river Nile. It had nothing to do with America. They persist because they want America to be in Bible prophecy and I don't think we are. Here is the second one which they actually put America in the Gog and Magog war.

Ezekiel 38:13 "Sheba and Dedan and the merchants of Tarshish and all her villages will say to you, 'Have you come to plunder? Have you gathered your hordes to loot, to carry off silver and gold, to take away livestock and goods and to seize much plunder?"

Some say right there is proof that America is in Bible prophecy, right there in the Gog and Magog battle. They say it's talking about us because Tarshish has to be England and therefore the village mentioned there has to be talking about England's colonies like the United States. That's us. That is called grasping at straws.

But this is really their rationale. If you do your homework, the people in Ezekiel's time, when this was written, Tarshish was Spain and that means these colonies or villages, if that is what they are talking about, would be South or Central America. It's a joke. It has nothing to do with America whatsoever. The third one is this one:

Revelation 12:13-14 "When the dragon saw that he had been hurled to the earth, he pursued the woman (Israel) who had given birth to the male child (Jesus). The woman was given the two wings of a great eagle, so that she might fly to the place prepared for her in the desert, where she would be taken care of for a time, times and half a time, out of the serpent's reach."

Well, they say right there, the great eagle, and we all know that is the prominent symbol of our nation. The eagle, there it is, it's got to be America. We are the one who rescues Israel. No, not at all. First, if you do your homework, and I highly recommend reading the Bible, you are going to see in Exodus 19 that God carried Israel on eagles' wings, so they use the same phraseology that they did the first time that he rescued them in the Exodus on eagles' wings. He going to do it again in the 7-year Tribulation. It has nothing to do with the United States. Now this is probably the most popular one on the internet, still wrong. America is the great harlot.

Revelation 17:1-2 "One of the seven angels who had the seven bowls came and said to me, 'Come, I will show you the punishment of the great prostitute, who sits on many waters. With her the kings of the earth committed adultery and the inhabitants of the earth were intoxicated with the wine of her adulteries."

So, there you have it right there. The great prostitute, they would say, is America, because we rule over many waters, and we export all kinds of rotten adulterous materials. Well, no I don't think so. Now granted, unfortunately we do export a lot of junk, I'll give you that. Pornography, Hollywood, and all that baloney. Abortion, homosexuality, all that stuff, I give you that, but the context is speaking about Babylon the great, the One World Religion harlot system.

The Bible is clear that it comes against Israel in conjunction with the political system of the antichrist. Granted with this current administration, which is showing signs of going against Israel, but we are not the antichrist empire that controls the whole world. The Bible is very clear. The antichrist does not rise out of the United States. The antichrist rises out of the revised Roman Empire. In other words, Europe, as we are going to see in just a second, which is being formed right before our very eyes. So, this has nothing to do with America.

Here's the point, it would appear, if you study the Bible, that America, even as close as we are to the 7-year Tribulation and we leave prior in the Rapture, we're not around. Yet, we are pretty big right now on the global scene, something is going to happen to us. It's going to radically take us out. What is it? Well first of all I think we are going to be swallowed up. I think the Bible tells us what happens to us ultimately. We are going to be swallowed up into one of the ten economic kingdoms, that the planet is going to be split up into and then handed over to the antichrist. That is what we see here:

Revelation 17:9-13 "This calls for a mind with wisdom. The seven heads are seven hills on which the woman sits. They are also seven kings. Five have fallen, one is, the other has not yet come but when he does come, he must remain for a little while. The beast who once was, and now is not, is an eighth king. He belongs to the seven and is going to his destruction. The ten horns you saw are ten kings who have not yet received a kingdom, but who for one hour will receive authority as kings along with the beast. They have one purpose and will give their power and authority to the beast."

So according to the Bible, in the 7-year Tribulation, at some point, the whole world will be partitioned off into ten chunks ruled by ten kings and at one point they are going to give that whole power over to the antichrist. And it's a good thing we don't see any signs of that happening. That has been happening for a long time.

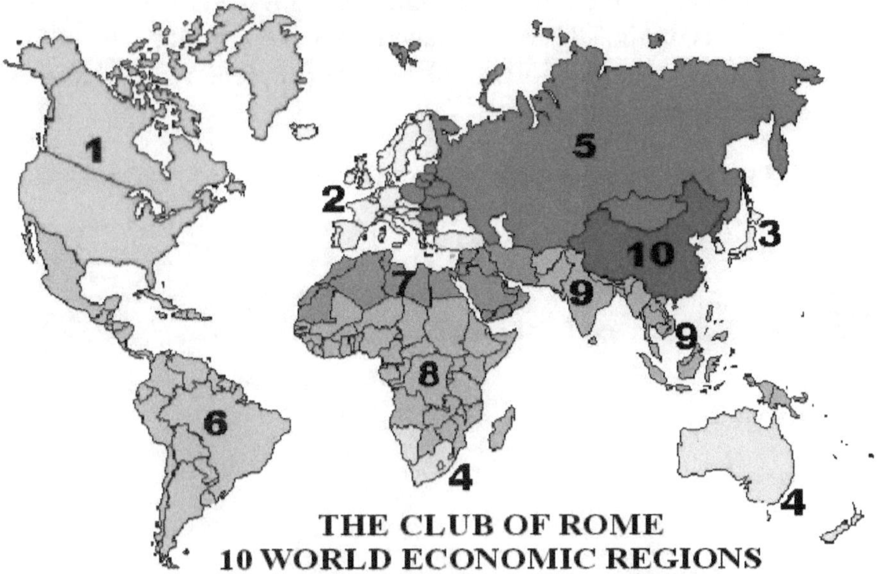

THE CLUB OF ROME
10 WORLD ECONOMIC REGIONS

Let's do a little recap on that from our prophecy studies. Back in 1968, I believe it was, and the early 70s the Club of Rome, they split up the world into, guess how many chunks? Ten, not five, not nineteen, not one hundred and thirty-three, it just happened to be ten. It's kind of like somebody is following a script or something.

I did a screen shot and I learned that if you see something on the internet you had better screen shot it, download it, PDF it and get it on your computer or it will get scrubbed. I learned that after 911 the hard way. But I took this shot while I was still in New York, and I just happened to be on the European Union website, and it showed their map of the world and if you scroll down, they just happen to have the world split up into what?

You can count them there, ten chunks. I got the next screen shot in 2009 but this was on the UN website, and they talked about an event that happened unbeknownst probably to the bulk of the planet, that what these elites are doing behind the scenes.

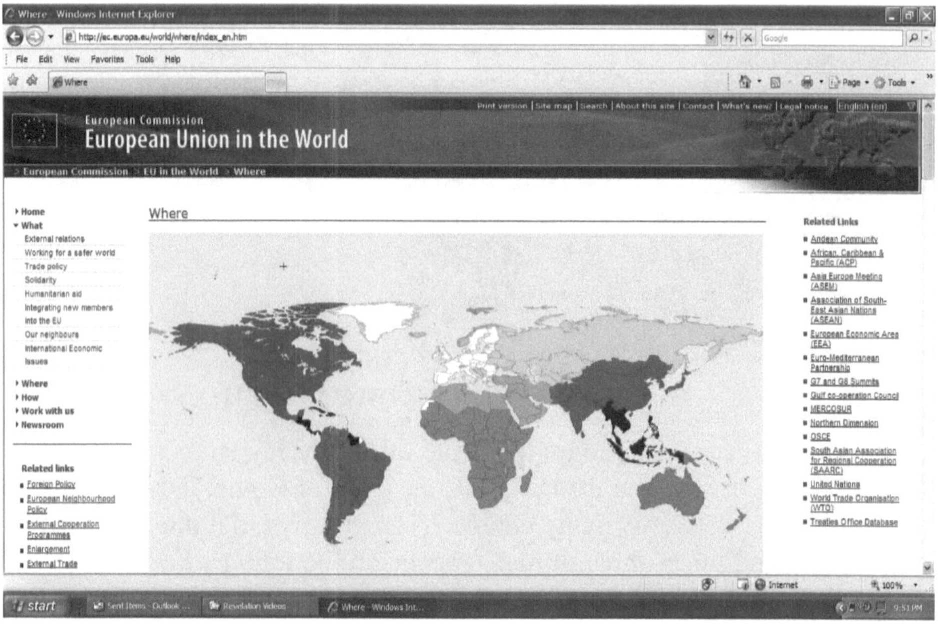

Here's what they did in 2008. As you can see here, March 11, 2009, they are talking about what they did the previous year.

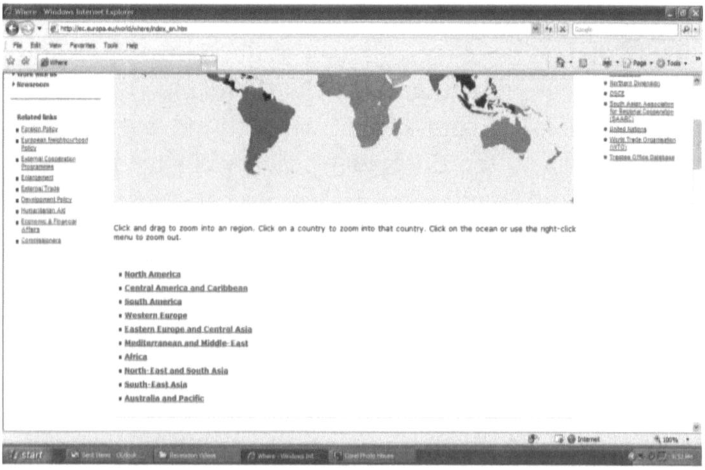

"A new research program on global democracy has been established. A global research program facilitated and coordinated through a convening group of ten persons based in ten world regions was established last year with core funding from the Ford Foundation."

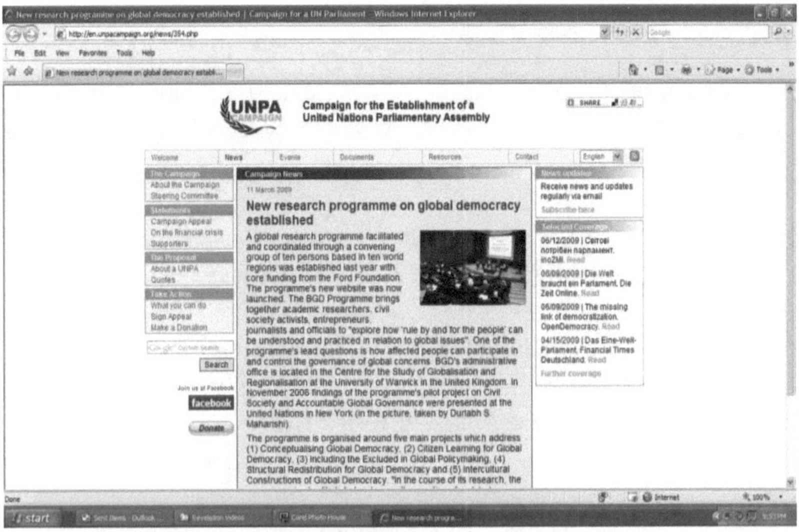

Not one hundred, not fourteen, not two, but ten persons, for global democracy, in ten world regions. They've been preparing for this. God told us 2,000 years ago that this was going to happen. We are going to be split up into ten chunks and at one point these ten rulers of these ten chunks of the country are all going to give their power over to the antichrist. What was the big experiment? The EU. What is the EU, still to this day? It's a conglomeration of nations that is coming under one chunk being ruled by a ruler, over many nations.

Then we saw the African Union, the South American Union, the Asian Union, the Mediterranean Union, the Central Asian Union, the Pacific Union, it's like somebody is following a map from 1968. And then the biggest one, and a lot of people think this is dead. It has never died. It's called the North American Union. And the plan is, and I think this is where it's going, America gets swallowed up, to merge the United States of America with Canada and Mexico. This has been a plan that has been going on for a long time, in fact, way back in Bush Jr.'s years. It has never gone away.

Lou Dobbs: *"New concerns tonight about moves that some call the North American Union. A number of high-level government meetings are taking place in Mexico to discuss North American integration of Mexico, the United States and Canada. More meetings are scheduled. It is an aggressive agenda proposed at the highest levels of our government and US Commerce. Without Congressional or voter oversight. Lisa Sylvester reports."*

Lisa Sylvester: *"A caravan of cars travels along the Arizona desert. Homeland Security Secretary, Michael Chertoff was visiting the US/Mexican border. Last week he was in Mexico City. Commerce Secretary Carlos Gutierrez visited Mexico February 1st, Attorney General Alberto Gonzales on January 11th and President Bush, himself, will travel there next month. The high-level meetings are to advance North American integration, also known as the Security Prosperity Partnership."*

Jim Edwards, Numbers, USA: *"There are several ways it could go. One is modeled after the EU; one is modeled after sort of an economic community. It's beyond the scope of just a trade free trade zone, which we fairly well have already with those two countries."*

It's not about trade, it's about merging the countries together, into one of these ten economic chunks, it's been on the books for a long time. It's has not gone away. Bush Jr. really advanced it, we got snookered with him. It continued through the Obama years. Trump got in and freaked them out. He not only pulled out of a lot of these treaties, but he wanted secure borders. This is why these people want open borders because they want it to be one big giant country. There is another issue going on with that. And then here comes sleepy Joe and I'm sure he's going to resist. No, he's a part of this program, with the Great Reset and all of these global elites, his slogan "Build Back Better" which he got from the World Economic Forum. But here's the point.

If I didn't know better, I'd think the world is being split up just like God said in the last days there would be ten different economic kingdoms, before our very eyes. It says they are going to give their power over, ultimately to the antichrist and this is what these elites admit they are doing to break America's backbone to get us to go along with this. And number one is to destroy our economy. And they admit that is what Covid is helping them to do, is to get American into such a state that just out of survival we have got to merge.

Klaus Schwab admitted that is exactly what they are doing. And Covid is the excuse for them to do it. They are deliberately doing this around the world. Oh, and by the way speaking of Mr. Klaus Schwab, he says he also wants to not just merge all these countries under total economic control and break down the people who are resisting the economy, so that they, under total desperation, will go along with this, he also said he wants to microchip people into this new global system.

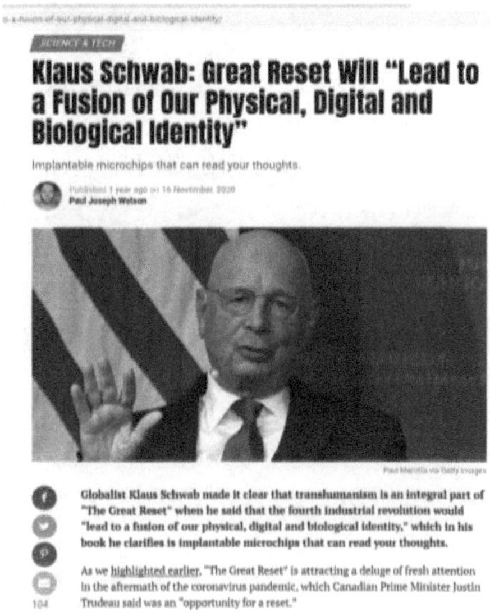
SCIENCE & TECH

Klaus Schwab: Great Reset Will "Lead to a Fusion of Our Physical, Digital and Biological Identity"

Implantable microchips that can read your thoughts.

Paul Joseph Watson

Globalist Klaus Schwab made it clear that transhumanism is an integral part of "The Great Reset" when he said that the fourth industrial revolution would "lead to a fusion of our physical, digital and biological identity," which in his book he clarifies is implantable microchips that can read your thoughts.

As we highlighted earlier, "The Great Reset" is attracting a deluge of fresh attention in the aftermath of the coronavirus pandemic, which Canadian Prime Minister Justin Trudeau said was an "opportunity for a reset."

What does that sound like? So, the merging of the ten economic kingdoms is just the first part. Now you have to tie all the citizens together in this New World Order. And he says in this article and in his book, he clarifies, *"These implantable microchips can read your thoughts."* Try resisting, and if you don't think that is possible, get our documentary "Hybrids, Super Soldiers and the Coming Genetic Apocalypse." The brain chip is the latest thing they are wanting. He wants them in your head as well. Here he is talking about Covid being the way to get the job done. Just get the planet to bow a knee, including America, into this new global system.

Klaus Schwab: *"At the end, what the 4th Industrial Revolution will lead to is a fusion of our physical, our digital, and our biological identities."*

"The difference in the 4th Industrial Revolution is that it doesn't change what you are doing, it changes you, take genetic editing just as an example. It's you who are changing. And of course, it has a big impact on your identity."

"It is important to use the Covid-19 virus as a timely opportunity."

"The people assume we are just going back to the good old world which we had, and everything will be normal again, in how we are used to normal in the old fashion, this is, let's say, fiction, it will not happen, the cut which we have now is much too strong in order not to leave traces."

In other words, Covid is the excuse, we are in it too far, we're not backing down, we're all in on this. This is what's really going on. He admits it. The only thing missing in that is the "SS" on his shoulder and him doing a "Hail Hitler"! He certainly has the accent there. It's being repeated on a massive scale, which is why Australia is even admitting that Covid is bringing about the New World Order.

NSW Government: *"Will they be put back in place to be listed once we are reopening?"*

Dr. Kerry Chant, Chief Medical Officer: *"We will be looking at what contact tracing looks like in the New World Order."*

Brad Hazzard, Australian Health Minister: *"And that's just the way it is, they'll accept this is the New World Order."*

They are admitting it. Isn't this wild? And what is the excuse to bring about this New World Order? Covid. Speaking of the New World Order, the revised Roman Empire, the antichrist that comes out of it and they give the ten sections over to him, we are also seeing right now that

Europe is wanting a president over this revised Roman Empire and not just any president.

A new super president who would be the overall powerful leader of Europe with the responsibility over Europe's economic matters, all foreign policies, and any European military operations. "Total Control" over the revised Roman Empire. Then talk about being ripe for the antichrist to take charge of this revised Roman Empire, Europe has been saying this for a long time. *"I don't care who this guy is, if he can give us what we want, we'll worship him even if he is the devil in disguise."*

Paul-Henri Spaak, former Belgian Prime Minister and the President of the Consultative Assembly of the Council of Europe: *"We do not want another committee. We have too many already. What we want is a man of sufficient stature to hold the allegiance of all people and to lift us out of the economic morass in which we are sinking. Send us such a man and, be he God or the devil, we will receive him."*

Do you think they are ripe for an antichrist figure, a Mr. Fixit? Yeah, I'll get you out of all this. This is going on now in Europe. Now speaking of Europe, this is crazy. The COP26 Summit that was happening recently at the UN Climate Change Conference, Prince Charles, one of the global elitists, population control people, he was there, and he made a speech. You will see Sleepy Joe there too. In this speech he talks about, out of the blue, and it's not a slip of the tongue because he is reading his notes, and he mentions this "He" who is going to be given more money than anybody in the world and more power. Who's "He"? This was from last month.

Prince Charles: *"Your Excellencies, ladies and gentlemen, the Covid-19 Pandemic has shown us just how devastating a global cross border threat can be. Climate change and viruses are no different, in fact they impose an even greater existential threat to the extent that we have to put ourselves on what might be called a warlike footing. Having myself, the opportunity of consulting with you over the last 18 months I know you all carry a heavy burden on your shoulders.*

You do not need me to tell you that the eyes and hopes of the world are upon you to act with all dispatch and decisively because time has quite literally run out. We also know that countries, many of whom are burdened by growing levels of debt simply cannot afford to go green. Here we need a vast military style campaign to martial the strength of a global private sector. With trillions at his disposal, far beyond global GDP, and with the greatest respect beyond even the governments of the world leaders, he offers the only real prospect opportunity of fundamental economic transition."

Did you catch that? Economic transition for the whole planet. I don't know maybe … I quote, *"Here we need a vast military type of campaign."* That sounds a little threatening. *"To martial the strength of a global private sector."* We are going to war. *"With trillions at his disposal."* Who's that? Who's "his"? He's reading his notes. *"Far beyond the global GDP"* he has more money than anybody on the planet. *"And with the greatest respect beyond even the governments of the world leaders"* in other words he will supersede all the governments around the world and have more power than anyone.

Who does that sound like? I'm not saying, thus saith the Lord, but that was just last month. So, you can see the world is already being split up into ten economic kingdoms. There is a revised Roman Empire occurring and it's being put into place and, not saying thus saith the Lord, but people are sure making some weird comments like Prince Charles about a possible, "his" global leader, somebody behind the scenes ready to save the planet. And what is being used as the excuse? Covid and climate change. So, this is what I believe is going to happen to America. We are going to get merged into one of these economic unions and could very well be with Canada and Mexico and so America as we know it will no longer exist. That's what happens to us. That's where I am on that aspect, we are swallowed into that.

My question is, come on man, how are you going to get America? I get the economic aspect of it, that's where they are trying to destroy our economy, just out of desperation, we have to merge with Canada and

Mexico just to survive this economic morass that we are sinking into. Hopefully somebody will arise and take this ship, but is that really going to be enough? I don't think so. There is too much red-blooded backbone left in our country.

So how are you going to do it? Well, let's go back to what I call the "Crone theory", what's going to push us over the edge to get us to literally walk away from our national sovereignty and merge with this global system. Well, let's go back to the Covid issue and the Covid delayed death issue. Maybe it's also, and not just sheer economic desperation but survivability desperation that we go along with this because so many people in America have died now from the Covid death shot. Remember we ain't seen nothing yet. They said the fallout is coming in a couple of years.

So, could this be the long-standing plan of other nations, including communist nations who have always wanted to take America down? Now for those of you who haven't learned their history, you need to. This is a warning from Nikita Khrushchev back in 1956, he warned way back then during the height of the Cold War, we will take America without firing a shot. That will never happen. And he goes on to say we do not have to invade the US; we will destroy you from within.

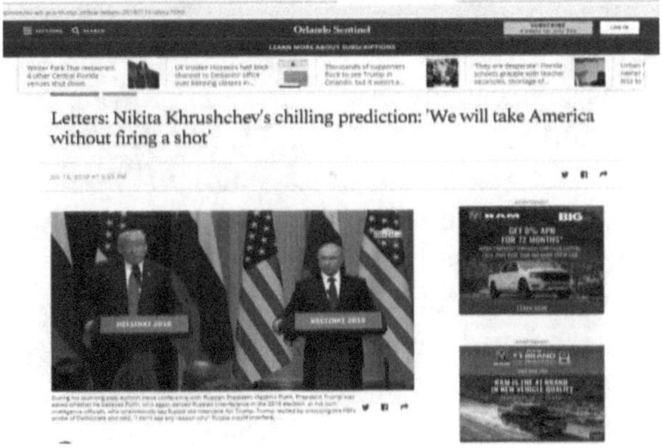
Orlando Sentinel

Letters: Nikita Khrushchev's chilling prediction: 'We will take America without firing a shot'

Alright, so that was a warning from 1956 from countries that want to take us down.

Let's go back to another communist country that rhymes with China and let's go back to this Covid issue which came from where? China, specifically a Chinese lab called the Wuhan Institute of Virology where they make what? Bioweapons and it is now out that Fauci is the one who helped them to do it. Covid then spread from China to around the world including the U.S. China, who many believe, is actually controlling the World Health Organization, making all these recommendations for the planet.

China controls our media; you do the research. I'm convinced of that. China also now owns most of our real estate in the United States of America, they have been buying it up for the past couple of decades. China owns a lot of our corporations in the United States of America. China owns most of our politicians and I'm convinced China has got China Joe in office, who isn't going to resist any of this stuff.

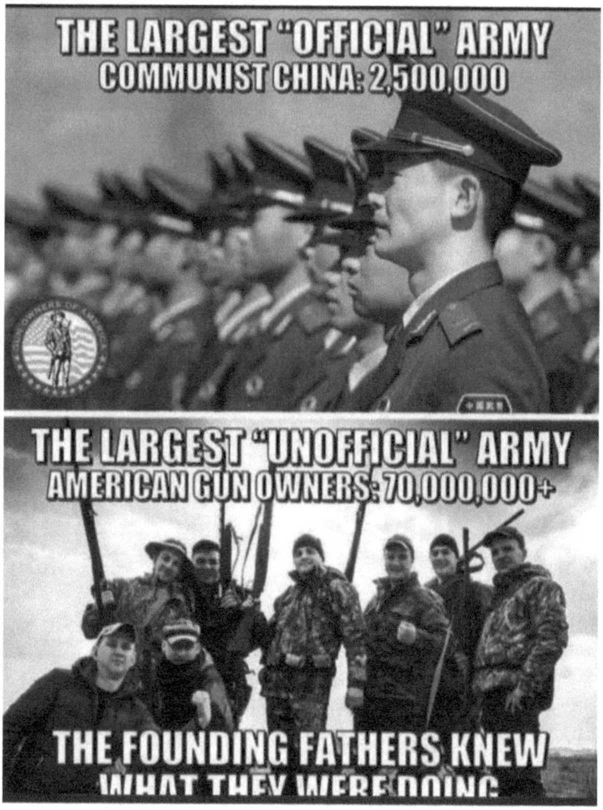

But here's the problem. You still have one problem. Nobody wants to invade, with a physical invasion, the United States of America.

And the reason why is our founding fathers were geniuses with the second amendment. The largest official army on the planet is China with 2.5 standing military. Ours is about 1.5, but outside of that we have the largest unofficial army, the American gun owner with 70 plus million. The founding fathers were geniuses. That's why we have been so well protected. They know this, do not invade

America. You will never survive. So, they have to find a different way to do it. Well, how are you going to do it?

What if you created a bioweapon, and released that into the American populace? Is that why Dr. Zelenko is saying that we are in WWIII? We need to wake up. And it isn't just a theory that they admit, it's coming out, even from people escaping from China, that Covid was, a bioweapon.

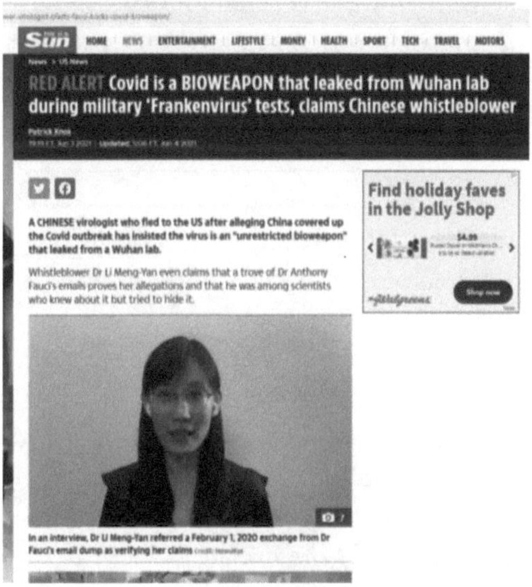

Sun HOME NEWS ENTERTAINMENT LIFESTYLE MONEY HEALTH SPORT TECH TRAVEL MOTORS

RED ALERT Covid is a BIOWEAPON that leaked from Wuhan lab during military 'Frankenvirus' tests, claims Chinese whistleblower

A CHINESE virologist who fled to the US after alleging China covered up the Covid outbreak has insisted the virus is an "unrestricted bioweapon" that leaked from a Wuhan lab.

Whistleblower Dr Li Meng-Yan even claims that a trove of Dr Anthony Fauci's emails proves her allegations and that he was among scientists who knew about it but tried to hide it.

In an interview, Dr Li Meng-Yan referred a February 1, 2020 exchange from Dr Fauci's email dump as verifying her claims

Covid is a bioweapon that leaked from Wuhan lab claimed Chinese whistleblower, a doctor. A Chinese virologist who fled to the U.S. insisted that the virus is an unrestricted bioweapon that was leaked from the Wuhan lab. Whistleblower, Dr. Li Meng-Yan even claims that a trove of Dr. Anthony Fauci's emails prove her allegations and that he was among the scientists that knew about it.

In the old days he would be considered a traitor and be hung. So, go back to the communist goal. Wait a second. We are going to take over America without even firing a shot? Oh, come on, how are you going to do that? First of all, what you do is release a bioweapon. Now the bioweapon, Covid, isn't what is going to kill people. It's the next stage. That just becomes the excuse to get the jab. The jab is what is going to kill people. And of all the entities being forced, if you look at it from a military point of view, who is being forced to take the jab? It's the U.S. military. And we ain't seen nothing yet but wait for the fallout. And wonder of wonders, people are saying, this is the takeover of the U.S. military.

Tucker Carlson: *"Another senior commander in the space force, Lieutenant Colonel Matthew Lohmeier lost his job, and we know why. His crime was criticizing Marxism. It's a fireable offense now. Then in August, Lloyd Austin came up with a new political purity test. This one was specifically designed to separate the obedient from the free. We can't have any of the latter category.*

Austin said he planned to fire anyone in the entire armed services who would not submit to the Covid-19 vaccination shot. It didn't matter whether they had natural immunity or not, as many in the military do. Their personal, moral, or religious exemptions were totally irrelevant. The point was to bow to his authority and the authority of the Democratic party. No excuses, no exception."

Lloyd Austin: *"I have determined that mandatory vaccination against coronavirus disease 2019 (Covid-19) is necessary to protect the Force and defend the American people."*

Tucker Carlson: *"Period, no debate. So, what is the scientific justification for this, well of course there isn't any. There is zero scientific basis for any of this. The fighting strength of the military is the young healthy people, virtually all of them are at extremely low risk of dying from covid, in fact to this day only 46 members of the entire US military have died from the coronavirus over the last year and a half.*

Suicides, by contrast have killed many, many times more. In just a few months last year 156 servicemen killed themselves. The military suicides are an actual crisis. Something he might want to address; he might want to look into that, but no that would get the Democratic party nothing. The point of mandatory vaccination is to identify the sincere Christians in the ranks, the free thinkers, the men with high testosterone levels and anyone else who does not love Joe Biden and make them leave immediately. It's a takeover of the U.S. military."

And I would agree, which is why one person said this: *"We are running some of the best people out of medicine, out of the military, and out of the defense industry. These people are both brilliant and talented 'and' the more freedom-minded of Americans. That should scare us all."*

Now if you think China isn't preparing for war, you better wake up. Ever since Sleepy Joe got into office, they have been pushing their boundaries in the South China Sea, Taiwan, Hong Kong. Russia right now, the communist nations, Ukraine. You think it's by chance? This guy's not going to resist. Maybe do some fumbling, bumbling thing and get us into WWIII, because that is what they want.

If you don't think China is preparing for war, I'm going to give you contrast. I am going to share with you first a commercial, a modern commercial from China to their citizens, about their military and then I'm going to show a current military commercial from the United States. All I can say is, we're in trouble!

The commercial is all spoken in Chinese. It begins with a man sitting in the lobby of a hospital. His name is called, and he immediately stands up straight at attention. It's like it has been drilled into him so hard that even in his personal life he jumps to attention. The next scene is showing 4 Chinese soldiers standing out in the middle of the desert. One left the group and had to walk a few steps, but he didn't walk. His legs were stiff, he looks like he has been made to march like this for so long that he can't walk naturally.

Then we come to a crowd of military men all standing at attention. They are all identical, uniforms are perfect, they are so stiff standing there you can hardly see them breathe. The commanding officers come in and proceed to yell commands. They still do not move. At perfect attention, then they salute. Every word that comes out of their mouths is a yell, like they are mentally abusing the soldiers as they stand there at perfect attention. Even when one is being spoken to individually the tone is loud and abusive. The scene then changes to what looks like a career that can be obtained through the military from medical to space travel to weapons to war battles with tanks, guns, parachutes and underwater scuba attire.

And here's a recent U.S. commercial:

This commercial isn't actual people playing the parts, it is a cartoon message. The scene opens about a female soldier who operates the patriot missile defense system. The girl's story, as she is telling it, begins in California about a little girl raised by two moms. *"Although I had a fairly typical childhood, I took ballet, played violin, I also marched for equality. I like to think I was defending freedom from an early age.*

When I was 6 years old one of my mom's had an accident and was paralyzed. The doctors said she might never walk again. But she worked to get back on her feet, eventually standing at the altar marrying my other mom. With such powerful role models, I finished high school at the top of my class. I then attended UC Davis and joined the sorority with other strong women."

Do you think that is just by chance? Do you think China has a big influence on our media? That was their commercial and full of some serious testosterone and then your feminizing the U.S. military? And it's not just that, it's the socialist agenda mindset which is the codeword for communism. Which is also being done in our school system. So, if communism were to come over here to America do you think people would resist? No. But that's our military, we're in trouble.

So, go back to the communist takeover plan. "We're going to take over America without firing a shot." Can they do that? Well after you decimate the military patriots and you force the rest of them to get the jab, most of them are going to die off, according to the doctors, if that were to take place. So, whatever is left of the military in the U.S., is people who are into socialism like that who will go along with it and think it's great. Then the next thing you know we are completely decimated. That's just the military, just that one entity, who's being forced to get the jab.

Now the rest of the American population, why would you want the American population? Because you have 70 million plus gun owners that are standing in your way, but not if they get the jab. Anybody putting this together? Like me maybe. Again, I can't say, thus saith the Lord, but it's starting to stack up for me. You just wait a couple of years and voila! Maybe that's why America gets merged into one of these economic kingdoms.

There aren't enough people left. They destroyed our economy, they destroyed our military, they destroyed America's people. And then they will come over here without firing a shot and they will act like our savior. Sounds like a plan. Oh, and for those of you who are doing the swab test, you might want to do the research, that too is coming from China, and you know what? It also causes cancer.

"Hi, this is Kassandra, you favorite registered nurse, coming to you live from an undisclosed location. I just wanted to let everybody know that not only am I a registered nurse for several decades, almost three, I am also a medical investigator. I am bringing you information today about the swab, the swab that is used to test for the current claimed pandemic. Facebook took down my previous video, it just happened to disappear, so I am bringing you another one.

So, the swabs that are used for testing, I have two of them here made by different manufacturers. The first one is made by Ningbo HLS Medical products, and it's made in China. On it, it says sterile/EO. Keep that in mind because I'm going to give you more information about what the EO stands for. The other one is made by Miraclean Technology, and it also is made in China. It also says sterile/EO.

So, these are two sterile swabs that are used deep into the nasal cavity, halfway up to your skull to test for the current pandemic. I don't want to say the name of it because I don't want to be banned again from Facebook.

So, what is EO? EO stands for Ethylene Oxide. So, these swabs are saturated with, coated with EO. So, what is ethylene oxide? Per the United States Environmental Protection Agency, the EPA classified ethylene oxide as a human carcinogen in December 2016. The EPA as well as the

International Agency for Research on cancer and the national toxicology program classifies ethylene oxide as a carcinogen to humans.

Evidence in humans indicate that exposure to ethylene oxide by inhalation increases the risk of lymphoma cancers, Myeloma and leukemias and for female's breast cancer. Ethylene oxide is mutagenic which means it can change the DNA in your cells. Children may be more susceptible to the harmful effects of mutagenic substances."

So, if China doesn't get you with the jab, they're going to get you with the swab. And don't forget they are making the bulk of the masks too. They are making a ton of money. Anyone see a pattern here? If that's the case, not saying thus saith the Lord but maybe that is what happens to America. Maybe that is why we don't see America in Bible prophecy.

And if you think they are going to come over here and be our heroes … You decimate the economy, you decimate the population, whoever is left, the non-patriots, they are going to welcome them. Believe it or not, this has been the plan for a long time. I want to share with you, this is the map from the World Association of Parliamentarians. The World Government Army Map from as far back as 1952. You can check it out for yourself. Let me break down that map. The plan is to have foreign troops stationed in foreign countries to help control the world. Now why? Well, common sense, you would think it would be very hard for an American soldier to kill a fellow American, so you have to fix that.

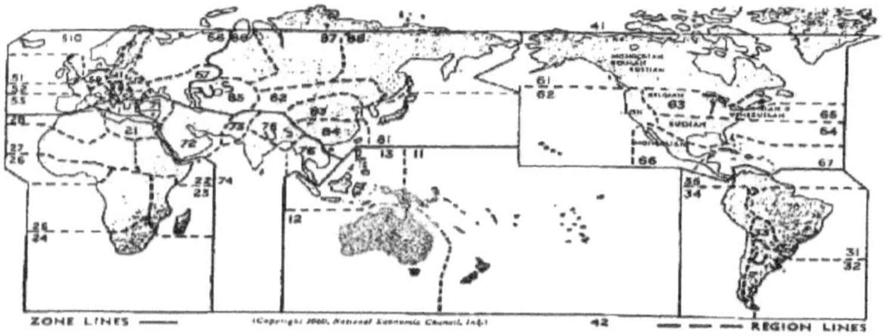

United States troops to be stationed:
Region 12. Australia
Region 32. Uruguay, Argensine
Region 55. Yugoslavia, Greece, Albania, Roumania, Bulgaria.
Region 58. Austria, Hungary, Czechoslovakia
Region 75. India, Nepal, Bhutan, Tibet, E. Pakistan.
Region 85. Kazak SSR, Turkmen, Usbeg, Tadshik, Kirghiz SSR.

This map, adopted in 1952 in London by the *World Association of Parliamentarians for World Government*, shows what alien troops would occupy and police the six regions into which the United States and Canada would be divided.

The ruling body or World Parliament would consist only of appointed members. It would reflect population strengths, so Asia would dominate it.

There would be a World Director, 8 zone directors and 51 regional directors. None of the zone or regional directors would ever serve in their own countries. So an alien would command troops stationed in the U. S. and through them enforce World Government law, and prevent Americans from "sheltering behind national allegiance."

That's what this map is all about. It's been on the books since 1952. But not if you had Chinese soldiers over here. And that actually is what this map delineates, and I quote:

"The details of having Chinese, Russian, Columbian, Venezuelan, and Belgium troops stationed in the United States of America."

They wouldn't have a problem with shooting American's. And then American troops will be stationed in Europe to help control things over there. If they go down, at least it's not a fellow American. Do you see what they are doing? And then that brings Henry Kissinger's fatal surreal comment into play:

Henry Kissinger: *"Today America would be outraged if UN troops entered Los Angeles to restore order. Tomorrow they will be grateful. When presented with this scenario, individual rights will be willingly relinquished for the guarantee of their well-being granted to them by the World Government."*

You know after a Covid delayed death issue, the complete decimation of our economy, and you know what? You never once fired a shot. And you took over America. Where have I heard that before? So, again, is that what happens to America? Could be! But what we do know is that this leads up to the antichrist kingdom. What we are talking about tonight occurs during the 7-year Tribulation and we leave at the Rapture.

So, that tells me the Rapture has to be getting close. So, I want to leave you with what the Bible says so you don't ask "What do I do? What do I do with all of this? I thought the last chapter was bad. No, we need to get back to what I call Plan A. Did you know there has never been a Plan B for the Church? Never, we just need to get back to Plan A. In fact, God specifically tells us what to do, specifically for the day that we live in, as we await the Rapture.

He tells us what we are supposed to do. It's not to cry and whine, it's not to freak out and get afraid, it's not to comply, it's not to obey our overlord masters, it's to resist! Put up a fight! Now I didn't say that God did. God tells us exactly what we do. The man of lawlessness, the antichrist, God tells us to await the rapture, especially as we see the signs of this coming kingdom in the 7-year tribulation arise all around us.

2 Thessalonians 2:1-10 "Concerning the coming of our Lord Jesus Christ and our being gathered to him (the Rapture), we ask you, brothers, not to become easily unsettled or alarmed by some prophecy, report or letter supposed to have come from us, saying that the day of the Lord has already come. Don't let anyone deceive you in any way, for that day will not come until the rebellion occurs and the man of lawlessness is revealed, the man doomed to destruction. He will oppose and will exalt himself over everything that is called God or is worshiped, so that he sets himself up in God's temple, proclaiming himself to be God. Don't you remember than when I was with you I used to tell you these things? And now you know what is holding him back, so that he may be revealed at the proper time. For the secret power of lawlessness is already at work; but the one who now holds it back will continue to do so till he is taken out of the way (the church). And then the lawless one will be revealed, whom the Lord Jesus will overthrow with the breath of his mouth and destroy by the splendor of his coming. The coming of the lawless one will be in accordance with the work of Satan displayed in all kinds of counterfeit miracles, signs and wonders and in every sort of evil that deceived those who are perishing. They perish because they refused to love the truth and so be saved."

As we dealt with in our Rapture study, the day of the Lord starts at the beginning of the 7-year Tribulation and moves forward. So basically, when some say you are already in the 7-year Tribulation, no. How will we know when the lawless one, the antichrist, will appear? **Daniel 9:27** when he makes the peace treaty, covenant with Israel. That's the event that starts the 7-year Tribulation.

Then he sets himself up in the Temple in the middle of the 7-year Tribulation. The Bible tells us exactly what we are supposed to do. You don't have to pray, what am I supposed to do? He tells you. You are to restrain, resist. The Greek word means to hold back, to restrain, to hinder the course of progress thereof. You know why these guys haven't nailed it in the coffin yet? It's because we are still here. Because there are faithful people and dare I say Christians that are speaking up against this.

And the Bible says when we are out of here there is nothing holding him back. But he tells us, in the meantime while we are still here, we need to restrain, not comply, not deny, not condone, not go along with this. We need to fight back. We need to restrain. We need to speak up. That's what we are supposed to do on this Covid issue. We need to resist! This is WWIII, like Dr. Zelenko said. And this is why these people said this.

"Stop receiving advice from people who are not being advised by God!"

Christian, hello. One guy said this, If Facebook existed in 1776, and someone said, "the British are coming, the British are coming, nope, false information, not all the British are coming, only part of the British are coming." Another guy said this, are you kidding me? I guess that is why Rodney Dangerfield said this. And somebody wouldn't

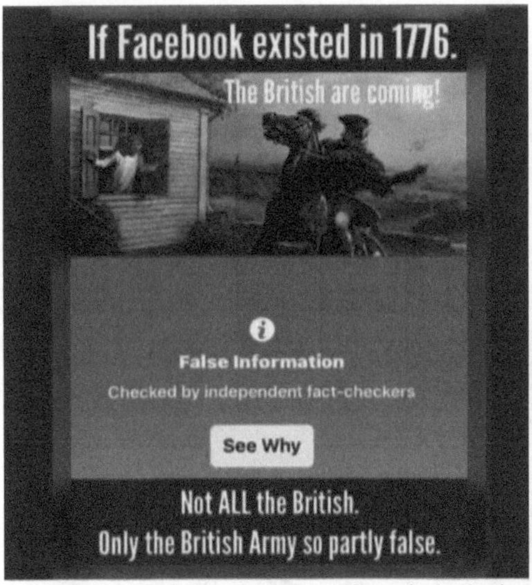
If Facebook existed in 1776.
False Information
Checked by independent fact-checkers
See Why
Not ALL the British.
Only the British Army so partly false.

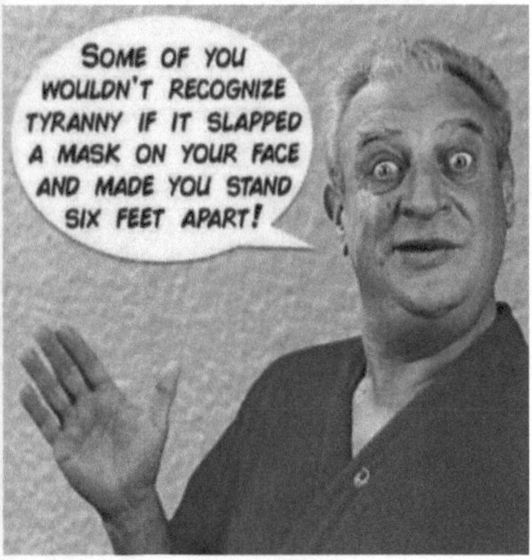
SOME OF YOU WOULDN'T RECOGNIZE TYRANNY IF IT SLAPPED A MASK ON YOUR FACE AND MADE YOU STAND SIX FEET APART!

even recognize tyranny when it is being broadcast live on TV.

Hitler/Biden: *"I will sign an executive order that will now require all executive branch, federal employees to be vaccinated. ALL! Then I will sign another executive order that will require federal contractors to do the same. If you want to work with the federal government and do business with us? GET VACCINATED!"*

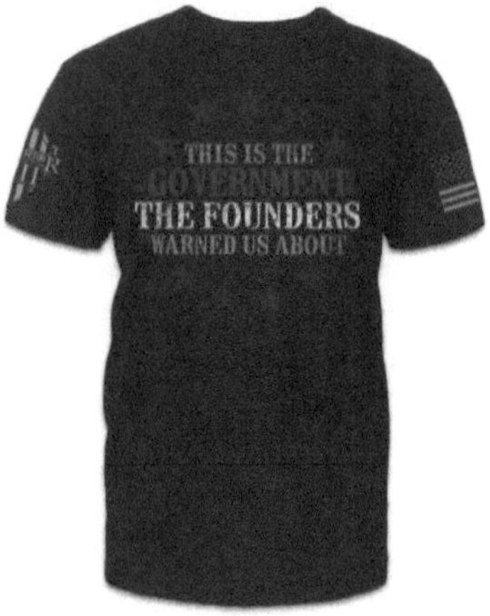

Yeah, that is called a tyrant. And can I tell you what, this is the government that the founding father warned us about.

You just saw it on TV, in fact another person said this. The mask that could end it all.

If we would speak up and get motivated on this issue. We are not to roll back. We are not to be afraid. We are to resist. We are to restrain. Are you restraining? Speak up and stop being a bunch of chickens. We need to get our American backbone back. I'm telling you our founding fathers must be rolling over in their graves. We need to speak up! They will give me back my freedom if I just keep complying. Freedom isn't a reward for good behavior, that's how prisons operate. Freedom comes from God! It's a violation.

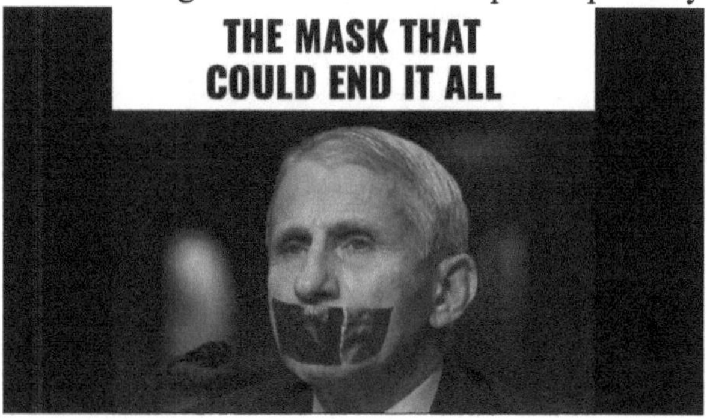

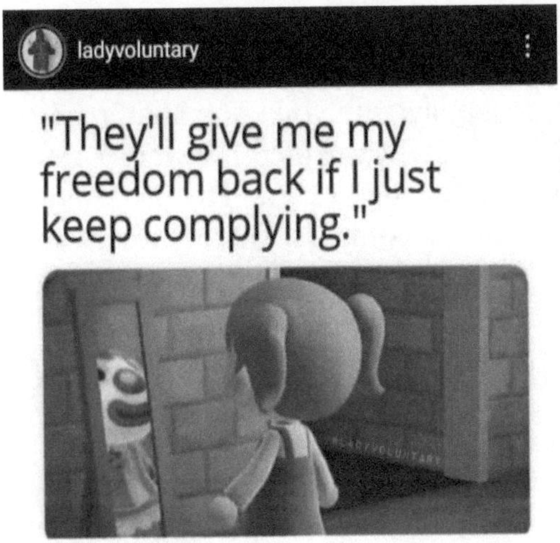

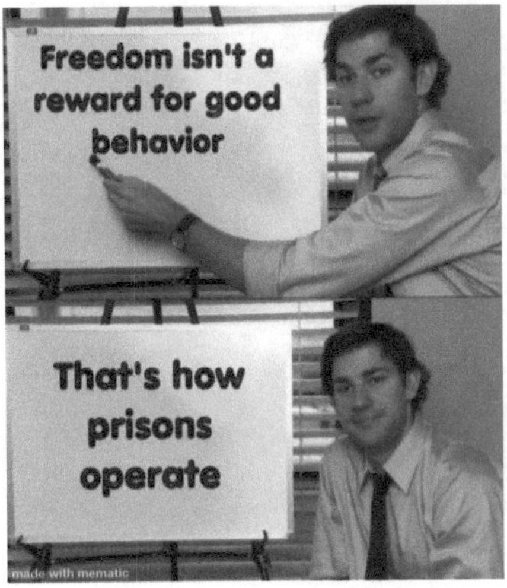

And this is where it's headed. You're hiding unvaccinated people under your floorboards, aren't you? It's coming.

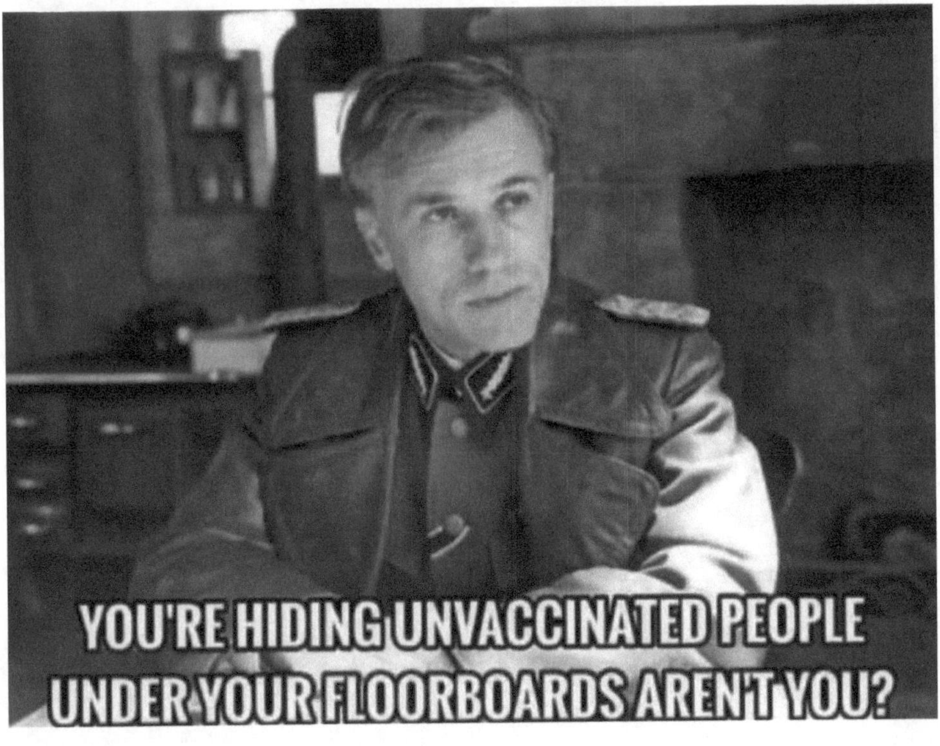

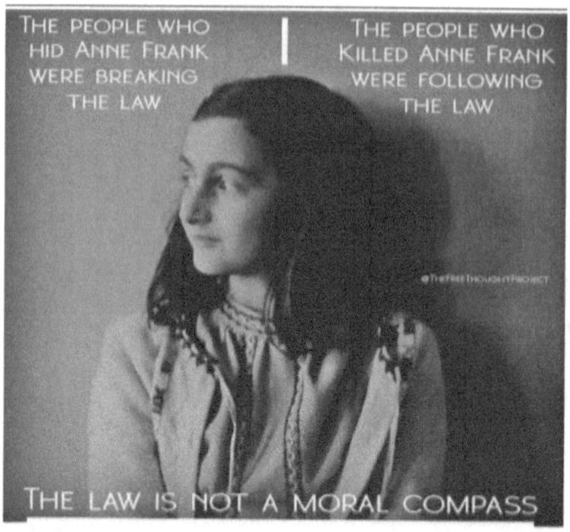

By the way, the people who were hiding Anne Frank were breaking the law, did you know that? The people who killed her were following the law. The law is not a moral compass. God is. If you've ever wondered whether you would have complied during 1930s Germany, now you know. Let that sink in.

And it's better to walk alone than with a crowd going in the wrong direction. You need to be that guy and stop being afraid. You need to speak up, I don't care how much they are going in the wrong direction.
That's what we are supposed to do.

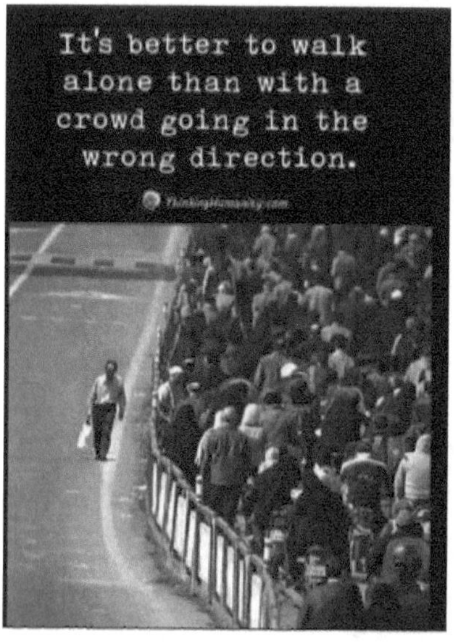

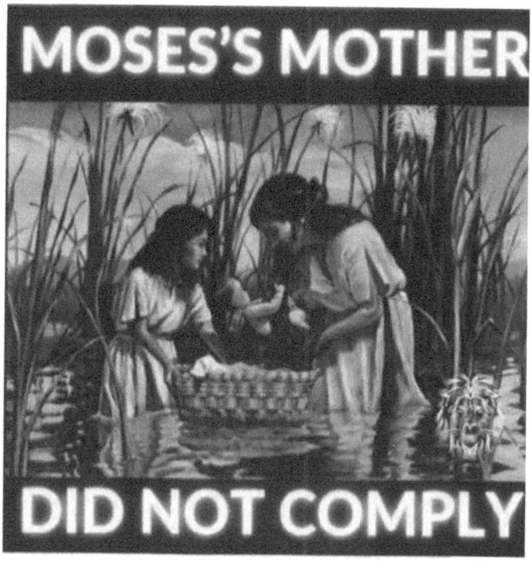

Oh, by the way, Moses' mother didn't comply, read your Bible. Read the Bible, resist! Do not comply, speak up! That's what God says we need to do. And if you don't think this junk is going to come here, like in Canada, now you can't have food if you don't get the jab. I'm telling you;

Canada and Australia, I'm convinced, are the pretext of what they plan to do to America if we don't speak up and resist and get motivated. Australia right now is sending people, if you don't get the jab, to a concentration camp, I mean a Covid Camp, this is happening right now.

Stew Peters: *"You may have noticed that we have been talking a lot about Australia over the last couple of weeks and we are doing that for a reason. Because as bad as things have been in America, Australia shows how things can still get worse in the direction that we could be headed. Two years ago, Australia wasn't some dictatorship like China, it was a regular democracy, with regular elections that were fairer than ours. Australia isn't some alien culture like South Korea, it speaks English, it's a former British colony with English derived laws.*

Australia was, until Covid, a relatively free country, but now it's a horrifying dystopia. It's a hellscape where police will inspect your Starbucks cup to make sure it has coffee in it. It's a country where you can be fined thousands of dollars for violating the ever-changing health rules. How did this happen to Australia?

It's a country whose heritage is a lot like America. Its early settlers were pioneers who had to fend for themselves and carve out a living in a hostile country. This is a country with nine of the world's ten deadliest snakes plus the worlds most poisonous spiders and some of its most dangerous plants. It's a hard country. But now it is forced to submit. Why?

Well for one the public has been substantially disarmed. After a mass shooting in Port Arthur Tasmania, the government has made one of the most aggressive gun grabs in human history. In just a few years the government seized and destroyed more than a million guns. About one-third of all guns in the country.

Now to own a gun in Australia you need a license. To get that license you have to convince the government that you have a valid reason to have it. And no, self-defense is not considered a valid reason. Nor is, I'm afraid my government might be taken over by a totalitarian psychopath.

So, in short, Australian's are no longer citizens, they are subjects. They don't get their rights from Almighty God; they get them from their almighty government which can strip them away whenever it feels like it."

This is from an actual Australian Covid Camp: A man or guard, dressed in a white gown with gloves and mask is standing outside the window talking to a lady that is in confinement sitting on her porch.

Lady in confinement: *"Am I allowed to go to the laundry?"*

Guard: *"You are allowed to go to the laundry, but you've got to wear a mask. You definitely can't go up to the fencing rails. But you're allowed to go to the laundry, yeah. That's always been the case."*

Lady in confinement: *"So if I was sitting right here,* (she points to a table and chair at the other side of her porch but next to the fencing rails) *right next to the fence, why do you put the cabin right next to the fence? It makes no sense. Does it?"*

Guard: *"Yeah, but you can't leave your balcony to go to the fence to talk to somebody else. That's just obvious. Again, it doesn't have to make sense. There has to be lines everywhere drawn, yeah. And one of the lines is you cannot leave your balcony and you cannot go to someone else. When it makes no sense or doesn't seem right to you, that is the line, and that's what the law is, and that's how it goes. That's the law."*

Lady in confinement: *"That the law allows?"*

Guard: *"Yep, there's a CHO direction on how the behavior must be done, especially in this area because it's much more highly infectious and likely to have infected people here."*

Lady in confinement: *"Highly infectious when all of us people are negative."*

Guard: *"So far, the risk is still very high."*

Why are you in a camp if you are negative? It has nothing to do with that. Look at this. An Australian man was arrested for escaping from one of these camps.

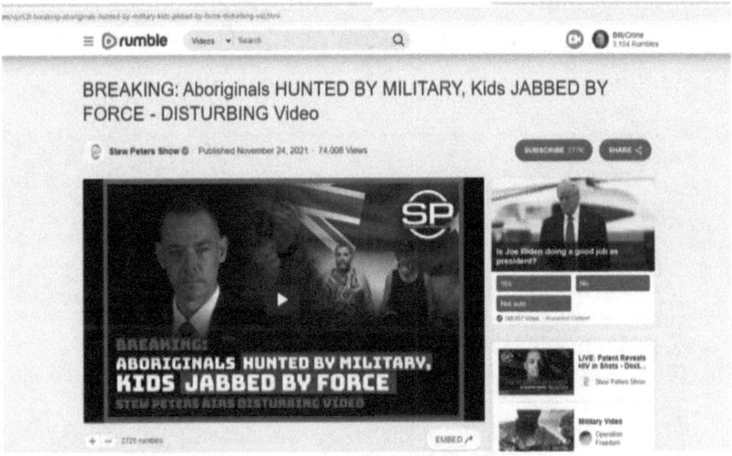
rumble
BREAKING: Aboriginals HUNTED BY MILITARY, Kids JABBED BY FORCE - DISTURBING Video
SP
BREAKING:
ABORIGINALS HUNTED BY MILITARY,
KIDS JABBED BY FORCE
STEW PETERS AIRS DISTURBING VIDEO
EMBED

"After a large-scale manhunt ensued following his escape from a Quarantine Camp, testing negative for the virus."

This has nothing to do with Covid. This is actually going on as we sit here. Which is why one guy sent me this email last week. This is what is going on down there. He said:

"Hey Billy, I love your ministry. There is currently no ministry related to Jesus in Australia. I have a wife and a young son, and I am attempting to plan our escape. We got passports, not Covid passports obviously, but I currently have my house on the market and I'm going to buy a yacht. I don't know how to sail, but I am going to learn, thank you Jesus."

He's going to buy a boat to get out of there!

"I'm planning to come to the states before the Rapture as it will be good to be around Christians that pray again. I believe your church is in Nevada. I'm going to aim for Florida, but I am confident that I can assist Jesus if I can get to your church and support your ministry, however I can. Love you, Bro. Cheers in Jesus."

It's the same stuff that went on in Germany. It's happening again and if we don't start resisting as the church, it's just going to come that much faster here. Down there they are doing forceful jabs on the people including the Aboriginals. It's sick! They are chasing them down and jabbing them. And it's getting closer to Canada. Canada's Covid jails are termed worse than ever.

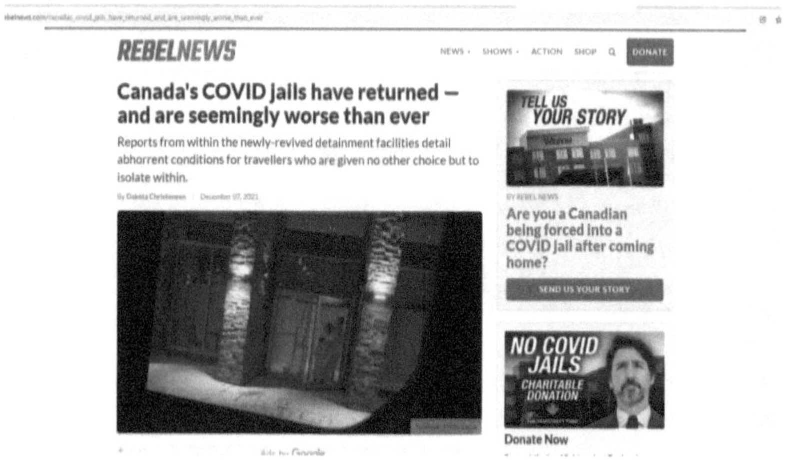
REBELNEWS

NEWS · SHOWS · ACTION SHOP DONATE

Canada's COVID jails have returned — and are seemingly worse than ever

Reports from within the newly-revived detainment facilities detail abhorrent conditions for travellers who are given no other choice but to isolate within.

TELL US YOUR STORY

Are you a Canadian being forced into a COVID jail after coming home?

SEND US YOUR STORY

NO COVID JAILS

CHARITABLE DONATION

Donate Now

And by the way, if you don't think history isn't repeating itself, how many have ever said, Gesundheit whenever someone sneezed? We assume that's German for God Bless You. It's not. You know what it is? It's German for good health. And it comes from back in Hitler's days. Here is a picture of one. It goes back to the Nazis first step of locking the Jews up. They gave people what was called a Gesundheit pass. A "good health" passport so they could continue to walk around and work in society, for those who were deemed healthy. One guy said this:

"The Nazi Germany had a health pass too. It was called the Gesundheit pass. The Nazis also used their methods to

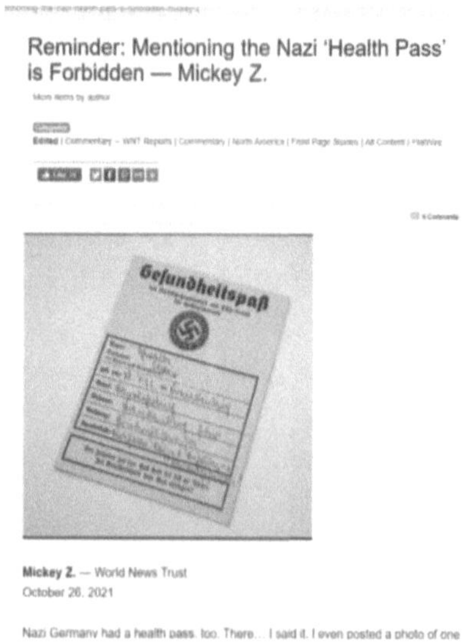
Reminder: Mentioning the Nazi 'Health Pass' is Forbidden — Mickey Z.

Mickey Z. — World News Trust
October 26, 2021

Nazi Germany had a health pass, too. There... I said it. I even posted a photo of one *segregate their own population with such methods. Try mentioning this in the context of Covid-19 vaccine passport and be prepared for the onslaught."*

We say Gesundheit and we don't even know what it means. It's happening again. You know why they are doing it? Because those who don't know their history are doomed to repeat it. We have a school system today where kids don't even know who Hitler is. They don't even believe there was an actual holocaust. Now they want to merge those passports into microchips. Just like Klaus Schwab said was coming with this new Great Reset.

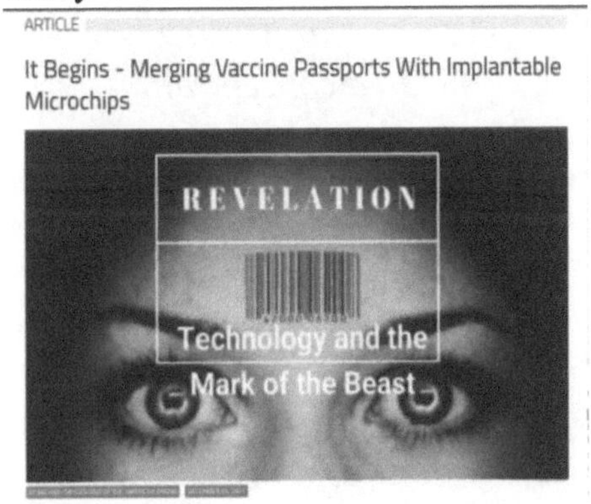

Merging vaccine passports with implantable microchips and watch, people are doing this willingly to themselves. They are putting microchips that contain your vaccine passport information into their hands and they are raving about how convenient it is. I don't know about you but the last time this kind of stuff went on, you know how much of a hassle it was when people would approach you and say show me your papers. It's no different. It's happening again.

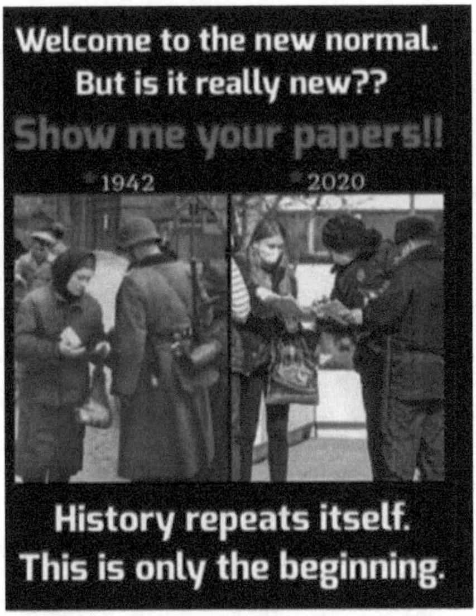
Welcome to the new normal.
But is it really new??
Show me your papers!!
1942
2020
History repeats itself.
This is only the beginning.

And speaking of this, while this was going on, these Gesundheit passports, "good health" passports, at the same time, they were making the Jewish people look bad, dirty and unclean. They would show posters like this. This is one of them. "They've

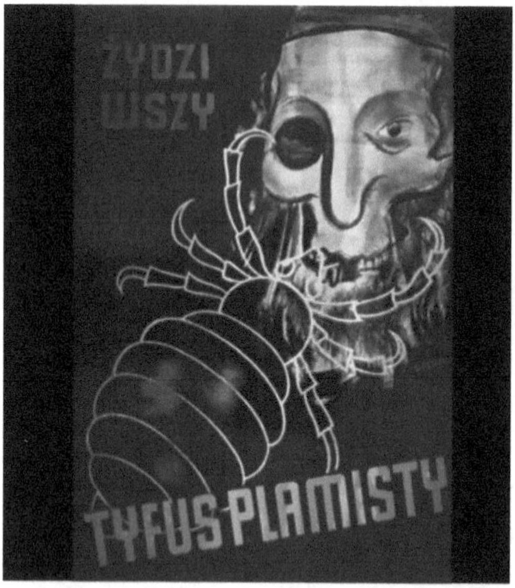

got lice, dirty, get rid of them!" They used the German propaganda to make the Jewish people look dirty and unclean. One Jewish lady said, *"You better wake up, it's the same thing!" "I was only three and a half when my family and I were evicted from our homes and deported to a concentration camp. Here our infectious epidemics are exactly what the Nazis used to dehumanize Jews as spreaders of disease. Today, the unvaccinated are being accused of being spreaders of disease."*

In other words, it's the same tactic. They can do it because we don't even know our own history. And dare I say we have lost our American backbone. Lest you doubt that they are spreading the propaganda, making us who have not gotten the jab, look like the bad guys, the unclean, the vermin. You better start reading some headlines. It's all over the place.

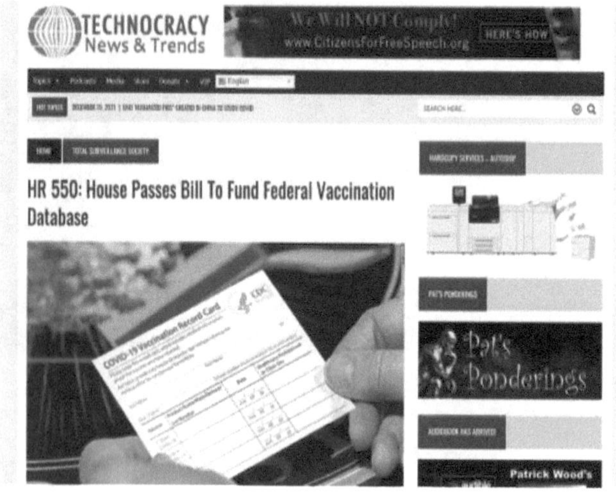

HR bill passes to fund federal vaccination database. Why would you want to do that? Because they are going to track who got it and who didn't.

This just happened. Pfizer CEO says people who spread misinformation on Covid vaccines are criminals.

Just today, the governor of a state here in America is calling people that don't get the shot not only criminals, but they are terrorists. We are terrorists, right?

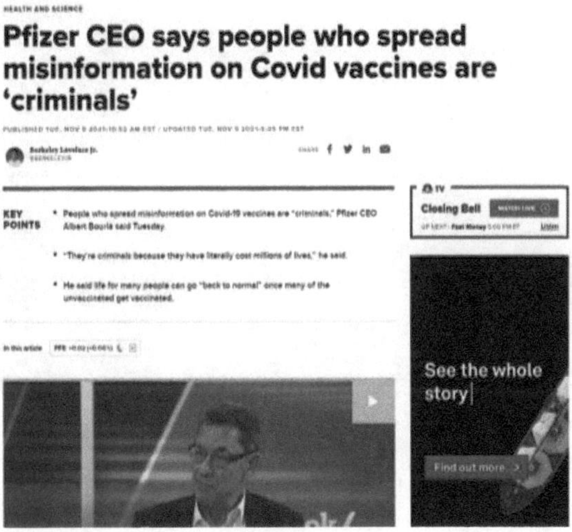

HEALTH AND SCIENCE

Pfizer CEO says people who spread misinformation on Covid vaccines are 'criminals'

KEY POINTS

- People who spread misinformation on Covid-19 vaccines are "criminals," Pfizer CEO Albert Bourla said Tuesday.
- "They're criminals because they have literally cost millions of lives," he said.
- He said life for many people can go "back to normal" once many of the unvaccinated get vaccinated.

Closing Bell

See the whole story

Find out more

Nevada becomes the first state to impose a surcharge on unvaccinated workers.

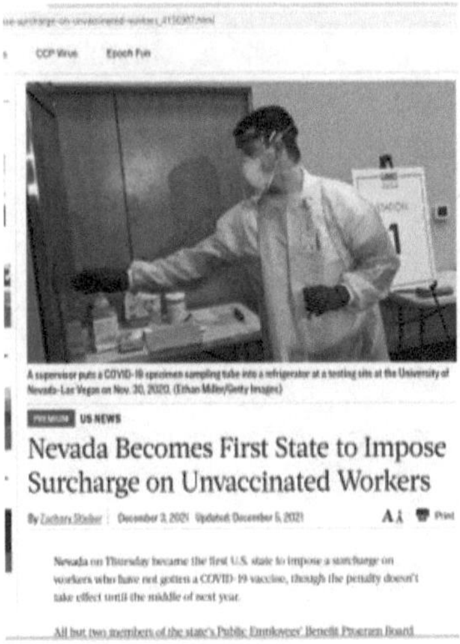

A supervisor puts a COVID-19 specimen sampling tube into a refrigerator at a testing site at the University of Nevada-Las Vegas on Nov. 30, 2020. (Ethan Miller/Getty Images)

US NEWS

Nevada Becomes First State to Impose Surcharge on Unvaccinated Workers

December 3, 2021 Updated: December 5, 2021

Nevada on Thursday became the first U.S. state to impose a surcharge on workers who have not gotten a COVID-19 vaccine, though the penalty doesn't take effect until the middle of next year.

All but two members of the state's Public Employees' Benefit Program Board

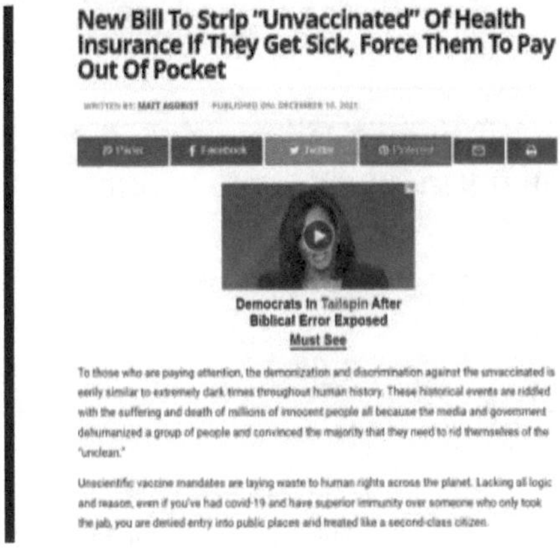

New Bill To Strip "Unvaccinated" Of Health Insurance If They Get Sick, Force Them To Pay Out Of Pocket

Democrats In Tailspin After Biblical Error Exposed

Must See

To those who are paying attention, the demonization and discrimination against the unvaccinated is eerily similar to extremely dark times throughout human history. These historical events are riddled with the suffering and death of millions of innocent people all because the media and government dehumanized a group of people and convinced the majority that they need to rid themselves of the "unclean."

Unscientific vaccine mandates are laying waste to human rights across the planet. Lacking all logic and reason, even if you've had covid-19 and have superior immunity over someone who only took the jab, you are denied entry into public places and treated like a second-class citizen.

A new bill to strip the "Unvaccinated" of health insurance if they get sick and force them to pay out of pocket.

Military takeover: Fired unvaccinated nurses being replaced by National Guard troops. Why are you inviting the military in on that?

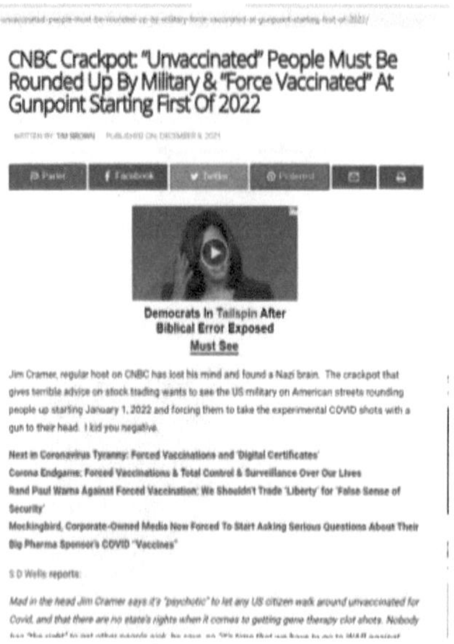

CNBC Crackpot: "Unvaccinated" People Must Be Rounded Up By Military & "Force Vaccinated" At Gunpoint Starting First Of 2022

Democrats In Tailspin After Biblical Error Exposed
Must See

Jim Cramer, regular host on CNBC has lost his mind and found a Nazi brain. The crackpot that gives terrible advice on stock trading wants to see the US military on American streets rounding people up starting January 1, 2022 and forcing them to take the experimental COVID shots with a gun to their head. I kid you negative.

Next in Coronavirus Tyranny: Forced Vaccinations and 'Digital Certificates'
Corona Endgame: Forced Vaccinations & Total Control & Surveillance Over Our Lives
Rand Paul Warns Against Forced Vaccination: We Shouldn't Trade 'Liberty' for 'False Sense of Security'
Mockingbird, Corporate-Owned Media Now Forced To Start Asking Serious Questions About Their Big Pharma Sponsor's COVID "Vaccines"

S D Wells reports:

Mad in the head Jim Cramer says it's "psychotic" to let any US citizen walk around unvaccinated for Covid, and that there are no state's rights when it comes to getting gene therapy clot shots. Nobody

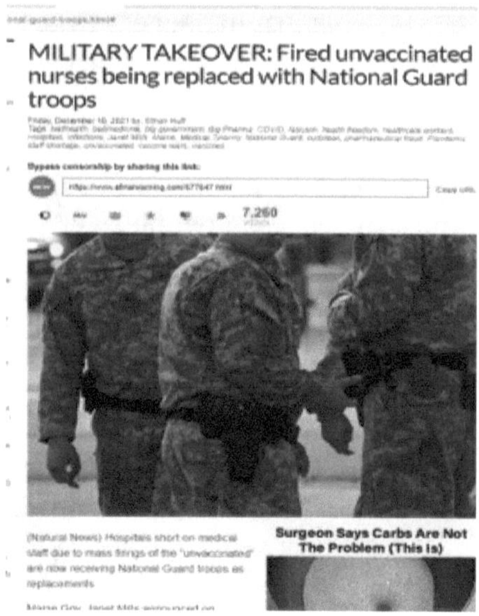

MILITARY TAKEOVER: Fired unvaccinated nurses being replaced with National Guard troops

Bypass censorship by sharing this link:

7,260

(Natural News) Hospitals short on medical staff due to mass firings of the "unvaccinated" are now receiving National Guard troops as replacements

Surgeon Says Carbs Are Not The Problem (This Is)

Another one says that unvaccinated people must be rounded up by the military and forced vaccinated at gunpoint starting the first of 2022.

CNBC Pundit calls unvaxxed people "psychotic' demands U.S. military hunt them down, force vaccine or force quarantine.

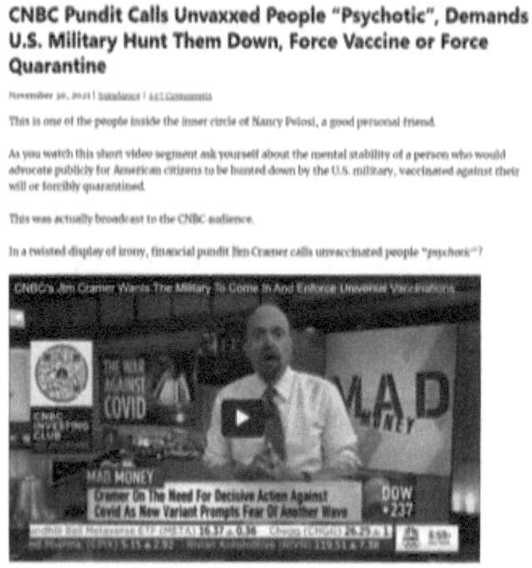

CNBC Pundit Calls Unvaxxed People "Psychotic", Demands U.S. Military Hunt Them Down, Force Vaccine or Force Quarantine

This is one of the people inside the inner circle of Nancy Pelosi, a good personal friend.

As you watch this short video segment ask yourself about the mental stability of a person who would advocate publicly for American citizens to be hunted down by the U.S. military, vaccinated against their will or forcibly quarantined.

This was actually broadcast to the CNBC audience.

In a twisted display of irony, financial pundit Jim Cramer calls unvaccinated people "psychotic"?

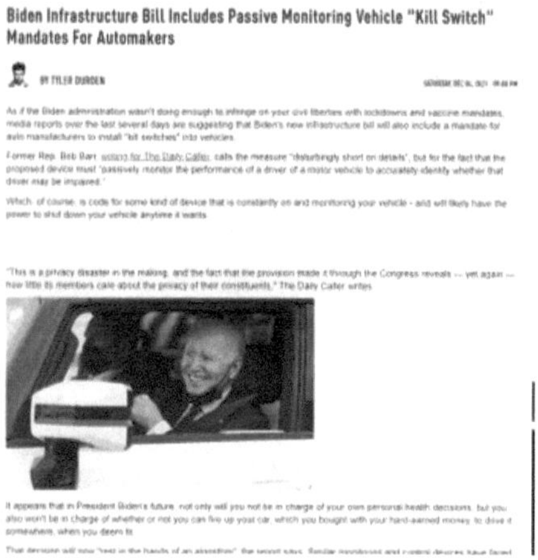

Biden Infrastructure Bill Includes Passive Monitoring Vehicle "Kill Switch" Mandates For Automakers

BY TYLER DURDEN

As if the Biden administration wasn't doing enough to infringe on your civil liberties with lockdowns and vaccine mandates, media reports over the last several days are suggesting that Biden's new infrastructure bill will also include a mandate for auto manufacturers to install "kill switches" into vehicles.

Former Rep. Bob Barr, writing for The Daily Caller, calls the measure "disturbingly short on details", but for the fact that the proposed device must "passively monitor the performance of a driver of a motor vehicle to accurately identify whether that driver may be impaired."

Which, of course, is code for some kind of device that is constantly on and monitoring your vehicle - and will likely have the power to shut down your vehicle anytime it wants.

"This is a privacy disaster in the making, and the fact that the provision made it through the Congress reveals — yet again — how little its members care about the privacy of their constituents," The Daily Caller writes.

Biden snuck this into the
infrastructure bill that includes passive monitoring vehicle "kill switch"

mandates for automakers. So, if you try to run away, you won't be able to run. Germany announces national lockdown for who? The unvaccinated.

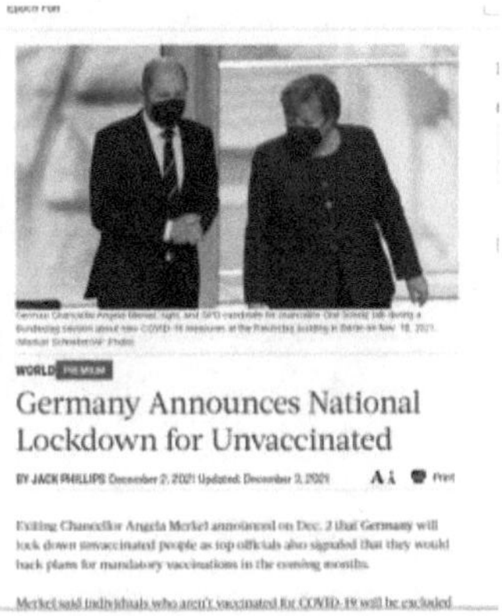

WORLD

Germany Announces National Lockdown for Unvaccinated

BY JACK PHILLIPS December 2, 2021 Updated: December 3, 2021

Exiting Chancellor Angela Merkel announced on Dec. 2 that Germany will lock down unvaccinated people as top officials also signaled that they would back plans for mandatory vaccinations in the coming months.

Merkel said individuals who aren't vaccinated for COVID-19 will be excluded

Austria and Germany locking down the unvaccinated, EU leader calls for throwing out the Nuremberg Code in favor of forced vaccinating all dissenters. They even admit what they are doing. They are just throwing that thing out; it doesn't work with their agenda.

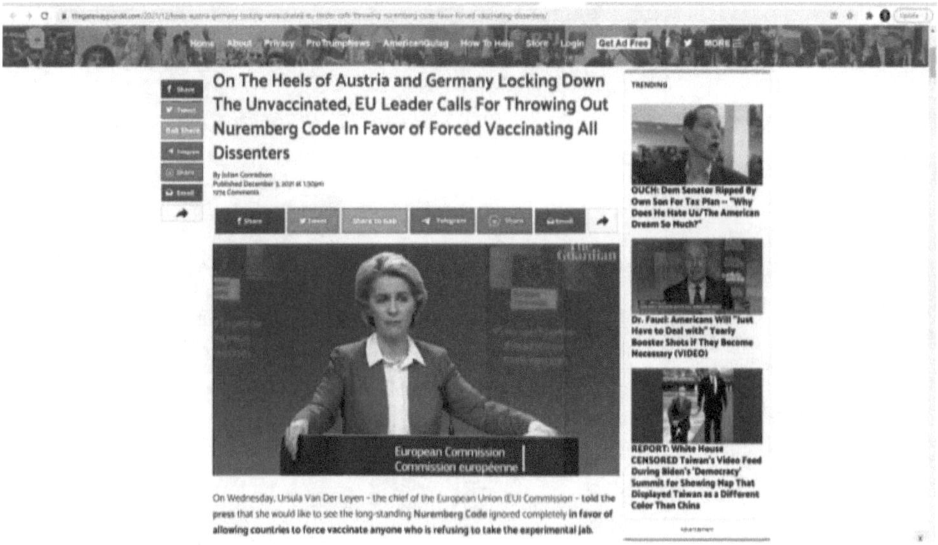

On The Heels of Austria and Germany Locking Down The Unvaccinated, EU Leader Calls For Throwing Out Nuremberg Code In Favor of Forced Vaccinating All Dissenters

On Wednesday, Ursula Van Der Leyen - the chief of the European Union (EU) Commission - told the press that she would like to see the long-standing Nuremberg Code ignored completely in favor of allowing countries to force vaccinate anyone who is refusing to take the experimental jab.

TRENDING

OUCH: Dem Senator Ripped By Own Son For Tax Plan – "Why Does He Hate Us/The American Dream So Much?"

Dr. Fauci: Americans Will "Just Have to Deal with" Yearly Booster Shots If They Become Necessary (VIDEO)

REPORT: White House CENSORED Taiwan's Video Feed During Biden's 'Democracy' Summit for Showing Map That Displayed Taiwan as a Different Color Than China

Oh, and by the way, now they are developing mRNA vegetables so that grocery stores can hide the 'vaccines' in your food.

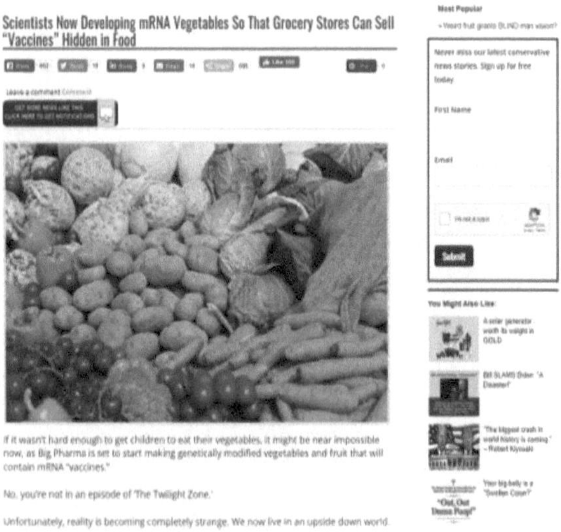
Scientists Now Developing mRNA Vegetables So That Grocery Stores Can Sell "Vaccines" Hidden in Food

If it wasn't hard enough to get children to eat their vegetables, it might be near impossible now, as Big Pharma is set to start making genetically modified vegetables and fruit that will contain mRNA "vaccines."

No, you're not in an episode of 'The Twilight Zone.'

Unfortunately, reality is becoming completely strange. We now live in an upside down world.

We're going to get it in you one way or the other. Now people are saying that you better wake up America because we are going to have to publicly resist Covid quarantine camps.

Aw, come on, there are not Covid camps in America. Yes, there is. I just checked it out this week. Go to the CDC, of course they don't call it Covid camps, it would freak people out. It's called the shielding approach. It's still up on the CDC website and let let me share with you the definition.

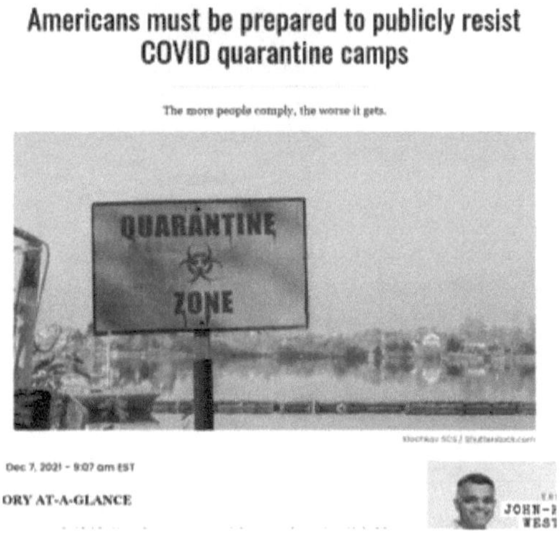
Americans must be prepared to publicly resist COVID quarantine camps

The more people comply, the worse it gets.

Dec 7, 2021 - 9:07 am EST

"The shielding approach aims to reduce the number of severe Covid-19 cases by limiting contact between individuals at higher risk of developing severe disease (high-risk) and the general population (low-risk). High-risk individuals would be temporarily relocated to safe or

'green zones' established at the household, neighborhood, camp/sector or community level depending on the context and setting. They would have minimal contact with family members and other low-risk residents."

If you don't think the Nazi socialist propagandist aren't working on some of the people in America, watch what this girl did. Pray for her. She said,

"Hoping and praying that those lost to the violence in Waukesha just now were unvaccinated."

Then a few hours later she posted:

"Glad to see people starting to understand what must be done to the unvaccinated. We always win!"

Folks, we better get busy doing what God says to do. It's not a time to freak out. It's not a time to be afraid. Don't go AWOL or hide out in the hills. You need to resist. And God told us what to do in the meantime. Restrain against this. Speak up, fight back. We need to get a true backbone like Christians, like this Canadian Polish Pastor did when they came to his church.

As the six police are coming in, he confronts them and he says.

"Please get out. Get out of this property immediately. Immediately get out! Get out of this property immediately! Out! I don't want to see you in this property. I don't want to hear a word. Out! Out! Out of this property. Immediately! You come back with a warrant. Out! Out!"

Every time one of the officers starts to speak, he speaks louder and says out. This officer cannot say one word. They can't say anything they are just standing there looking at him. Now he is screaming.

"Out! Out! Out of this property. Immediately, out! Immediately, go out and don't come back! I don't want to talk to you, not a word. Out! Out of

this property immediately. I don't care what you have to say. Out of this property, you Nazis. Out! Out! Gestapo is not allowed here! Immediately, Gestapo is not allowed here. Out! Do you understand English? Get out of this property! Go, Go, Go, and don't come back without a warrant. Out Nazis. Out! Do you understand? Nazis are not welcome here. Out, and don't come back without a warrant. Do not come back without a warrant. Do you understand that you are not welcome? Nazis are not welcome here. Gestapo is not welcome here. Do not come back you Nazi psychopaths! Unbelievable, sick, evil people, intimidating people in the church, during the Passover. You Gestapo, Nazi, fascists!"

Gradually they turned around and left.

Now that is a shepherd. That shepherd is Pastor Artur Pawlowski.

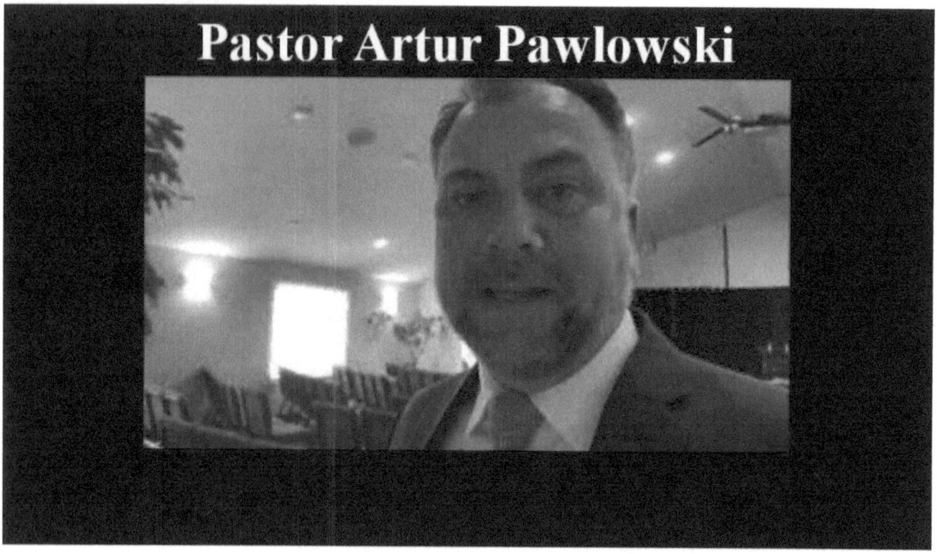

He is doing this amidst what is going on in Canada. He is formerly from Poland. He knows what it can get like. And I love the way he said, "We are lions, and we eat hyenas for breakfast." That's how you stop it. That's how you exist in the last days that we have left. Not comply. Not be afraid. Stand up! And you resist. And you eat those hyenas.

The good news is there are some people here in America who still have American backbone. Like this pilot. Here's how you put a stop to this stuff.

Female Passenger: *"Thank you. Then, move him!"*

Stewardess: *"This is a full flight; I can't move him"*

Female Passenger: *"I don't want to sit there. So, you want me to call the cops? Because I will. I'll call them right now."*

Stewardess: *"We can't move people because they don't want to sit next to someone."*

Female Passenger: *"He's violating our rights and our safety. I asked him for his vaccine card. And he doesn't have one. Because he's not vaccinated! If you want to travel, you have to have a mask and be vaccinated."*

Stewardess: *"You're not exactly wearing a mask."*

Female Passenger: *"I'm not wearing a mask because I have asthma! I have a health condition; I have children and I'm fully vaccinated to protect them. You are intentionally putting my health at risk right now!"*

Stewardess: *"Ma'am, if you wish to be on this flight, I need you to take a seat. That is the seat you paid for and it's the only one available."*

Female Passenger: *"I know the law! You are violating the law right now. You are completely breaking the law. You have to find me another seat."*

Stewardess: *"It's not the law to be vaccinated to come on this flight."*

Female Passenger: *"You can't make me breathe his oxygen because he's not vaccinated. You're not listening to me!"*

Stewardess: *"If you wish to be on this flight, I need you to take your seat."*

Female Passenger: *"I'm not sitting there! You're putting my life in danger right now. I cannot be made to breathe his oxygen, that's not fair."*

Stewardess: *"Ma'am, this is the seat you paid for."*

Female Passenger: *"Do you want me to see my children again? You're putting them at risk now!"*

Stewardess: *"It's the only one available."*

Female Passenger: *"I don't want to sit there. He's not vaccinated. You're intentionally putting my life in danger."*

Stewardess: *"Ma'am we're not putting your life in danger."*

Female Passenger: *"I'm not gonna sit there!"*

Stewardess: *"Ma'am please take your seat."*

Female passenger: "No, I'm not sitting there! (She turns around when she hears a voice behind her.)

Captain: *"Ma'am, I know how challenging air travel is these days, but there will be no discrimination on my aircraft."*

Female Passenger: *"It's not discrimination."*

Captain: *"Vaccinated or unvaccinated we should respect each other and as it seems you have trouble doing that. Please, exit the aircraft."*

Everyone applauds, and the female passenger stands there with her mouth open. He takes her hand and escorts her off the plane.

That's how you stop it. Rise up, resist, not on my plane, not in my house, not in my school, not in my town, not in my church, not in my city, not in my business. GET OUT! We eat hyenas for breakfast. Christian lions do. And that is what God has called us to do in the last days as we await the Rapture. We are not going to stop the 7-Year Tribulation. My number one premise is to be obedient to the word of God. He says to resist, I need to resist.

Number two, if I don't resist it's all going to come down that much faster. And I'm trying to maintain as much freedom as I can even in the United States of America to do what God has called me to do. But if I don't resist, I'm going to lose it. We need to obey God and realize what is on the line. In fact, there are all kinds of victories. The media is never going to tell you this but there are people, including non-Christians who are rising up against this. Being lions all over the world and I'm going to share a few of those with you.

Join the Resistance!

Attorney – Justice will not come through the courts by the people rising up!

One medical professional resignation – I'm not afraid of losing every last comfort that I have to stand up for what is right.

Teens Stand up – I will not wear the mask. I will not take the vaccine, I will resist evil, I will submit to God, I will defy tyrants.

Nurses speak out and protest mandatory shots.

More than 3,000 doctors & scientists sign Declaration accusing Covid Policymakers of 'Crimes Against Humanity.'

Groups standing up against minors being jabbed shut down vaxx centers.

Mass walkouts against vaccine mandates begin NOW.

Massive protests explode in Greece as response to banning unvaccinated from social life.

Massive protests are happening worldwide against vaccine passports.

Nearly 20,000 people demonstrate in Trieste, Italy against the government's vaccine.

Despite horrifying state violence, brave Australia continues to resist Covid Police State.

20,000 Australians shut down Melbourne Highway in massive lockdown protest and it's glorious.!

Aussie Truckers victorious – south Australia drops mandatory jab for interstate drivers following blockade protest.

Belgium – Dairy farmers rise up! Protest with tractors and farm equipment – sling cow slurry over agents of the state.

France – Health caregivers burn their diplomas in protest against compulsory vaccinations.

French police lay down shields – join 100,000 protesters marching against vaccine passport.

Millions pour out onto the streets in London to protest Covid tyranny and it's spectacular!

Protests break out in England, Paris, Portugal and around the world against CONvid-1984 tyranny.

Massive Protests all throughout France against Macron's tyrannical apartheid Health Passports.

The people of France and Italy are engaged in massive protests against COVID Health Pass.

These are the resistance – Canadian nurses walk out, US students walk out, Greek medics protest Aussie truckers' blockade and more!

Massive European protests against Covid-19 lockdowns, vaccine mandates erupt into a 'war zone'.

When nearly 300,000 French Protest Covid tyranny.

Massive protests erupt in Italy as tyrants reveal health passports.
NY Supreme Court delivers crushing blow to mayor Bill de Blasio's vaccine mandate.

Federal Court blocks Biden administration's private business Covid-19 vaccine mandate.

Florida unveils tools for reporting employers who violate restrictions on vaccine mandates.

Biden's vaccine mandate suffers another blow, it is now unlawful and blocked in all 50 states.

In other words, KEEP RESISTING like God said to. IT'S WORKING!

And remember, YOU ARE NOT ALONE, as Christine Anderson a member of the European Parliament reminds us! That is the lie that is being perpetrated in the media. They act like there is no excuse, you are all alone, you're in the minority, and that's not true. There are enough Americans that still have a backbone that are speaking out, but you never hear about them, there is a blackout in the media. And we need to frankly, join the resistance. She said this in their face, at the European Parliament.

Christine Anderson: *"Whenever a government claims to have the people's interest at heart, you need to think again. In the entire history of* *mankind there have never a political elite sincerely concerned about the well-being of regular people. What makes any of us think that it is any different now? If the age of enlightenment has brought forth anything, it's certainly this. Never take anything any government tells you at face value."*

Biden: *"The only pandemic we have is among the unvaccinated."*

Christine Anderson: *"Always question everything any government does or does not do. Always look for ulterior motives and always ask 'cui bono', who benefits."*

MSNBC reports: *"The voluntary phase is over. It's time for mandates."*

Christine Anderson: *"Whenever a political elite pushes this hard and resorts to extortion and manipulation to get their way, you can almost always be sure your benefit is definitely not what they have at heart."*

"You can ask the people to go home and if they didn't, arrest them."

Christine Anderson: *"As far as I am concerned, I will not be vaccinated with anything that has not been properly tested and is shown to have no scientific evidence that the benefit outweighs the disease itself, with long term side effects which to this day we don't know anything about. I will not be reduced to a mere Guinea Pig by getting vaccinated with an experimental drug. And I will most assuredly not be vaccinated because my government tells me to and promises in return, I will be granted freedom."*

Global National News: *"If you have travel plans there is one more thing to add to your travel list, proof of vaccination."*

Christine Anderson: *"Let's be clear about one thing, no one grants me freedom for I am a free person."*

Arnold Schwarzenegger: *"No, s**** your freedom."*

CNN Live: *"It has nothing to do with freedom, it has to do with liberty."*

Christine Anderson: *"So I dare the European Commission and the German Government to throw me in jail, lock me up, and throw away the key for all I care. But you will never be able to force me into being vaccinated, if I am free citizen, then I choose not to be vaccinated."*

You are not alone! No more shots, the resistance is worldwide and growing. *"We don't want more shots, no cards, no tyranny, otherwise take the Statue of Liberty back to France."*

We are not alone, man what has happened to us, and if it doesn't start with the church, we're in a heap of trouble. We need to stand up as Christians, we need to resist, we need to get back that American spirit, that American backbone. We need to buy as much time as we can to do what God has called us to do and be those resisters/restrainers in these last days. We need to be Christian lions. We need to eat these hyenas. Remember these two things:

1. Normal isn't coming back. Jesus is!
2. In the End, Jesus wins! And we belong to Him.

How to Receive Jesus Christ:

1. Admit your need (I am a sinner).
2. Be willing to turn from your sins (repent).
3. Believe that Jesus Christ died for you on the Cross and rose from the grave.
4. Through prayer, invite Jesus Christ to come in and control your life through the Holy Spirit. (Receive Him as Lord and Savior.)

What to pray:

Dear Lord Jesus,

I know that I am a sinner and need Your forgiveness. I believe that You died for my sins. I want to turn from my sins. I now invite You to come into my heart and life. I want to trust and follow You as Lord and Savior.

In Jesus' name. Amen.

Notes

https://twitter.com/AnonymeCitoyen/status/1441747083770351624?s=19
https://twitter.com/ElectionWiz/status/1441738231385661440?s=19
https://sonsoflibertymedia.com/20000-australians-shut-down-melbourne-highway-in-massive-lockdown-protest-its-glorious-video/
https://www.lifesitenews.com/opinion/americans-must-be-prepared-to-publicly-resist-covid-quarantine-camps/
https://sonsoflibertymedia.com/americas-frontline-doctor-reveals-how-to-detoxify-from-graphene-oxide-video/
https://sonsoflibertymedia.com/americas-frontline-doctor-you-can-detoxify-yourself-from-graphene-oxide-much-more-video/
https://rumble.com/vq7l2z-artur-pawlowski-speaks-out-on-major-victory-over-nazi-tyranny-in-canada.html
https://sonsoflibertymedia.com/attorney-justice-will-not-come-through-the-courts-but-by-the-people-rising-up/
https://beforeitsnews.com/health/2021/10/attorney-thomas-renz-releases-data-from-never-before-seen-vaccine-injurydeath-tracking-system-its-absolutely-horrifying-3042024.html
https://sonsoflibertymedia.com/aussie-cops-launch-manhunt-checkpoints-as-teens-escape-from-covid-internment-camp/
https://sonsoflibertymedia.com/aussie-truckers-victorious-south-australia-drops-mandatory-jab-for-interstate-drivers-following-blockade-protest/
https://sonsoflibertymedia.com/belgium-dairy-farmers-rise-up-protest-with-tractors-farm-equipment-sling-cow-slurry-over-agents-of-the-state-video/
https://www.zerohedge.com/markets/biden-infrastructure-bill-includes-passive-monitoring-vehicle-kill-switch-mandates
https://newspunch.com/bill-gates-predicts-the-date-the-pandemic-will-suddenly-end/
https://www.naturalnews.com/2021-09-29-attorney-thomas-renz-nearly-50k-medicare-patients-died-soon-after-getting-covid-shot.html
https://rumble.com/vpr53l-breaking-aboriginals-hunted-by-military-kids-jabbed-by-force-disturbing-vid.html

https://beforeitsnews.com/politics/2021/10/breaking-developments-stew-peters-dr-jane-ruby-rip-the-killer-jab-whistleblower-moabs-by-project-veritas-3245918.html
https://www.cnbc.com/2021/08/10/breakthrough-covid-cases-why-fully-vaccinated-people-can-get-covid.html
https://sonsoflibertymedia.com/california-bribed-boy-with-pizza-to-get-covid-shot-without-parents-consent-told-him-to-keep-it-secret/
https://www.rebelnews.com/canadas_covid_jails_have_returned_and_are_seemingly_worse_than_ever
https://www.organiclifestylemagazine.com/cdc-admits-finacial-hospital-incentives-drove-up-covid-19-death-rates
https://covid.cdc.gov/covid-data-tracker/#datatracker-home
https://sonsoflibertymedia.com/cnbc-crackpot-unvaccinated-people-must-be-rounded-up-by-military-force-vaccinated-at-gunpoint-starting-first-of-2022/
https://theconservativetreehouse.com/blog/2021/11/30/cnbc-pundit-calls-unvaxxed-people-psychotic-demands-u-s-military-hunt-them-down-force-vaccine-or-force-quarantine/
https://www.cnbc.com/2021/06/25/covid-breakthrough-cases-cdc-says-more-than-4100-people-have-been-hospitalized-or-died-after-vaccination.html
https://www.cnbc.com/2021/11/09/covid-vaccines-pfizer-ceo-says-people-who-spread-misinformation-on-shots-are-criminals.html
https://saraacarter.com/covid-19-natural-immunity-more-effective-than-vaccine-research-suggests/
https://sonsoflibertymedia.com/despite-horrifying-state-violence-brave-australia-continue-to-resist-covid-police-state-video/
https://newswithviews.com/detroit-tv-asks-for-stories-of-unvaxxed-dying-from-covid-gets-over-180k-responses-of-vaccine-injured-and-dead-instead/
https://www.afinalwarning.com/558712.html
https://beforeitsnews.com/u-s-politics/2021/10/dr-david-martin-coronavirus-patents-prove-covid-fraud-illegal-dealings-the-people-demand-justice-video-2583489.html

https://beforeitsnews.com/u-s-politics/2021/10/every-medical-professional-american-should-read-this-hospitals-ct-technologists-resignation-im-not-afraid-of-losing-every-last-comfort-that-i-have-to-stand-up-for-what-is-right-2584062.html
https://sonsoflibertymedia.com/exclusive-artur-pawlowski-on-victory-over-canadian-nazis-we-are-lions-we-eat-hyenas-for-breakfast-video/
https://beforeitsnews.com/alternative/2021/11/exclusive-judy-mikovits-phd-antidote-for-vaxxine-toxin-and-warns-against-dangerous-fake-one-video-3761906.html
https://www.cdc.gov/nchs/fastats/leading-causes-of-death.htm
https://worldnationnews.com/fda-asks-court-for-55-years-to-release-full-data-on-pfizers-covid-19-vaccine/
https://aaronsiri.substack.com/p/fda-asks-federal-judge-to-grant-it?r=qrq5x&utm_campaign=post&utm_medium=web&utm_source=
https://www.theepochtimes.com/mkt_breakingnews/federal-court-blocks-biden-administrations-private-business-covid-19-vaccine-
https://www.theepochtimes.com/mkt_app/florida-unveils-tools-for-reporting-employers-who-violate-restrictions-on-vaccine-mandates_4141573.htmlmandate_4089942.html
https://www.bitchute.com/video/Oayn0rMLeWOB/
https://beforeitsnews.com/eu/2021/08/former-pfizer-biotech-analyst-karen-kingston-says-fda-approval-for-pfizer-is-checkmate-stew-peters-2676090.html
https://survivaldan101.com/former-pfizer-exec-children-are-50-times-more-likely-to-die-from-coronavirus-vaccine-than-from-the-virus-itself/
https://sonsoflibertymedia.com/france-health-caregivers-burn-their-diplomas-in-protest-against-compulsory-vaccinations-they-are-not-alone-
https://sonsoflibertymedia.com/french-police-lay-down-shields-join-100000-protesters-marching-against-vaccine-passport/video/
https://dailyexpose.uk/2021/12/04/4-in-5-covid-deaths-fully-vaccinated-november/
https://www.theepochtimes.com/mkt_morningbrief/germany-announces-national-lockdown-for-the-unvaccinated_4135243.html

https://beforeitsnews.com/health/2021/09/greg-hunter-covid-19-vaccines-are-poison-karen-kingston-top-pharmaceutical-analyst-must-video-3041720.html
https://beforeitsnews.com/health/2021/09/greg-hunter-unvaxed-at-risk-from-vaxed-in-coming-dark-winter-karen-kingston-must-video-3041950.html
https://sonsoflibertymedia.com/groups-standing-against-minors-being-jabbed-as-info-protests-shut-down-vaxx-centers-video/
https://www.factcheck.org/2020/04/hospital-payments-and-the-covid-19-death-count/
https://www.hfma.org/topics/news/2020/07/the-new-round-will-pay--50-000-per-covid-19-admission--compared-.html
https://www.technocracy.news/hr-550-house-passes-bill-to-fund-federal-vaccination-database/
https://www.thegatewaypundit.com/2021/12/huge-glenn-beck-tucker-carlson-us-doctors-reviewing-moderna-vaccine-december-2019-covid-hit-us-video/
http://medicine.news/2021-09-14-idaho-doctor-20times-increase-cancer-vaccinated-covid.html
https://www.cdc.gov/coronavirus/2019-ncov/global-covid-19/shielding-approach-humanitarian.html
https://patriotsbeacon.com/inventor-of-mrna-vaccine-calls-for-stop-of-covid-vaxx/?utm_source=BS-Mailer&utm_medium=email&utm_content=subscriber_id:42583243&utm_campaign=RM%201000%20Clickers%20Drop%2012-9%20papproach-
https://www.heraldscotland.com/news/19726487.investigation-launched-abnormal-spike-newborn-baby-deaths-scotland/
https://www.prophecynewswatch.com/article.cfm?recent_news_id=5100a
https://www.oann.com/jj-scientist-justin-durrant-dont-get-jj-covid-
https://www.naturalnews.com/2021-10-14-data-proves-vaccine-distribution-led-to-deaths.html
https://thetruedefender.com/just-in-india-doesnt-have-new-coronavirus-cases-after-implementing-ivermectin-protocol/deaths-

https://www.naturalnews.com/2021-11-08-mass-walkouts-against-vaccine-mandates-begin-now-november-8-
https://sonsoflibertymedia.com/massive-protests-explode-in-greece-as-response-to-banning-unvaccinated-from-social-life-vaccine passports
https://sonsoflibertymedia.com/massive-protests-worldwide-against-
https://naturalnews.com/2021-12-10-fired-unvaccinated-nurses-replaced-national-guard-troops.html
https://sonsoflibertymedia.com/millions-pour-out-onto-the-streets-in-london-to-protest-covid-tyranny-its-spectacular-video
https://sonsoflibertymedia.com/more-than-3000-doctors-scientists-sign-declaration-accusing-covid-policy-makers-of-crimes-against-humanity-video
https://www.theepochtimes.com/mkt_breakingnews/natural-immunity-more-protective-over-time-than-covid-19-vaccination-study_4149953.html
https://www.theepochtimes.com/nevada-becomes-first-state-to-impose-surcharge-on-unvaccinated-workers_4136987.html
https://sonsoflibertymedia.com/new-bill-to-strip-unvaccinated-of-health-insurance-if-they-get-sick-force-them-to-pay-out-of-pocket/
https://www.wfla.com/community/health/coronavirus/new-cdc-report-shows-94-of-covid-19-deaths-in-us-had-underlying-medical-conditions
https://beckernews.com/stunning-new-data-covid-case-rates-among-the-fully-vaccinated-are-now-higher-than-the-not-vaccinated-42727/
https://beforeitsnews.com/prophecy/2021/10/new-stew-peters-shocking-dr-carrie-madej-releases-first-look-at-pfizer-vial-contents-2524862.html
https://www.visiontimes.com/2021/12/04/no-jab-no-food-canada-new-brunswick.html
https://www.bitchute.com/video/UJpUn43T0cdu/
https://sonsoflibertymedia.com/nurses-speak-out-protest-mandatory-shots-plus-live-with-kate-shemirani-video/

https://www.dailymail.co.uk/news/article-10270025/Unvaccinated-Nevada-state-workers-pay-insurance-surcharge.html
https://trendingpolitics.com/ny-supreme-court-delivers-crushing-blow-to-mayor-bill-de-blasios-vaccine-mandate-knab/
https://www.thegatewaypundit.com/2021/12/heels-austria-germany-locking-unvaccinated-eu-leader-calls-throwing-nuremberg-code-favor-forced-vaccinating-dissenters/
https://populist.press/
https://sonsoflibertymedia.com/pfizer-tops-all-over-covid-shots-for-number-of-deaths-in-latest-vaers-report/
https://beforeitsnews.com/politics/2021/10/pfizer-whistleblower-leaks-execs-emails-exposing-suppression-of-covid-vax-info-from-public-project-veritas-3245853.html
https://www.businessinsider.com/sarco-machines-3d-printed-capsule-assisted-suicide-pod-booth-switzerland-2021-12
https://americasfrontlinedoctors.org/2/frontlinenews/poison-death-shot-dr-zelenko-testifies-before-israeli-rabbinical-court/
https://sonsoflibertymedia.com/protests-break-out-in-england-paris-portugal-around-the-world-against-convid-1984-tyranny-videos/
https://sonsoflibertymedia.com/refusing-the-truth-another-one-that-paid-the-ultimate-price-not-a-word-from-the-mainstream-media-as-to-how/
https://worldnewstrust.com/reminder-mentioning-the-nazi-health-pass-is-forbidden-mickey-z
https://thenationalpulse.com/exclusive/pfizer-board-member-is-former-facebook-director/
https://www.conservativenewszone.com/articles/scientists-now-developing-mrna-vegetables-so-that-grocery-stores-can-sell-vaccines-hidden-in-food/
https://uafreport.com/daniel/sen-johnson-we-do-not-have-an-fda-approved-vaccine-being-administered-in-the-u-s/
https://thepostmillennial.com/eu-chief-nuremberg-code
https://www.naturalnews.com/2021-12-02-smoking-gun-pfizer-document-exposes-fda-criminal-cover-up-of-vaccine-deaths.html#
https://beforeitsnews.com/alternative/2021/07/stew-peters-with-karen-kingston-bombshell-former-pfizer-employee-confirms-poison-in-covid-kill-shot-video-3755517.html

https://medicalxpress.com/news/2021-09-severe-breakthrough-cases-covid-.html
https://sonsoflibertymedia.com/teens-stand-up-i-will-not-wear-the-mask-i-will-not-take-the-vaccine-i-will-resist-evil-i-will-submit-to-god-i-will-defy-tyrants-video/
https://t.me/SidneyPowell/2533
https://t.me/c/1264699318/8706
https://vsecretscc.com/kirsh?_kx=2QLOyRCQVLSR-DyJ04StwFUENQFBOdpm5JOTYF4638I%3D.WXNMR7
https://beforeitsnews.com/alternative/2021/10/the-ai-organization-founder-nano-tech-vaccines-are-extinction-agenda-stew-peters-3759641.html
https://www.icandecide.org/ican_press/the-fda-now-asks-judge-to-grant-it-until-2096-to-fully-release-pfizers-covid-19-vaccine-data/
https://sonsoflibertymedia.com/the-french-just-arent-having-macrons-tyrannical-apartheid-health-passports-massive-protests-all-throughout-france-video/
https://www.thelastamericanvagabond.com/great-narrative-metaverse-dystopian-vision-future/
https://www.stridentconservative.com/the-parallel-between-covid-vaccine-passports-and-nazi-germany/
https://sonsoflibertymedia.com/the-people-of-france-italy-are-engaged-in-massive-protests-against-covid-health-pass-video/
https://www.naturalnews.com/2021-10-04-the-vaccine-death-report.html
https://www.thegatewaypundit.com/2021/11/now-365-studies-prove-efficacy-ivermectin-hcq-treating-covid-19-will-anyone-confront-fauci-medical-elites-deception/?utm_source=Telegram&utm_medium=PostSideSharingButtons&utm_campaign=websitesharingbuttons
https://sonsoflibertymedia.com/these-are-the-resistance-canadian-nurses-walk-out-us-students-walk-out-greek-medics-protest-aussie-truckers-blockade-more-videos/
https://www.rjmilitaria.com/product/third-reich-gesundheitspass-arbeitsbuch-irma-klob/
https://thekylebecker.substack.com/p/this-unlawful-mandate-is-now-blocked

https://beforeitsnews.com/health/2021/08/toxic-graphene-oxide-in-pfizer-vaxx-karen-kingston-3041354.html
https://www.worldometers.info/coronavirus/country/us/
https://vernoncoleman.org/articles/how-many-people-are-vaccines-killing
https://www.israel365news.com/199600/us-army-accused-of-promoting-satanism-to-troops-watch/
https://alexberenson.substack.com/p/vaccinated-english-adults-under-60
https://sonsoflibertymedia.com/vaers-report-study-indicates-nearly-2-million-americans-may-have-died-following-covid-shot-video/
https://originalrebel.net/2021/05/04/vaers-system-is-only-recording-fewer-than-1-of-covid-19-vaccines-side-effects-and-deaths/
https://gnigh-66270.medium.com/vaers-underreporting-and-the-mysterious-1-5b4f9b109145
https://resistthemainstream.org/watch-massive-european-protests-against-covid-19-lockdowns-vaccine-mandates-erupt-into-an-war-zone/?utm_source=telegram
https://www.forbes.com/sites/worldeconomicforum/2016/11/10/shopping-i-cant-really-remember-what-that-is-or-how-differently-well-live-in-2030/?sh=e3522ec17350
https://sonsoflibertymedia.com/when-nearly-300000-french-protest-covid-tyranny-you-know-the-jig-is-up-video/
https://sonsoflibertymedia.com/whoa-official-data-confirms-fully-vaccinated-account-for-9-out-of-every-10-covid-19-deaths-since-august/
https://sonsoflibertymedia.com/yep-its-happening-in-italy-too-massive-protests-erupt-as-tyrants-reveal-health-passports/
https://dnyuz.com/2021/12/07/your-face-is-or-will-be-your-boarding-pass/
https://www.youtube.com/watch?v=lv1QT085QEg
https://www.youtube.com/watch?v=R9DUt_QCxxw
https://regia-marinho.medium.com/how-to-take-over-the-world-real-or-fake-cartoon-1ffeb1ba6b10
https://www.youtube.com/watch?v=xwA4k0E51Oo
https://www.youtube.com/watch?v=GukIoZ8d3Ew
https://www.youtube.com/watch?v=JQulGSF18OM&list=UUAwylBbx8RiRD3VsaYdwNTw&index=67
https://www.youtube.com/watch?v=_JtZ1e78ITE

https://www.businessinsider.com/video-biden-said-december-2020-wouldnt-make-vaccine-mandatory-2021-9
https://www.c-span.org/video/?c4962333/senator-paul-dr-fauci-clash-research-funding-wuhan-lab
https://www.youtube.com/watch?v=Es9OOh-UIRw
https://www.youtube.com/watch?v=8CG8aI4XCGw
https://www.youtube.com/watch?v=iF3sKVX6L_4
https://www.youtube.com/watch?v=cJEz8Xfq9iU
https://www.youtube.com/watch?v=zCxFAAwI6yw
https://www.youtube.com/watch?v=mP9iHyj1uiU
https://www.youtube.com/watch?v=99q-2G3HX6A
https://www.youtube.com/watch?v=Ux-KrMygrzA
https://www.youtube.com/watch?v=F0e2t43gMSs
https://www.youtube.com/watch?v=0u304OYDDlA
https://www.cdc.gov/coronavirus/2019-ncov/vaccines/effectiveness/index.html
https://www.independent.co.uk/news/world/americas/us-politics/vaccine-covid-fauci-deaths-b1808878.html
https://www.cnbc.com/video/2021/07/21/fauci-vaccines-are-safe-and-effective-against-delta-variant.html
https://www.nih.gov/news-events/nih-research-matters/experimental-coronavirus-vaccine-highly-effective
https://www.nytimes.com/2021/03/31/health/pfizer-biontech-vaccine-adolescents.html
https://www.the-sun.com/news/2923136/coronavirus-news-uk-lockdown-vaccine-indian-variant-latest/
https://www.cnn.com/2021/04/09/health/covid-vaccines-adverse-reaction-rare-trnd/index.html
https://apnews.com/article/covid-19-vaccine-us-study-highly-effective-57cde25de803c98503c5ff9937598420
https://www.vumc.org/health-policy/covid19-vaccine-effective-study-cdc
https://www.statnews.com/2020/12/08/fda-scientists-endorse-highly-effective-pfizer-biontech-covid-19-vaccine-ahead-of-key-panel/

https://newsroom.ucla.edu/releases/vaccines-preventing-symptomatic-infection-health-workers-covid19
https://www.urmc.rochester.edu/news/story/astrazeneca-covid-vaccine-is-100-effective-at-preventing-severe-disease
https://www.yalemedicine.org/news/covid-19-vaccine-comparison
https://www.nebraskamed.com/COVID/novavax-vaccine-results-how-effective-is-it-against-variants
https://www.cnbc.com/2021/05/25/covid-vaccine-moderna-says-shot-is-100percent-effective-in-teens-plans-to-seek-fda-ok-in-june.html
https://www.astrazeneca.com/content/dam/az/covid-19/media/factsheets/COVID-19_Vaccine_AstraZeneca_Real-World_Evidence_Summary.pdf
https://news.sky.com/story/covid-19-novavax-jab-100-effective-in-protecting-against-moderate-and-severe-disease-trial-results-suggest-12332248
https://www.webmd.com/vaccines/covid-19-vaccine/news/20211123/pfizer-covid-vaccine-effectiveness-adolescents-study#:~:text=Nov.,months%20after%20the%20second%20dose.
https://www.mcknights.com/news/clinical-news/jj-asks-for-booster-go-ahead-says-second-vaccine-dose-provides-100-percent-covid-protection/
https://www.astrazeneca.com/media-centre/press-releases/2021/covid-19-vaccine-astrazeneca-confirms-protection-against-severe-disease-hospitalisation-and-death-in-the-primary-analysis-of-phase-iii-trials.html
https://www.cnbc.com/2021/03/31/covid-vaccine-pfizer-says-shot-is-100percent-effective-in-kids-ages-12-to-15.html
https://westerntoday.wwu.edu/inthemedia/moderna-says-its-covid-vaccine-is-100-effective-in-teens-plans-to-seek-fda-ok-in-early
https://www.ucsf.edu/news/2021/03/420071/how-effective-johnson-johnson-covid-19-vaccine-heres-what-you-should-know
https://www.usatoday.com/story/news/health/2021/05/25/moderna-covid-19-vaccine-safe-children-study/7422896002/
https://www.fox13news.com/news/real-world-vaccine-study-shows-99-effective-rate

https://www.columbusjewishnews.com/jns/israeli-health-ministry-pfizer-vaccine-close-to-99-percent-effective/article_5d7b7993-f8a5-5681-8f62-7e674886b691.html
https://www.ukrinform.net/rubric-society/3230630-pfizer-coronavirus-vaccine-is-98-effective-expert.html
https://www.cbsnews.com/news/pfizer-vaccine-covid-97-effective-symptomatic/
https://www.timesofisrael.com/pfizer-vaccine-96-7-effective-at-preventing-covid-deaths-israeli-data-shows/
https://www.dailymail.co.uk/health/article-10021541/Moderna-vaccine-effective-against-COVID-19-infection-96-compared-Pfizer-shot-89.html
https://www.hindustantimes.com/india-news/one-covid-vaccine-jab-96-6-effective-in-averting-deaths-two-97-5-centre-101631211897726.html
https://www.webmd.com/vaccines/covid-19-vaccine/news/20201118/updated-pfizer-data-shows-vaccine-is-95-effective
https://www.nytimes.com/2021/04/28/health/pfizer-moderna-vaccine-hospitalization.html
https://www.reuters.com/business/healthcare-pharmaceuticals/moderna-says-its-covid-19-shot-remains-93-effective-4-6-months-after-second-dose-2021-08-05/
https://www.astrazeneca.com/media-centre/press-releases/2021/covid-19-vaccine-astrazeneca-effective-against-delta-indian-variant.html
https://www.wric.com/health/coronavirus/new-cdc-study-shows-two-dose-vaccines-are-91-effective-at-reducing-infection-risk/
https://www.axios.com/mrna-covid-vaccines-effective-real-world-conditions-492ac016-1220-4276-aacc-967492a4e117.html
https://www.heraldscotland.com/news/19048284.novavax-covid-vaccine-approved-use-uk/
https://pharmaphorum.com/news/novavax-confirms-efficacy-of-covid-19-jab-against-uk-variant/
https://www.beckershospitalreview.com/pharmacy/pfizer-vaccine-88-effective-against-delta-variant-uk-study-

finds.html#:~:text=Two%20doses%20of%20Pfizer's%20COVID,England%20Journal%20of%20Medicine%20found.
https://mainichi.jp/english/articles/20211006/p2a/00m/0na/002000c
https://www.jpost.com/health-science/pfizer-covid-vaccine-86-percent-effective-after-third-shot-maccabi-677053
https://www.foxnews.com/health/pfizer-covid-19-vaccine-85-effective-after-single-dose-israeli-researchers-find
https://www.cnbc.com/2021/07/28/pfizers-ceo-says-covid-vaccine-effectiveness-drops-to-84percent-after-six-months.html
https://www.marketwatch.com/story/pfizer-says-immunity-drops-to-83-within-six-months-in-people-who-got-its-covid-19-shot-further-bolstering-the-company-case-for-a-booster-11627579817
https://indianexpress.com/article/india/pune/one-dose-of-covid-vaccine-82-effective-in-preventing-death-2-doses-95-effective-icmr-nie-study-7370899/
https://www.pharmaceutical-technology.com/news/bharat-biotech-vaccine-efficacy/
https://www.cnbc.com/2021/03/29/cdc-study-shows-single-dose-of-pfizer-or-moderna-covid-vaccines-was-80percent-effective.html
https://www.cnbc.com/2021/03/22/astrazeneca-coronavirus-vaccine-79percent-effective-in-us-trial.html
https://www.cidrap.umn.edu/news-perspective/2021/07/pfizer-covid-vaccine-shows-78-efficacy-pregnancy#:~:text=Two%20doses%20of%20the%20Pfizer,was%20published%20yesterday%20in%20JAMA.
https://www.cnbc.com/2021/09/17/moderna-vaccine-more-effective-than-pfizer-jj-especially-after-4-months-cdc.html
https://southernmarylandchronicle.com/2021/03/25/astrazeneca-says-covid-19-vaccine-76-effective-in-new-analysis-to-seek-u-s-approval/
https://www.publichealthontario.ca/-/media/documents/ncov/covid-wwksf/2021/04/wwksf-vaccine-effectiveness.pdf?la=en
https://www.statnews.com/2021/02/02/comparing-the-covid-19-vaccines-developed-by-pfizer-moderna-and-johnson-johnson/

https://www.audacy.com/kcbsradio/news/national/j-and-j-booster-waiting-on-approval-1st-dose-only-71-effective

https://www.channelnewsasia.com/singapore/covid-19-vaccine-protection-against-infection-delta-variant-1987586

https://www.bloomberg.com/news/articles/2021-07-01/first-dna-covid-vaccine-found-67-effective-in-clinical-trials#:~:text=The%20drugmaker%20applied%20for%20emergency,of%2067%25%2C%20Cadila%20said.

https://khn.org/morning-breakout/pfizer-covid-shots-effectiveness-falls-to-64-in-israel/

https://www.gov.uk/government/news/covid-19-vaccines-highly-effective-in-most-people-in-clinical-risk-groups

https://www.biospace.com/article/australian-researchers-say-best-covid-19-vaccines-58-percent-effective-at-250-days/

https://www.cnbc.com/2021/08/17/covid-vaccine-booster-shots-nih-director-says-new-israel-data-is-building-case-in-the-us.html

https://www.yahoo.com/now/novavax-vaccine-96-effective-against-210200537.html?guccounter=1&guce_referrer=aHR0cHM6Ly93d3cuZ29vZ2xlLmNvbS8&guce_referrer_sig=AQAAAKuhAfgL8a8pCYu9HMSqt0ZzPvUx18OTJBZLciTQt5MGz9SOXkCUsaWnYN-JXhp0xF1rrBzgiB7yv6604wH8uCqhCqwWZQKZdqCTF66Zj2vDwaNgasmS9mjJkNEIWxEWa68pv3o_NtHaE53gdwMt37YCZ7820kDtQOBjBAistV9l

https://www.forbes.com/sites/roberthart/2021/07/23/pfizer-shot-just-39-effective-against-delta-infection-but-largely-prevents-severe-illness-israel-study-suggests/?sh=434765fb584f

https://www.reuters.com/business/healthcare-pharmaceuticals/novavax-vaccine-shows-43-efficacy-against-south-african-variant-study-finds-2021-05-05/

https://www.npr.org/sections/health-shots/2020/09/12/911987987/a-covid-19-vaccine-may-be-only-50-effective-is-that-good-enough#:~:text=Despite%20all%20these%20remaining%20unknowns,good%20possibility%20of%20being%20protected.

https://www.npr.org/sections/health-shots/2020/09/12/911987987/a-covid-19-vaccine-may-be-only-50-effective-is-that-good-enough#:~:text=Despite%20all%20these%20remaining%20unknowns,good%20possibility%20of%20being%20protected.
https://www.business-standard.com/article/current-affairs/moderna-covid-vaccine-76-effective-against-delta-pfizer-42-study-121081201173_1.html
https://www.timesofisrael.com/israeli-uk-data-offer-mixed-signals-on-vaccines-potency-against-delta-strain/
https://www.cnbc.com/2021/07/23/delta-variant-pfizer-covid-vaccine-39percent-effective-in-israel-prevents-severe-illness.html
https://www.dailymail.co.uk/news/article-10064291/Pfizers-Covid-efficacy-against-infection-plunges-20-six-months-data-Qatar-shows.html
https://www.cbsnews.com/news/pfizer-covid-19-vaccine-booster-shots-seniors-cdc-endorse/
https://www.kpcc.org/npr-news/2021-09-28/for-people-who-got-the-j-j-vaccine-some-doctors-are-advising-boosters-asap
https://www.cnbc.com/2021/04/15/pfizer-ceo-says-third-covid-vaccine-dose-likely-needed-within-12-months.html
https://www.yahoo.com/now/israel-tightened-covid-vaccine-pass-102710216.html
https://www.bloomberg.com/news/articles/2021-07-25/fauci-says-u-s-moving-in-wrong-direction-in-combating-covid#:~:text=The%20U.S.%20is%20moving%20in,nation's%20top%20infectious%20disease%20expert.
https://www.reuters.com/business/healthcare-pharmaceuticals/pfizer-ask-fda-authorize-booster-dose-covid-vaccine-delta-variant-spreads-2021-07-08/
https://thehill.com/changing-america/well-being/prevention-cures/572700-breakthrough-data-outlines-need-for-booster
https://www.bbc.com/news/health-58499863
https://bestlifeonline.com/pfizer-booster-news/
https://ktla.com/news/coronavirus/fauci-says-quite-possible-americans-may-need-covid-19-vaccine-booster-in-coming-months/

https://nypost.com/2021/12/11/dr-fauci-says-omicron-booster-may-not-be-necessary-for-vaccinated/
https://www.foxnews.com/health/us-halts-johnson-johnson-covid-19-vaccine-shipments-report
https://theprint.in/health/india-serum-institute-halts-clinical-t
https://guardian.ng/news/sweden-halts-use-of-moderna-vaccine-for-young-adults/
https://www.cnbc.com/2021/08/26/japan-pulls-1point6-million-moderna-vaccine-doses-over-contamination-concerns-.html
https://khn.org/morning-breakout/tennessee-no-longer-encouraging-vaccines-of-any-kind-for-minors/
https://nypost.com/2021/04/07/uk-halts-astrazeneca-vaccine-kid-trials-amid-blood-clot-concerns/
https://www.bbc.com/news/world-africa-55975052
https://www.forbes.com/sites/forbesdigitalcovers/2021/05/14/virus-book-excerpt-nina-burleigh-how-the-covid-19-vaccine-injected-billions-into-big-pharma-albert-bourla-moncef-slaoui/?sh=578dfd27d806
https://www.cnn.com/2021/05/21/business/covid-vaccine-billionaires/index.html
https://www.nytimes.com/2021/06/16/us/emergent-biosolutions-covid-vaccine.html
https://www.youtube.com/watch?v=YLnkOJw7t8Q
https://www.doctorswithoutborders.org/what-we-do/news-stories/news/moderna-posts-billions-profit-covid-19-vaccine-wont-share-technology
https://nypost.com/2021/10/07/moderna-founders-make-forbes-list-of-400-richest-americans/
https://www.alarmcall.org/society/as-covid-vaccines-drive-record-profits-ceos-get-ultra-rich-off-massive-pay-packages-questionable-stock-sales/99/
https://abcnews.go.com/Health/wireStory/pfizers-posts-49b-1q-profit-vaccine-strategy-pays-77492171
https://www.citizensjournal.us/stunning-study-reveals-how-ineffective-pfizer-vaccine-actually-is/

https://medicine.wustl.edu/news/past-vaccine-disasters-show-why-rushing-a-coronavirus-vaccine-now-would-be-colossally-stupid/
https://www.nytimes.com/interactive/2021/world/covid-cases.html
https://pagesix.com/2021/07/13/rob-schneider-blasts-covid-19-vaccines/
https://www.c-span.org/video/?515164-7/republican-senators-covid-19-vaccine-mandates
https://americasbestpics.com/picture/ti-his-retired-california-rn-is-asking-the-question-we-SdQCJF4z8
https://defendingtherepublicpac.com/covid/
https://rumble.com/viw1nv-children-adolescents-and-the-covid-vaccine.html
https://www.usnews.com/news/politics/articles/2021-09-29/lawyer-new-york-governor-uses-god-unfairly-in-vaccine-fight
https://www.youtube.com/watch?v=Oz4X4LW5gP0
https://www.youtube.com/watch?v=G9US8tSwYWg
https://www.reuters.com/article/uk-factcheck-fauci-outdated-video-masks/fact-checkoutdated-video-of-fauci-saying-theres-no-reason-to-be-walking-around-with-a-mask-idUSKBN26T2TR
https://www.youtube.com/watch?v=PRa6t_e7dgI
https://www.youtube.com/watch?v=GfbH3oko9SA
https://www.youtube.com/watch?v=SWkmzcTM1rU
https://www.youtube.com/watch?v=OcQwPf2n2vA
https://www.youtube.com/watch?v=QrKTiYemH2c
https://www.youtube.com/watch?v=SVcvCPTANMI
https://rumble.com/vhzgm5-tucker-fauci-deserves-to-be-under-criminal-investigation-on-email.html
https://www.foxnews.com/opinion/tucker-carlson-biden-pentagon-military-wokeness-lloyd-austin
https://www.youtube.com/watch?v=e6QNsNMFH5s
https://www.reuters.com/video/watch/idOVEXC20RV
https://www.youtube.com/watch?v=s53xk4CBOWE
https://www.naturalblaze.com/2021/08/film-seeing-2020-the-censored-science.html

https://www.facebook.com/watch/live/?ref=watch_permalink&v=542588153590514
https://www.newsweek.com/video-nancy-pelosi-we-cannot-require-vaccinations-resurfaces-1627730
https://www.yahoo.com/now/last-fauci-said-cannot-force-212300017.html
https://www.bitchute.com/video/WjQlZ8y2PGlc/
https://rumble.com/vn482j-dr.-carrie-madej-first-u.s.-lab-examines-vaccine-vials-horrific-findings-re.html
https://www.sfchronicle.com/opinion/openforum/article/Vaccines-are-safe-and-effective-against-delta-16474170.php
https://www.c-span.org/video/?c4962333/senator-paul-dr-fauci-clash-research-funding-wuhan-lab
https://twitter.com/TheLeadCNN/status/1452770600993308677
https://denvergazette.com/news/fauci-stands-by-gain-of-function-research-denials-defends-collaboration-with-wuhan-lab/article_8ba272e2-2940-532c-9820-4b015465a246.html
https://www.youtube.com/watch?v=Tau6Or8Gy_c
https://www.biospace.com/article/1nih-awards-ecohealth-alliance-7-5-million-grant-despite-political-furor/
https://www.imdb.com/title/tt15512020/
https://www.projectveritas.com/news/federal-govt-whistleblower-goes-public-with-secret-recordings-government/
https://podtail.com/en/podcast/the-stew-peters-show/funeral-director-mass-vaccine-deaths-child-danger-/
https://www.foxnews.com/transcript/tucker-carlson-military-suicide-is-a-crisis-the-pentagon-should-address
https://www.facebook.com/Centralinswa/videos/260900825053596/
https://www.youtube.com/watch?v=ynZAGPlLOMg
https://www.cdc.gov/coronavirus/2019-ncov/daily-life-coping/participate-in-activities.html
https://www.cnbc.com/2021/01/25/dr-fauci-double-mask-during-covid-makes-common-sense-more-effective.html

https://www.google.com/search?q=demonstrations+in+france&sxsrf=AOaemvJX7h_T-433xmvUBVSmF4TAt62yGw:1640730167352&source=lnms&tbm=isch&sa=X&ved=2ahUKEwiv6a-WxIf1AhVZkWoFHaiWAx4Q_AUoAnoECAEQBA&biw=658&bih=720&dpr=1
https://www.google.com/search?q=demonstrations+in+switzerland+passports+for+restaurants&tbm=isch&ved=2ahUKEwid0a3kxIf1
https://www.youtube.com/watch?v=9HHW0mj2EDc
https://www.youtube.com/watch?v=JOWRembdPS8
https://www.youtube.com/watch?v=MIYGFSONKbk
https://www.youtube.com/watch?v=5sIWb9GTbbE
https://video.foxnews.com/v/6274513508001#sp=show-clips
https://www.oann.com/fauci-hhs-officials-discuss-using-new-virus-from-china-to-enforce-universal-vaccines-in-footage-from-oct-2019/
https://www.youtube.com/watch?v=eBXB6vbQq74
https://www.news4jax.com/news/local/2021/01/22/baker-county-high-student-hospitalized-after-collapsing-during-tennis-practice/
https://www.cnbc.com/2021/06/25/covid-breakthrough-cases-cdc-says-more-than-4100-people-have-been-hospitalized-or-died-after-vaccination.html
https://www.cnbc.com/2021/05/12/cdc-says-28-blood-clot-cases-3-deaths-may-be-linked-to-jj-covid-vaccine.html
https://www.wbtw.com/health/coronavirus/23-die-in-norway-after-receiving-covid-vaccine/
https://www.clarkcountytoday.com/news/seventeen-year-old-washington-female-dies-from-heart-attack-weeks-after-receiving-second-pfizer-vaccination/
https://www.cnn.com/2021/07/21/politics/full-president-joe-biden-cnn-town-hall-july-21/index.html
https://www.facebook.com/watch/?v=321151009368360
https://theweek.com/speedreads/974785/cdc-director-data-suggests-vaccinated-people-largely-not-carry-virus

https://www.goodmorningamerica.com/news/story/cdc-director-warns-delta-variant-dominant-coronavirus-strain-78354918
https://www.yahoo.com/lifestyle/bill-gates-evaluates-us-covid-143600103.html
https://www.youtube.com/watch?v=AK8OB8wlMGA
https://www.youtube.com/watch?v=5Gw3jiWOwm0
https://www.youtube.com/watch?v=qT9x5slXsFc
https://www.youtube.com/watch?v=ie6lRKAdvuY&t=529s
https://www.youtube.com/watch?v=RU43V0Zt2gA
https://www.youtube.com/watch?v=mh_kCOCTxH8
https://www.youtube.com/watch?v=0UHCFPDhrEI
https://www.youtube.com/watch?v=JhfXsPiRuAs
https://www.youtube.com/watch?v=CjzZOM6kGZg
https://www.youtube.com/watch?v=FSdUsOQgIn0
https://www.getalifemedia.com/
https://www.youtube.com/watch?v=sauuC9oUXQo
https://www.youtube.com/watch?v=DEDqsEjhQYk
https://rumble.com/vn8v7a-india-govt.-declares-most-populated-state-officially-covid-free-after-wides.html
https://www.youtube.com/watch?v=ie6lRKAdvuY
https://rumble.com/vnh8qk-fauci-hhs-officials-discuss-using-new-virus-from-china-to-enforce-universal.html
https://www.reddit.com/r/mississippi/comments/qmzizz/cody_flint_from_ms/
https://podcasts.apple.com/us/podcast/an-interview-with-dr-anthony-fauci/id1200361736?i=1000541591083
https://153news.net/watch_video.php?v=1H78N38W465X
https://www.youtube.com/watch?v=sli2Vn6Iiy4
https://www.youtube.com/watch?v=RGEOw_bAqkc
https://www.youtube.com/watch?v=4SkzTa8HRDk
https://www.youtube.com/watch?v=5dIsweN-YKo
https://www.youtube.com/watch?v=S-2nE6AK1OU
https://www.youtube.com/watch?v=zJIJXkRwve0

https://www.youtube.com/watch?v=x_ZX24j9jcE
https://www.youtube.com/watch?v=S-2nE6AK1OU&t=63s
https://www.youtube.com/watch?v=6Bt7cmxhb2g
https://www.youtube.com/watch?v=KAp1yB4T0fo
https://www.youtube.com/watch?v=WHVolB_L1JM
https://www.youtube.com/watch?v=AZ7N95IAlRg
https://www.youtube.com/watch?v=CVIy3rjuKGY
https://www.youtube.com/watch?v=ttyLlORGixg
https://www.youtube.com/watch?v=0DKRvS-C04o
https://www.youtube.com/watch?v=u27WKCnbeXc
https://www.youtube.com/watch?v=kCSWSpRaXfM
https://www.youtube.com/watch?v=dswaElkiRO8
https://www.youtube.com/watch?v=SkhRFcRFoVk
https://www.youtube.com/watch?v=02z6vkTtXkI
https://frankspeech.com/video/stew-peters-show-joined-dr-ariyana-love
https://www.youtube.com/watch?v=mGFdWcJU7-0
https://www.youtube.com/watch?v=Ia9nO-Jj4to
https://www.youtube.com/watch?v=BC1o4__XZM4
https://www.youtube.com/watch?v=Df5S14LLFaM
https://www.youtube.com/watch?v=ms9nTAfMnOA
https://www.youtube.com/watch?v=t_Q8Hjacn9c
https://www.youtube.com/watch?v=KVhP5FY7oeo
https://www.youtube.com/watch?v=874jNMd6Yu0
https://www.youtube.com/watch?v=ZJk7qLsCnWs
https://www.youtube.com/watch?v=GfUPiazbl8U
https://www.youtube.com/watch?v=4WaOq3wQlxI
https://www.youtube.com/watch?v=8P9ADta0lR8
https://www.youtube.com/watch?v=iVdsSsSnCCA
https://rumble.com/vq7p5d-friday-emergency-broadcast-biden-pledges-to-forcibly-inject-all-babies-full.html
https://ifunny.co/video/am-63-jarome-bell-romebellva-what-he-said-again-the-BgFgr1mv8
https://www.youtube.com/watch?v=PC5cEbecMqE

https://rumble.com/vqblvt-dr.-vladimir-zelenko-md-vszhelyzeti-figyelmeztets.html
https://rumble.com/vqn634-dr.-zelenko-covid-jab-causes-aids.html
dr.carrie-madej-first-u.s.lab-examines-quot-vaccine-quot-vials-horrific-findings-revealed.mp4.mpg.mpg
https://www.youtube.com/watch?v=6ai5ymSYQHI
https://www.youtube.com/watch?v=J1bhl_3Ztgw
https://www.youtube.com/watch?v=oMrak_oyaZI
https://www.youtube.com/watch?v=5FndgPKK9Lk
https://www.youtube.com/watch?v=8jsyzCwm1uU
https://www.nbclosangeles.com/news/local/mom-says-son-vaccinated-in-exchange-for-pizza-at-lausd-without-her-consent/2773619/
https://rumble.com/vml4sn-funeral-directer-john-olooney-blows-the-whistle-on-covid.html
https://rumble.com/vrpq4l-vax-induced-mass-death-funeral-director-predicts-covid-camps-and-jab-genoci.html
https://www.youtube.com/watch?v=LwNM2T39RSo
https://www.youtube.com/watch?v=ZFwbix_Kg_Q
https://www.youtube.com/watch?v=LwNM2T39RSo&t=121s
https://www.youtube.com/watch?v=KJ_RSP_EK0E
https://www.youtube.com/watch?v=btAqULdBObo
https://www.youtube.com/watch?v=mGFdWcJU7-0&t=648s
https://www.youtube.com/watch?v=nNXpcPUHCPw
https://www.youtube.com/watch?v=sli2Vn6Iiy4&t=58s
https://www.youtube.com/watch?v=HxuGcVfSoSw
https://www.youtube.com/watch?v=H5q34eDHBxg
https://www.youtube.com/watch?v=ooBiMBCJj1c
https://www.youtube.com/watch?v=Mn3L2Tvd90Q
https://www.youtube.com/watch?v=-YQ1uKNDuNw
https://www.youtube.com/watch?v=O_8HHfTEiXc
https://www.youtube.com/watch?v=C98PAdpp9Vc
https://www.youtube.com/watch?v=i8yM-ECtqk0

https://www.theatlantic.com/technology/archive/2021/02/vaccine-influencers-covid-anti-vax-instagram/618052/
https://ktla.com/news/nationworld/dr-fauci-keep-wearing-masks-for-several-several-months-while-vaccines-roll-out/
https://www.usnews.com/news/health-news/articles/2021-10-25/moderna-says-its-vaccine-is-safe-and-effective-in-kids-6-11
https://www.youtube.com/watch?v=d45qFYOc_3Y
https://www.youtube.com/watch?v=aZ-U8yO9yjc
https://encyclopedia.ushmm.org/content/en/article/martin-niemoeller-first-they-came-for-the-socialists
https://rumble.com/vqpc2n-dr.-rand-paul-joins-unfiltered-with-dan-bongino-december-11-2021.html
https://www.youtube.com/watch?v=CxGTl7BaDAI
https://www.youtube.com/watch?v=S3TH5if8h7s
https://rumble.com/vqrrz4-dr.-robert-malone-healthy-children-should-not-be-vaccinated-for-covid-19.html
https://rumble.com/vrlgdb-the-real-reason-so-many-flights-are-being-cancled-worldwide.html
https://rumble.com/vr1gv4-dr.-peter-mccullough-the-vaccines-will-cause-more-deaths-than-covid.html
https://rumble.com/vrckcg-lithuania-vilnius-protest-against-the-government-and-vaccine-passports-augu.html
https://rumble.com/vrv326-update-nurse-mrs.-skelton-covid-vaccine-5-months-later.-is-she-better-you-b.html